Collins

BTEC NATIONAL

Health & Social Care

Level 3

Mark Walsh

Published by Collins Education
An imprint of HarperCollins Publishers
77-85 Fulham Palace Rd
Hammersmith
London
W68JB

Browse the complete Collins Education catalogue at
www.collinseducation.com

10 9 8 7 6 5 4 3 2 1

ISBN 978 0 00 741849 7

British Library Cataloguing in Publication Data.
A Catalogue record for this publication is available from the British Library.

Commissioned by Charlie Evans
Project Managed by Jo Kemp
Design and typesetting by Joerg Hartsmannsgruber and Thomson Digital
Cover design by Angela English
Index by Indexing Specialists Ltd
Printed and bound by L.E.G.O.S.p.a

This material has been endorsed by Edexcel and offers high quality support for the delivery of Edexcel qualifications. Edexcel endorsement does not mean that this material is essential to achieve any Edexcel qualification, nor does it mean that this is the only suitable material available to support any Edexcel examination and any resource lists produced by Edexcel shall include this and other appropriate texts. While this material has been through an Edexcel quality assurance process, all responsibility for the content remains with the publisher. Copies of all official specifications for all Edexcel qualifications may be found on the Edexcel website – www.edexcel.com

Contents

Photo Acknowledgements

Advertising Archives: 131, 181, 386
Alamy: 2, 6, 11, 13, 15, 19, 22, 24, 26, 40, 45, 50, 61, 63, 64, 67, 68, 71, 74, 80, 83, 106, 111, 114, 119, 124, 141, 146, 147, 164, 165, 167, 179, 202b, 202c, 204a, 204b, 204c, 204d, 204e, 225a, 225b, 235, 239, 258, 285, 290, 292, 309, 322, 355, 389, 394
Corbis: 379
Getty Images: 15, 19, 24, 33, 37, 45, 122, 202a, 208, 311, 315, 320, 341, 349, 351, 359, 362
Istockphoto: 4, 8, 9, 10, 11, 12, 14, 17b, 17c, 18, 21, 29, 32, 36, 42a, 48, 52, 56, 58, 62, 65, 91, 92, 100, 112, 144, 148, 149, 160, 169, 180, 183, 187, 190, 202d, 207, 214, 247, 256, 264, 268, 273, 274, 276, 278, 287, 288, 289, 300, 305, 307, 308, 317, 325, 332, 338a, 346-7, 348, 354, 368a, 354, 368b, 373, 376, 378, 380, 384a, 384b, 385, 392
Photolibrary: 49
Policy Press: 75
Science Photo Library 198, 217, 231a, 231b
Shutterstock: 3, 4, 6, 7a, 7b, 7c, 7d, 10, 16, 17a, 21, 26, 27, 28, 30, 32a, 32b, 34, 39, 42b, 44, 47a, 47b, 47c, 47d, 69, 72, 76, 77, 82, 84, 86, 88, 98, 103a, 103b, 108, 109, 110, 121, 125, 127, 128, 136, 138, 145, 150, 153, 156, 158, 166, 170, 174, 182, 186a, 186b, 196-7, 215, 218, 223, 226, 231c, 232, 240, 242, 246, 261, 282, 298-9, 302, 303a, 303b, 303c, 303d, 306, 312, 313, 323, 324, 326, 328a, 328b, 330, 338b, 343am 343b, 343c, 343d, 350, 365, 366, 368a, 370, 374, 387, 393, 396, 397
Topfoto: 369

Introduction

Welcome to BTEC Level 3 National Health and Social Care!

This course book is written for students aiming to achieve one of the following BTEC Level 3 National Health and Social Care awards:

BTEC Level 3 National Certificate in Health and Social Care	(30 credits)
BTEC Level 3 National Subsidiary Diploma in Health and Social care	(60 credits)
BTEC Level 3 National Diploma Health and Social Care	(120 credits)
BTEC Level 3 National Extended Diploma Health and Social Care	(180 credits)

The material in this book covers eight units of the BTEC Level 3 National Health and Social Care award. All of the units that you need to complete to obtain a certificate or subsidiary diploma award are contained in this book. Most of the mandatory units required for the diploma and extended diploma awards in health and social care are also covered in this book. A number of additional specialist mandatory and option units are covered in an additional course book that focuses on options needed to achieve the specialist pathways (social care, health studies, health sciences) that are part of the Diploma and Extended Diploma awards.

Each chapter of the book covers a specific BTEC Level 3 National unit. You will see that the chapters are divided into topics. Each topic provides you with a focused and manageable chunk of learning and covers all of the content areas that you need to know about in a particular unit. You should also notice that the material in each topic is clearly linked to the unit's pass, merit and distinction grading criteria. This mapping of the content against the grading criteria should help you to prepare for your assignments. The assignments that you are given by your tutor will require you to demonstrate that you have the knowledge and are able to do the things which the pass, merit or distinction criteria refer to.

Overall this course book provides a comprehensive resource for units 1 to 8 of the BTEC Level 3 National Health and Social Care programme. You can be sure that the content is closely matched to the BTEC specification and is designed and presented to help you achieve the grades you are aiming for and which you are capable of. There is a strong vocational focus to the materials in the book, using case studies, activities and realistic examples to develop your interest in and understanding of health and social care practice and the range of settings in which care professionals work.

Students often begin a BTEC National Health and Social Care course with the aim of undertaking further professional training or to get a job in a care setting. I hope that the material in the book is accessible, interesting and inspires you to pursue and achieve this goal. Good luck with your course!

Mark Walsh

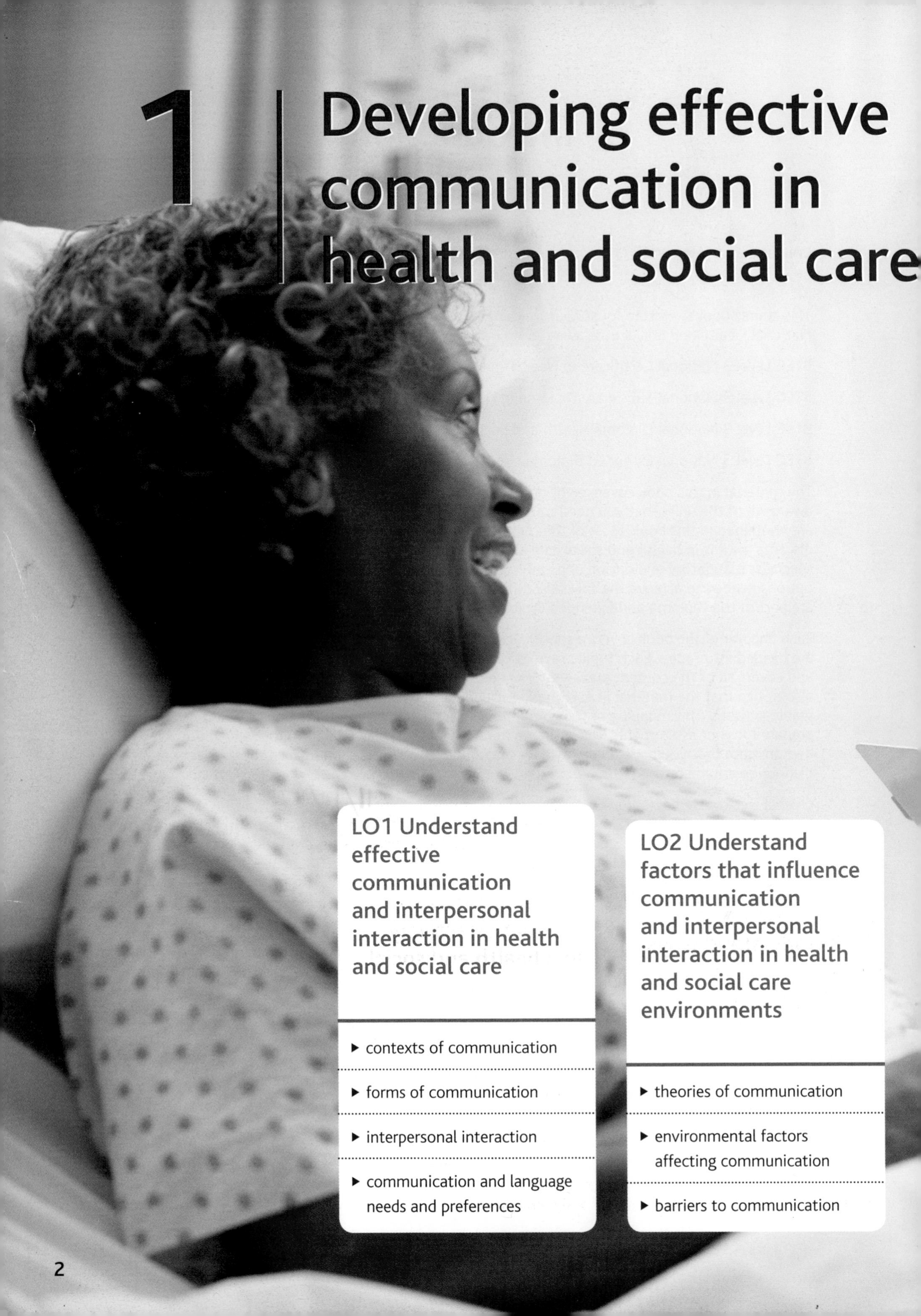

1 Developing effective communication in health and social care

LO1 Understand effective communication and interpersonal interaction in health and social care

- contexts of communication
- forms of communication
- interpersonal interaction
- communication and language needs and preferences

LO2 Understand factors that influence communication and interpersonal interaction in health and social care environments

- theories of communication
- environmental factors affecting communication
- barriers to communication

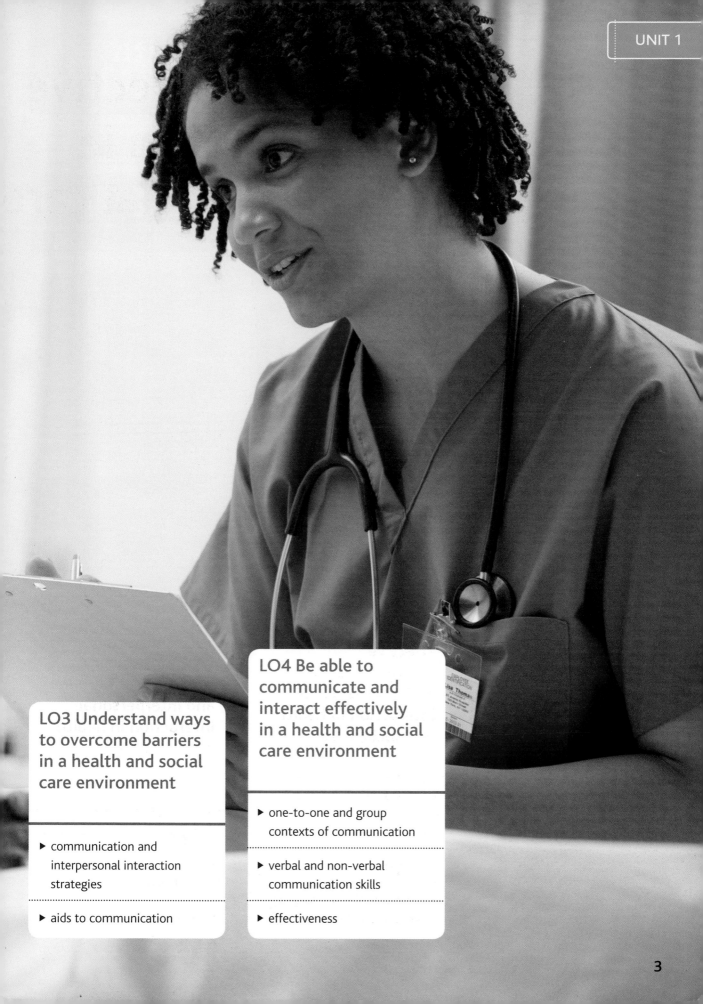

LO3 Understand ways to overcome barriers in a health and social care environment

- communication and interpersonal interaction strategies
- aids to communication

LO4 Be able to communicate and interact effectively in a health and social care environment

- one-to-one and group contexts of communication
- verbal and non-verbal communication skills
- effectiveness

Contexts of communication in health and social care

Your assessment criteria:

P1 Explain the role of effective communication and interpersonal interaction in a health and social care context

Health and social care professionals have to develop effective communication skills in order to work with the diverse range of people who use and work within care services. The two contexts, or types of circumstances, in which communication and interaction occur are *one-to-one* and *group* contexts.

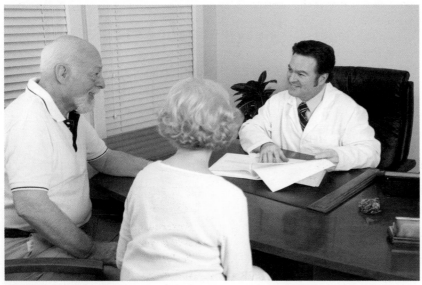

Effective communication is an important feature of care practice.

P1 One-to-one communication

One-to-one communication occurs when one person speaks with or writes to another individual. This happens when a care professional meets with a person who has health worries or personal concerns, such as during a doctor–patient appointment for example. Lots of one-to-one communication also occurs when care professionals meet with and talk to each other or with the partners, relatives or friends of people receiving care.

Communication in one-to-one situations is most effective when both parties are relaxed and are able to take turns at talking and listening. **Effective** communicators are good at:

- beginning the one-to-one interaction with a friendly, relaxed greeting
- focusing on the goal or 'business' of the **interaction**
- ending the interaction in a supportive, positive way.

Reflect

Who was your last one-to-one communication with? Did it follow the three phases of effective communication described on the left?

Key terms

Effective: *something that works or achieves a desired result or goal*

Interaction: *a two-way communication*

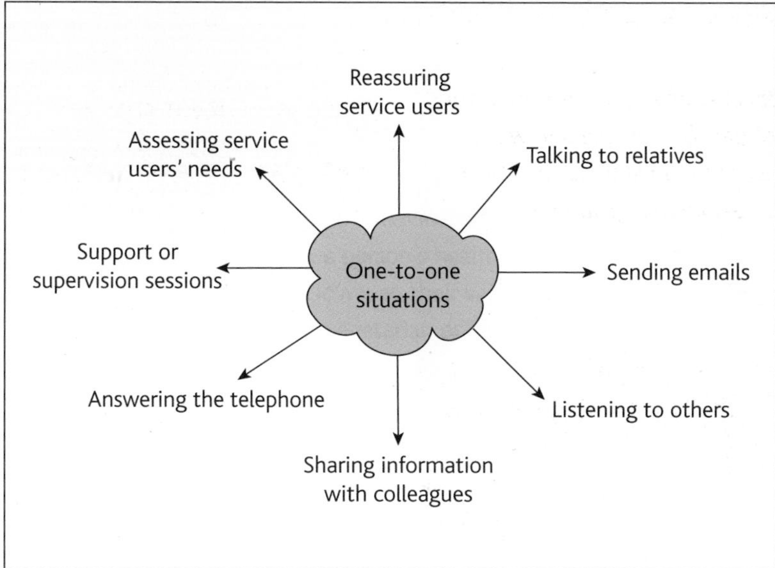

Figure 1.1 Examples of one-to-one communication situations.

Effective communication and interaction play an important role in the work of all health and social care professionals. For example, care professionals need to be able to use a range of communication and interaction skills in order to:

- work inclusively with people of different ages and diverse backgrounds
- respond appropriately to the variety of care-related problems and individual needs of people who use care services
- enable people to feel relaxed and secure enough to talk openly
- establish trusting relationships with colleagues and people who use care services
- ask sensitive and difficult questions, and obtain information about matters that might be very personal and sensitive
- obtain clear, accurate information about a person's problems, symptoms or concerns
- give others information about care-related issues in a clear, confident and professionally competent way.

If you have been to your doctors' surgery lately, your GP or practice nurse may have used their communication and interaction skills to find out about the symptoms of your health problems or may have given you advice or guidance on some aspect of your health behaviour or lifestyle. Establishing a good **rapport** with you, showing you respect, listening carefully and speaking clearly and in language you can understand would have contributed to the effectiveness of the interaction.

Discuss

What communication strengths and skills do you have that are relevant to health and social care work? Share your ideas with class colleagues and discuss ways in which the effectiveness of a person's communication skills can influence their care practice.

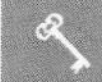

Key terms

Rapport: *this occurs when two people connect and are 'on the same wavelength'*

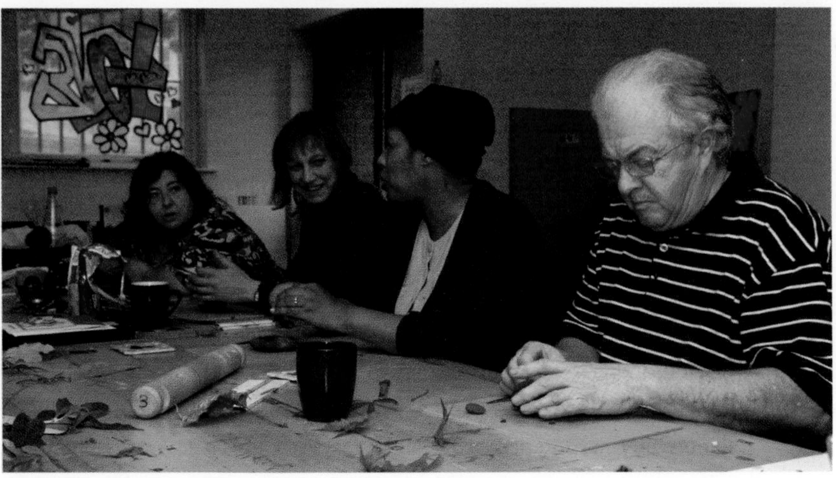

Creative activity sessions provide opportunities for group interactions.

Your assessment criteria:

P1 Explain the role of effective communication and interpersonal interaction in a health and social care context

P1 Group communication

Group communication follows slightly different 'rules' to communication in one-to-one situations. There is often more going on in a group, with a number of different people trying to speak, get their point across and their voice heard. Turn-taking can be more complicated; relationships and power issues between group members can also be more complex than in one-to-one contexts.

As a communication context, groups can have a number of benefits for participants:

- a group can be an effective way of sharing responsibilities
- groups can improve decision-making and problem-solving because they draw on the knowledge and skills of a number of people
- groups can improve members' self-esteem, social skills and social awareness, especially where the group has a therapeutic goal
- groups tend to command more respect and have more power than an individual acting alone.

However, groups can also limit the effectiveness of communication if:

- the power in a group is held by a single person or is misused by a small clique of people to dominate others and pursue their own agenda
- power struggles and battles break out within the group, resulting in a loss of purpose and effectiveness
- the group loses sight of its main goal or purpose, drifting into a pattern of ineffective activity that doesn't have a real benefit or outcome (holding meetings for the sake of meetings, for example)

Reflect

Have you ever been involved in a group where communication was difficult or ineffective? Why do you think this was?

- people find it hard to speak and contribute effectively or to challenge aspects of the group's thinking or practices. This can lead to poorly thought-out, unquestioned decisions being made.

Group communication is very common in the health and social care sector. This is largely because care professionals tend to work in teams and in partnership with service users and their families.

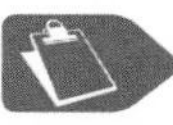

Case study

Teresa arrived for her interview on time but feeling a little nervous. She had worked hard to achieve the entry qualifications for nurse training and had gained experience as a health care support worker in a nursing home. Now she just had to pass the interview. Teresa was nervous because the selection day involved a group interview as well as an individual interview. Teresa and the seven other applicants were asked to discuss the following question:

'What makes a person a good care worker? Is it training, experience or their natural qualities?'

1. What kinds of skills will Teresa need to communicate effectively during the group interview activity?
2. Describe two reasons why the communication cycle may not always work effectively in a situation like this.
3. What could Teresa do to show that she has effective group communication skills?

What do you know?

1. Identify the two main contexts of communication and interpersonal interaction in health and social care settings.
2. Give two examples of situations in which group communication might occur in a health or social care setting.
3. Give two reasons why communicating in a group context requires different skills to communicating in one-to-one contexts.
4. How is effective communication different to ineffective communication?
5. Identify two reasons why communication in group contexts is sometimes ineffective.
6. Explain why a care professional needs to be able to communicate effectively.

Forms of communication in health and social care

Care professionals need to understand how communication and interpersonal interaction occur in both formal and informal contexts. Knowing when to communicate formally and when to use informal communication improves the effectiveness of a care professional's communication and interactions.

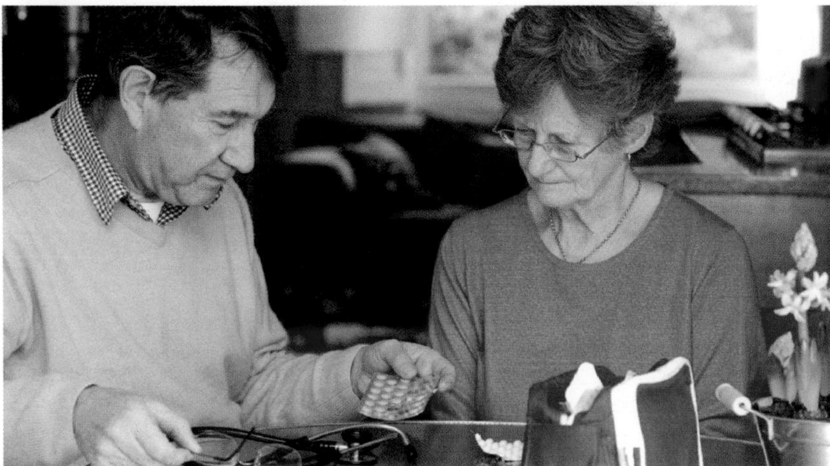

Many people rely on the information provided by health and social care practitioners.

Your assessment criteria:

P1 Explain the role of effective communication and interpersonal interaction in a health and social care context

P1 Formal and informal communication

Formal communication happens, for example, when somebody speaks or writes in an 'official' way because they are representing their care organisation or are contacting the organisation 'officially'. Answering the telephone by saying 'Good morning, Botley Medical Centre, how may I help you?' or writing a letter that begins 'Dear Sir or Madam' and that uses correct grammar and punctuation (while also avoiding **slang** or **jargon**) are both examples of formal communication.

Informal communication is more relaxed, more personal and 'looser' than formal communication. People use informal language when they speak with or write to their family, friends or close relatives. Answering the phone by saying 'Hey, how are you doing?', sending a text message with lots of **abbreviations** (LOL, L8R) or writing a letter that begins 'Hi Mum' are examples of informal communication. When people communicate in an informal way, they are less concerned about the 'proper' or 'correct' use of English. This doesn't mean that informal communication should be any less respectful or that it is necessarily less effective than formal communication.

The key issue for care professionals (and everyone else!) is to adjust the way they speak or write so that they choose a style that is appropriate for

Key terms

Abbreviations: *shortened forms of words or phrases (e.g. NHS for National Health Service)*

Formal communication: *official or correct forms of communication*

Informal communication: *doesn't stick to the formal rules of communication, for example a casual, relaxed conversation, written note or text message would be considered informal*

Jargon: *specialised, technical language used by a profession or group of people that may not be understood or used by others*

Slang: *informal, non-standard words used by members of a particular group (for example, 'innit' as used by some teenagers)*

the context in which the communication is occurring. A person who has health worries or personal concerns may think they are not being taken seriously or are being disrespected if a care professional speaks to them in a very informal way; they might feel that the care professional is patronising or 'talking down' to them. On the other hand, communicating with somebody in a way that is too formal might cause them to feel intimidated, belittled or that they are being treated in a cold and impersonal way. Care professionals have to learn to assess each person's communication needs and preferences and to understand the different contexts in which formal and informal communication are appropriate. Developing this understanding and flexibility enables a care professional to be respectful, sensitive and effective whenever they are communicating with others.

Communication between colleagues

Care professionals communicate with colleagues in many one-to-one and group contexts every day. Effective communication between colleagues requires:

- personal and professional respect for others
- trust in the judgement and values of colleagues
- good verbal and listening skills.

Care professionals may communicate formally and informally with colleagues. Effective communication and interactions enable people to work more efficiently and to collaborate with and support each other in teams.

Reflect

Can you think of examples from your work placement or personal experience where you have seen colleagues in a care setting communicating a) formally and b) informally?

Communication between professionals and people using services

Care professionals communicate with people using services very frequently and in a variety of ways. These can include formal meetings and appointments to assess and diagnose a person's health or wellbeing problems, in follow-up appointments to review a person's progress or recovery, in informal conversations during activity sessions and in brief interactions in the corridor or car park, for example.

To ensure that they communicate effectively, care professionals need to use language that isn't too technical, scientific or based on professional jargon. This can frustrate and intimidate people who use services, particularly if they feel they are being 'blinded by science' or that their concerns aren't being responded to in an appropriate manner. Effective communication and interaction enable people who use care services to feel more supported, are essential for identifying and responding to their individual care needs and form the basis of a trusting, respectful care relationship.

Investigate

What do the terms 'cerebrovascular accident', 'fractured tibia' and 'tachycardic' mean in plain, non-technical English?

P1 Communication with other professionals

Health and social care work is now based on **multi-professional** and **multi-agency working**. This means that care professionals need to be able to communicate effectively with colleagues from a variety of different care disciplines. A multi-professional mental health team might include mental health nurses, social workers, occupational therapists, clinical psychologists and psychiatrists, for example. Each of these care professionals has a particular disciplinary training and a range of specialist skills. They also share some core skills in working with people who are mentally distressed. Members of this team will need to be able to use their one-to-one and group communication skills flexibly so that they can talk to, share ideas and collaborate with their team colleagues in ways that benefit the people in their care.

Care professionals involved in multi-professional teams may communicate in both formal and informal contexts. When team members get to know each other very well, they may use more informal language at times. However, multi-agency working often requires care professionals to communicate more formally, using agreed plans and agendas to achieve specific goals. Formal communication may be used to ensure that the professionals and agencies involved in this kind of collaborative working are clear about each other's responsibilities and don't drift into miscommunication, compounding problems.

Your assessment criteria:

P1 Explain the role of effective communication and interpersonal interaction in a health and social care context

Key terms

Multi-agency working: *collaboration between different care organisations or agencies*

Multi-professional working: *usually involves different types of care professionals working together in a team*

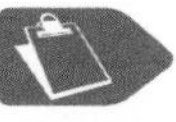

Case study

Sanjay, aged 8 years, has been neglected by his mother and Ricardo, his stepfather, for about a year. This began shortly after Ricardo moved into Sanjay's home. Ricardo often shouts at Sanjay, telling him to 'get out of the house' and threatening to beat him if he doesn't do as he's told. Quite late at night, Sanjay can sometimes be found wandering around the area where he lives, cold and hungry. The local social services department, the police and staff at Sanjay's primary school are all now aware that he is having a difficult time at home and that he is not being looked after very well. The mother of Sanjay's best friend at school wrote a letter to social services last week asking them to investigate what is happening to him. She did this after he came to her house in dirty clothes, asking if he could have something to eat early on Sunday morning.

1. Identify the form and type of communication that has alerted people to Sanjay's situation.

Investigate

Use the Internet to find out about the Every Child Matters *programme. Summarise the rationale for multi-agency working in children's services that it introduced.*

2. Explain why it is important that the different agencies dealing with Sanjay's case communicate effectively with one another.
3. What might happen in this situation if communication between the agencies is ineffective or breaks down?

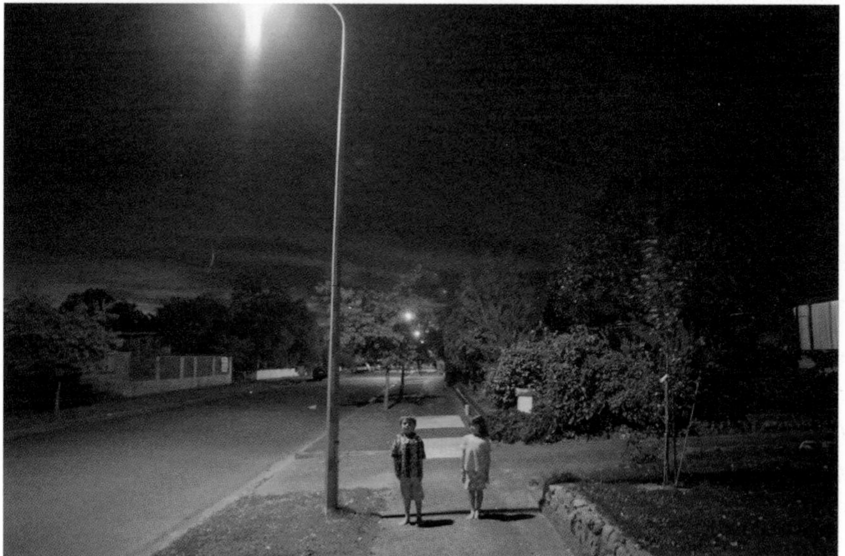

What do you know?

1. Identify one reason a care professional might communicate in a formal way.
2. Describe the difference between formal and informal communication.
3. Explain why a care professional might sometimes choose to communicate in an informal way.
4. Why can the use of jargon make a care professional's communication less effective?
5. What is multi-agency working and why are effective communication and interaction skills important in this way of working?
6. Describe three possible consequences of ineffective communication between health and social care professionals working in a multi-agency context.

Verbal communication skills

Care professionals communicate and interact with colleagues, other professionals and the people who use care services by using a variety of word-based (verbal) and non word-based (non-verbal) methods of communication. **Verbal** and **non-verbal communication** can be explored separately but occur simultaneously. You need to understand how the use of verbal and non-verbal skills contributes to the effectiveness of communication in care settings.

Your assessment criteria:

P1 Explain the role of effective communication and interpersonal interaction in a health and social care context

Key terms

Non-verbal communication: *forms of communication that do not use words (e.g. gestures)*

Verbal communication: *forms of communication that use words*

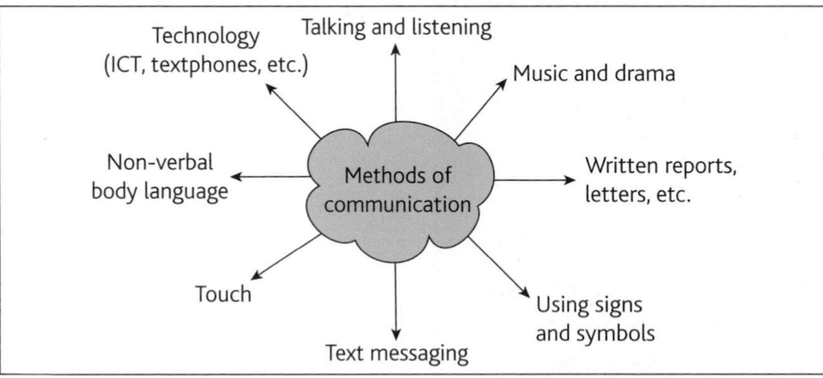

Figure 1.2 How do care professionals communicate and interact?

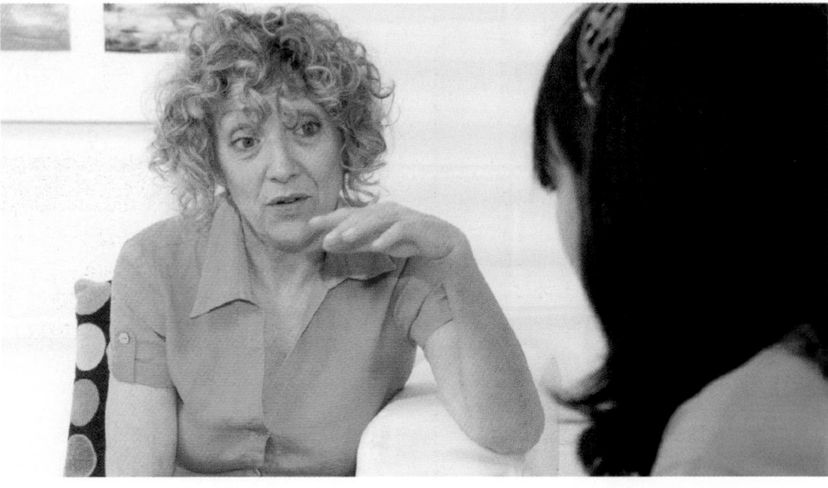

Effective communication involves both talking and listening skills.

P1 Interaction through verbal communication

Verbal communication is word-based. It can take a number of different forms including:

- oral or spoken communication
- text messaging or email communication
- written communication.

Care professionals may use some or all of these ways of communicating verbally, depending on their particular work role and the communication needs, skills and preferences of their colleagues and the people who use care services.

Issues that care professionals need to consider when communicating verbally with others include:

- the preferred language and the language support needs of the individual or group they are communicating with
- **dialect**
- slang
- the use of jargon and complex technical terms.

Key terms

Dialect: *a way of using language (e.g. English) that is associated with a particular region or group of people (e.g. London, cockney)*

Grammar: *the rules for speaking and writing a language*

Vocabulary: *the words known and used by an individual or group of people*

Effective verbal communication

Verbal communication is word-based, so it can involve written or spoken language. To communicate verbally a person needs to understand a **vocabulary** of words and a set of conventions – a **grammar** – that tells them how to put the words together. Every spoken and written language has its own vocabulary and grammar that needs to be learnt and understood in order for people to talk to others. Effective verbal communication occurs when one person speaks (or writes) and at least one other listens to (or reads) and understands the message.

Talking with service users, their relatives and with colleagues is a frequent, everyday occurrence for care professionals. For example, verbal communication skills are needed to:

- respond to questions asked by people who use services, their families and friends
- discuss the worries, concerns and distress of people who use care services
- ask questions when carrying out needs assessments or reviewing progress
- take part in team meetings
- break bad news and provide support to people
- form and maintain effective care relationships.

Because talking with others is such a familiar, everyday occurrence in care settings, care professionals may not spend much time thinking about or reflecting on their use of verbal communication skills. However, being aware of the language needs and preferences of the person you are speaking to, appreciating the impact of your own and their dialect, and being careful to minimise the use of slang and jargon can all help to make verbal communication more effective.

Reflect

How effective are your verbal communication skills now? Are they good enough to deal with the different situations listed on the left?

P1 Thinking about *how* you speak

A number of features of speech can affect the quality and effectiveness of verbal communication. These include the clarity, volume, **pace**, **tone** and **pitch** of a person's voice. For example, it isn't a good idea to shout, mumble, talk really fast or sound aggressive when having a conversation with a service user, their friends, family or your colleagues. Speaking in this way is unprofessional and is likely to draw attention away from what is being said; people will focus more on *how* you are speaking to them. This makes any communication ineffective. A care professional's speech should be clear, unambiguous and paced to suit the listener. Speaking in a measured, direct way enables the listener to hear and understand what is being said. Care professionals who use a relaxed, encouraging and friendly tone of voice are also able to convey warmth, sincerity and respect for the listener.

Case study

Laura, aged 17, had a work placement at a local nursery school last year. She says that she learnt a lot about how (and how not) to communicate during the 2 weeks she spent there. After a couple of days, she was asked to do some work on the phone. This involved answering early morning calls from parents whose children were unable to attend (because of illness) and also phoning a group of parents to tell them about the arrangements for a Forest School trip.

Initially, Laura was quite confident about her telephone skills but quickly got into difficulties. She was greeting one parent and their child in reception when she heard the telephone ring. She apologised and quickly ran to answer it. When she picked up the phone she said, 'Yep, Nursery, who is it? What's your child called?' without pausing for breath. The parent who was calling asked Laura to speak more slowly and in a friendlier tone. Laura felt told off and lost some confidence.

1. Which aspects of Laura's speech made her communication less effective than it should have been?
2. How could Laura have improved her approach when answering the phone?
3. What advice would you give to Laura to ensure she communicates the information about the Forest School trip as effectively as possible?

Your assessment criteria:

P1 Explain the role of effective communication and interpersonal interaction in a health and social care context

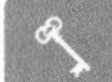

Key terms

Pace: *the rate, speed or tempo of speech*

Pitch: *the sound quality of a person's voice – 'She spoke in a low-pitched voice.'*

Tone: *the emotional quality of a person's voice – 'He used an aggressive tone.'*

Reflect

How do you think you sound when you speak? Is your voice quiet, loud, fast, slow, timid, aggressive? Ask some other people who know you well to comment on this too.

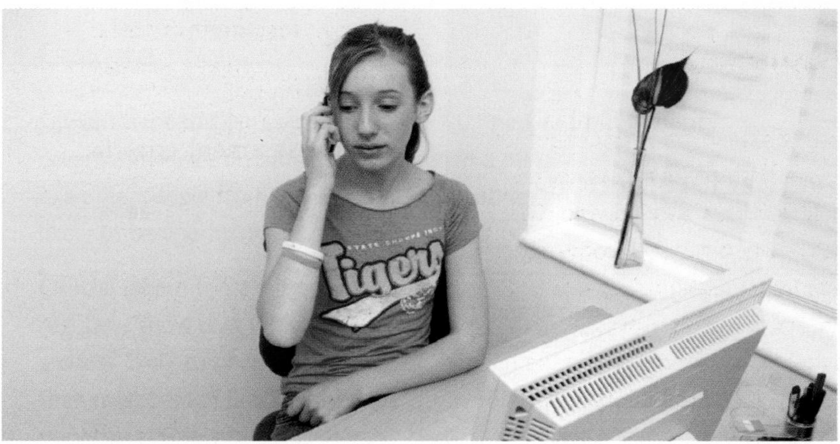

Pace, pitch and tone of voice are important in telephone conversations.

Written communication

Services users' records, organisational policies and procedures, official letters and memos, emails and text messages between care practitioners are all examples of verbal, or word-based, communication in written form.

Care practitioners spend a lot of time writing because they have to plan and document the care that they provide, evaluate their plans, produce reports and draft referral letters about service users. Many care organisations have official record-keeping systems, report procedures and standard forms, and employ administration staff to manage the large amount of paperwork that is involved in care provision. As a result, care professionals need to develop clear, effective writing skills and should have a good knowledge and understanding of ways of writing different kinds of document (such as patients' notes, reports and formal letters).

The specific writing skills needed by care professionals are generally learnt in practice and quickly become part of a care professional's skill set. However, it is important for care professionals to regularly review and reflect on their written communication skills to ensure they are using them as effectively as possible.

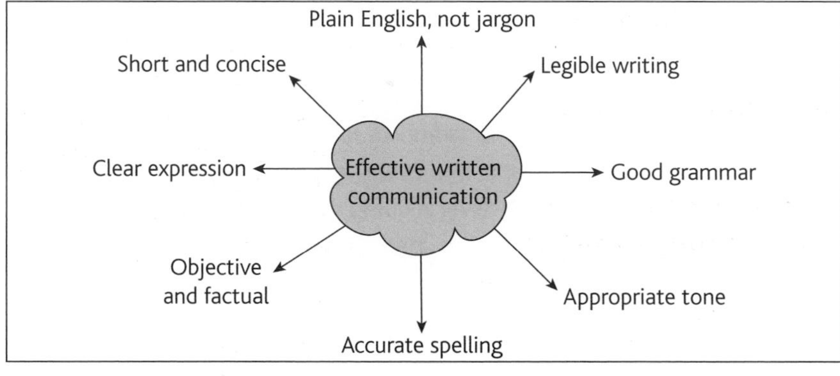

Figure 1.3 Features of effective written communication.

Non-verbal communication skills

P1 Being aware of non-verbal interaction

We don't have to talk to other people to communicate or interact with them. We also communicate non-verbally through **body language**, the way we dress and sometimes through the activities we take part in. As we will see, body language, art, drama and music, as well as specialist techniques such as **signing**, are all **non-verbal** methods of communication that are used within care settings.

Non-verbal communication happens continuously and, without realising it, most of us become skilled at 'reading' and interpreting it. Without doing so in a conscious way, you probably assess and make judgements about other people's moods and feelings, even their personality, on the basis of their body language. This is because you are able to receive and interpret the **'messages'** that other people send through their use of eye contact, posture, proximity, facial expression and touch, for example. Care professionals need to be aware of how both they and other people use non-verbal communication as this can have a very powerful impact on the effectiveness of communication and interactions.

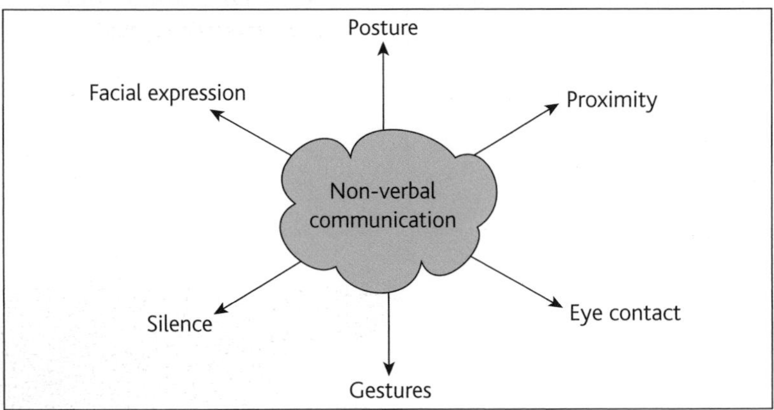

Figure 1.4 Forms of non-verbal communication.

Posture

A person's posture can communicate information about their attitude and feelings:

- For example, somebody who is sitting or standing in a very upright, stiff way may be seen by others as 'tense' in mood or as having a serious or aggressive attitude.
- Closed postures, in which a person has their arms or legs (or both) crossed, tend to suggest defensiveness, anxiety and tension.

Your assessment criteria:

P1 Explain the role of effective communication and interpersonal interaction in a health and social care context

Key terms

Body language: *the use of gesture, posture, facial expression and behaviour to communicate without using words*

Message: *the information (verbal message) or meaning (non-verbal message) that communication is about*

Non-verbal communication: *forms of communication that do not use words, such as body language*

Signing: *communicating using visible hand gestures*

Reflect

Look around you now. Are the people you can see sending messages non-verbally? What do you think they are 'saying'?

- Open postures, where the person has their arms by their sides and where they lean forward slightly, tend to indicate that the person is relaxed and comfortable.

Care practitioners can use their understanding of postural messages to read a person's mood and feelings. This can give useful information during assessment interviews and in one-to-one counselling sessions. Similarly, in everyday care situations a person's posture may indicate they are in pain, are unhappy or feel uncomfortable. However, it is always best to check your interpretation of a person's postural message with them before jumping to any conclusions. This can be done by sensitively asking the person a question about how they are feeling, to avoid reading too much into how they are standing or sitting.

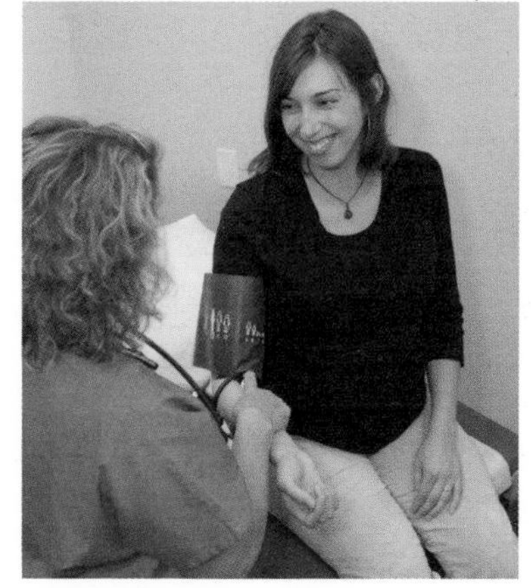

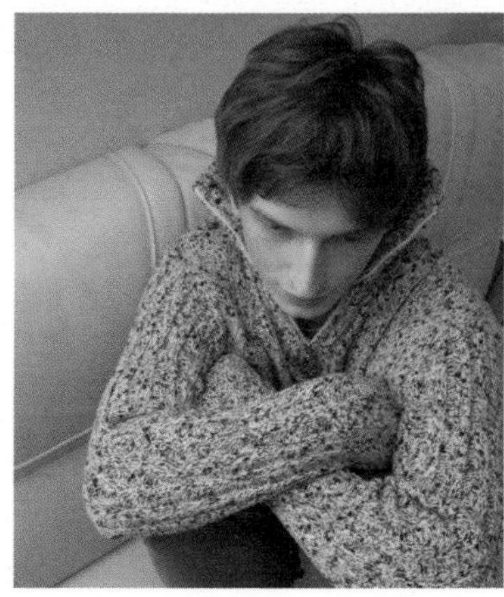

A person's posture sends messages about their feelings.

Reflect

Have a look around your school or college (or at home) and try to observe and interpret the meaning of one or two people's postures. What kinds of feelings or attitude do they seem to be communicating? What could you ask the person to check your interpretation of this?

Facial expression

The human face is very expressive and is an important source of non-verbal communication. When we read a person's facial expression we look at their:

- eyes – are the pupils dilated (large) or contracted (small)? Large, dilated pupils tend to suggest 'interest' or excitement.
- skin colour – is the person blushing or sweating?
- mouth – is the person smiling or frowning? Is the person's mouth dry?
- facial muscles – are the muscles in the face tight or relaxed?

Different facial expressions involve very subtle changes in each of these features. However, most people become very good at reading other people's facial expressions and at using their own to express their thoughts and feelings non-verbally. These facial messages can be used by care professionals to assess a person's mood and to judge their response or reaction to a situation, like being given the results of medical tests.

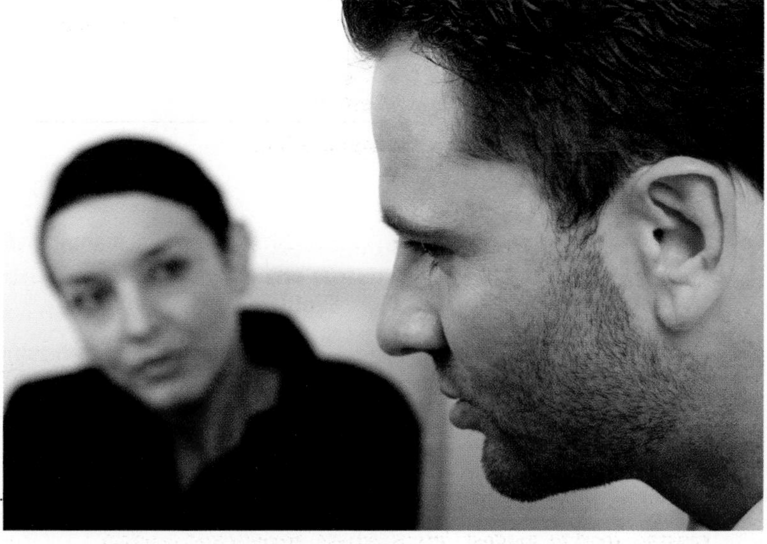

P1 Proximity

Proximity refers to the physical closeness between people during interactions. Another phrase that is sometimes used instead of proximity is 'personal space'. The amount of personal space that a person needs during an interaction tends to depend on their cultural background, upbringing and the type of relationship that they have with the other person. People from the Mediterranean, Middle East and South America, for example, tend to touch more and require less personal space when interacting than people from Western European and Scandinavian countries. The latter generally prefer only formal touching, such as brief handshakes, and plenty of personal space, unless they know the other person extremely well. We tend to require less personal space when our relationship with the other person is a close, intimate or personal one. Relationships that are more formal and less personal, such as with work colleagues, tend to require more personal space for interactions to be comfortable and effective.

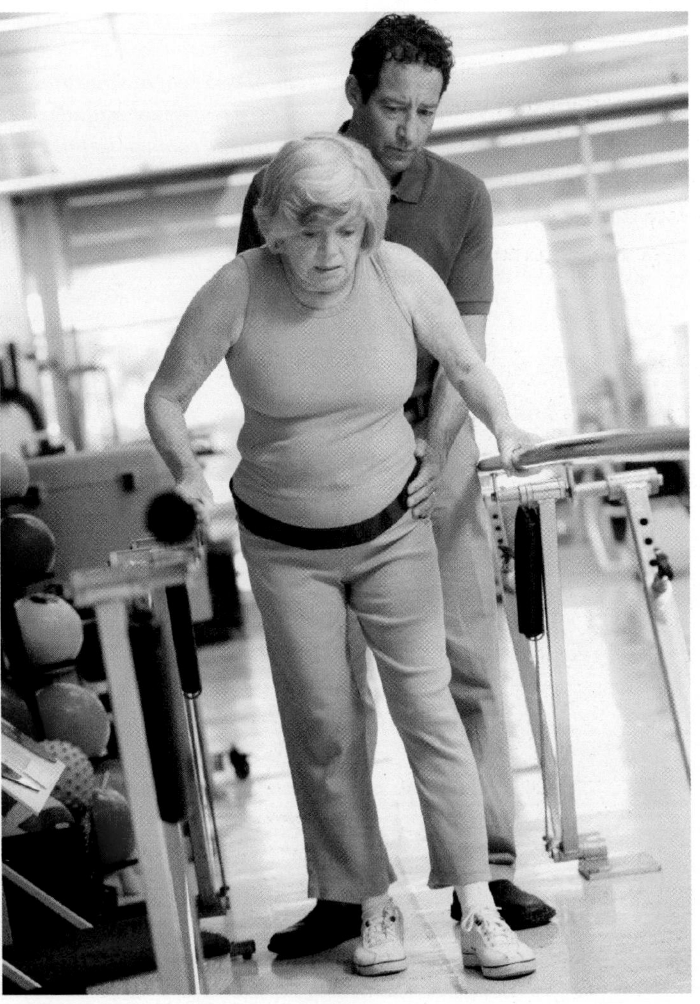

Your assessment criteria:

P1 Explain the role of effective communication and interpersonal interaction in a health and social care context

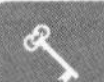

Key terms

Proximity: *another term for closeness or personal distance*

Reflect

Are you comfortable with close proximity when talking to new people or do you need a lot of personal space? Can you think of a situation where proximity affected your ability to communicate?

There are many different situations where a care practitioner needs to be aware of 'personal space' issues. For example, entering a person's room, touching them on the arm or simply sitting down next to them to have a conversation could feel intrusive or unsettling if the person thinks their personal space is being 'invaded'. A service user, if they are able, will usually adjust their proximity (by moving their chair or standing position, for example) to acquire the amount of personal space they need during an interaction. However, if the person is not physically able or lacks the confidence to do this, a care practitioner who adjusts their own proximity with sensitivity will improve the quality of the interaction and communication by doing so.

Touch

Care professionals are in a special position with regard to touching other people. In many settings where personal care is provided, the usual barriers that restrict where and how often we touch others in everyday life are suspended. Care professionals are generally allowed and expected to touch others as part of their work. In this context, care workers can use touch as a way of communicating reassurance, to carry out care procedures and to show concern for others; it is important that touch isn't misinterpreted or used as a way of communicating dominance or sexual desire. Asking whether it is okay to hold a person's hand or to touch them in another way – and explaining why this is necessary – can reduce anxieties and also ensure that the message that is communicated through touch is an appropriate one.

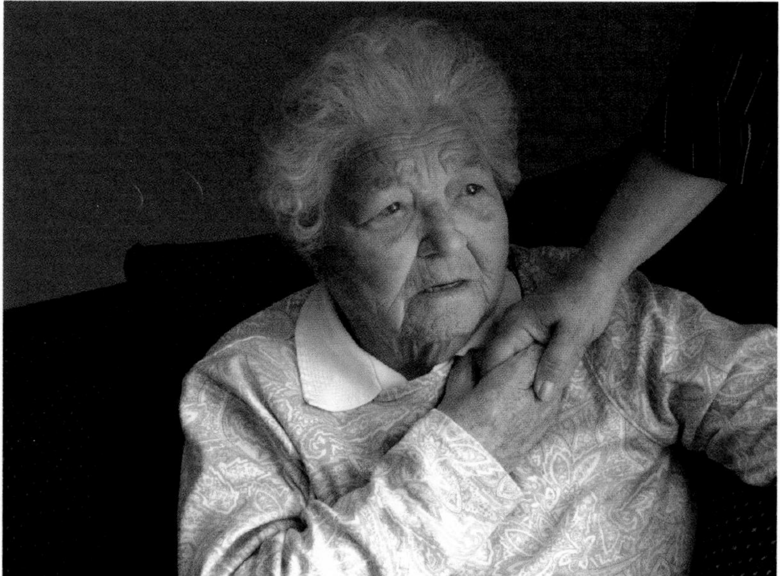

Touch is a way of communicating reassurance and empathy in care situations.

Discuss

Imagine that you are at a party and you meet somebody new who wants to talk with you. What are your 'rules' or expectations about touch and proximity in situations like this? Share your ideas with class colleagues, identifying what behaviours you would be comfortable with and what would make you feel uncomfortable. Think about the reasons why.

P1 Silence

Silence is an important part of many interactions in care settings. A care professional who can listen in silence is more likely to be listening actively to the other person than a care professional who interrupts or who doesn't allow the speaker time to pause and collect their thoughts. Care professionals who are unaware of the importance of silence sometimes interrupt conversations or fill any silences by talking themselves because they are embarrassed or feel nervous. Silence can be very helpful in enabling a person to disclose sensitive or very personal information; the care professional should use their body language to show they are interested in and respectful of the speaker.

Reflective listening

Reflective listening is sometimes called 'active listening'. It involves paying careful attention to a person's verbal and non-verbal communication and then reflecting back the messages you think they are sending as a way of checking your understanding. Reflective listening might involve:

- summarising what the person has said every now and then, to recap and check you are following their communication ('So, what happened was...')
- paraphrasing what they have been saying in your own words in order to clarify that you have understood them correctly ('You seem to be saying that...').

People who are able to use reflective listening:

- have the ability to pay attention
- use their own body language to show that they are interested and are listening
- hear and remember what the speaker says while also noticing and 'reading' the speaker's non-verbal communication
- can summarise and paraphrase appropriately
- ask questions to clarify their understanding.

Your assessment criteria:

P1 Explain the role of effective communication and interpersonal interaction in a health and social care context

Reflect

Are you good at active listening? How might improving your active listening skills help to make you a more effective care practitioner?

Case study

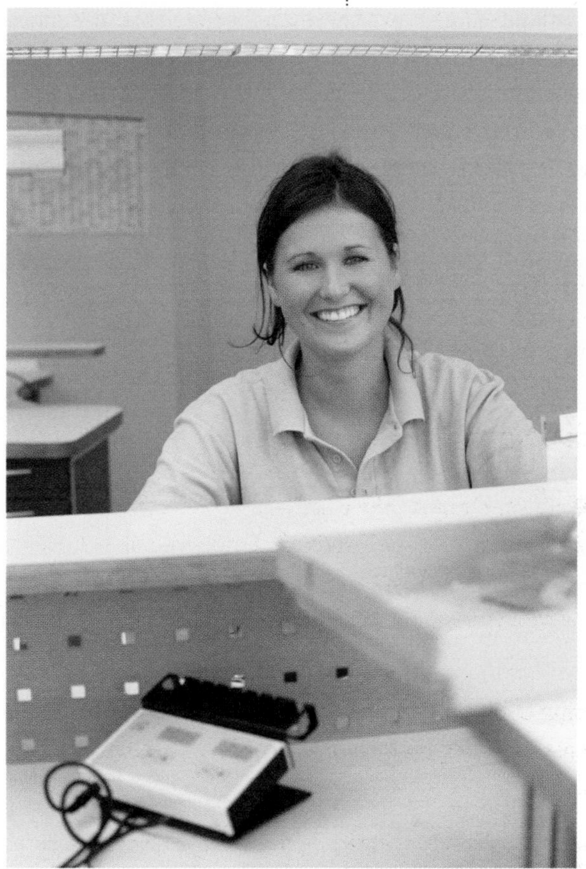

Daniella, aged 19, is a trainee dental nurse working in a busy practice with a diverse group of service users. Mr Ramesh, the dentist in charge, has told Daniella that the biggest problem for him is patient anxiety. He would like Daniella to calm patients and reassure them that their treatment will help rather than harm them. He has asked Daniella to think about ways of helping the patients to feel more relaxed and to be calm before he begins treating them.

1. Which aspects of Daniella's non-verbal communication are important in communicating reassurance and calmness?
2. Describe how Daniella might use touch in an appropriate way to reassure anxious patients.
3. Explain why the way Daniella speaks to patients can influence their anxiety levels.

What do you know?

1. Identify the two main forms of communication used in health and social care settings.
2. Describe three factors that influence the effectiveness of verbal communication.
3. Identify three factors that affect the way people communicate non-verbally.
4. How can silence contribute to the effectiveness of communication?
5. Explain what reflective listening involves.
6. How does reflective listening promote more effective communication?

Communication and language needs and preferences

Care professionals communicate effectively when they are able to 'connect' directly with other individuals. To be able to do this well, a care professional must adapt to the communication and language needs and preferences of others. This includes people who are unable to use spoken language and people who have sensory impairments that limit their communication and interaction abilities.

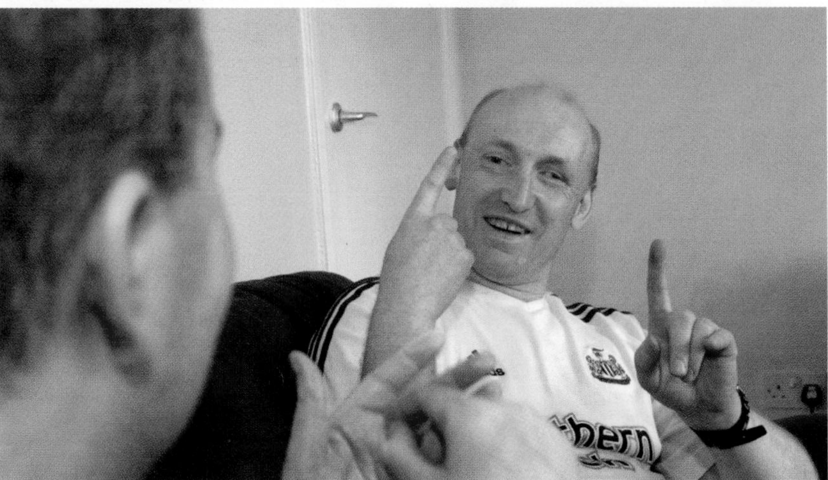

Signed languages are based on the use of gesture.

Your assessment criteria:

P1 Explain the role of effective communication and interpersonal interaction in a health and social care context

Reflect

Jot down some ideas about the ways that a speech or visual impairment could reduce the effectiveness of communication.

P1 Signed language

People who have hearing (or dual hearing and sight) impairments sometimes communicate through the use of specialist forms of non-verbal signing. Sign languages are often taught and used in settings where service users have limited ability to use verbal language due to learning disabilities. There are a number of different sign language systems including dactylography (finger spelling), British Sign Language and **Makaton**. The different gestures and symbols, and the grammar involved in putting together meaningful sequences of signs, have to be learnt before a person can use signing to communicate. It is useful, sometimes essential, for care practitioners to develop signing skills if some of the users of their care services communicate in this way.

Braille

Braille is a system of communication based on raised marks that can be 'read' by touch. It is named after Louis Braille, who invented and first published it as a blind 20-year-old in 1829. People who have a visual

Key terms

Braille: *a system of writing for visually impaired people in which patterns of raised dots represent letters and numbers*

Makaton: *a system of communication using simple hand signs, which is used by people with language and learning difficulties*

impairment that prevents them from reading handwritten or printed text use it. It is now possible to have computer-based text, such as emails, messages or reports, printed out in Braille using a specialist printer.

Use of signs, symbols and images

Signs, symbols and pictures are graphical or image-based ways of communicating small amounts of information in a direct way without using words. You can probably recall and understand the difference between the symbols for male and female toilets, for example. Many large care organisations, such as hospitals and local authorities, use lots of signs to direct people to various parts of their buildings and to impart other information; health and safety information is often communicated through the use of specific symbols. Signs, symbols and images that are used for communication purposes have to have a clear, easy-to-understand meaning to be effective.

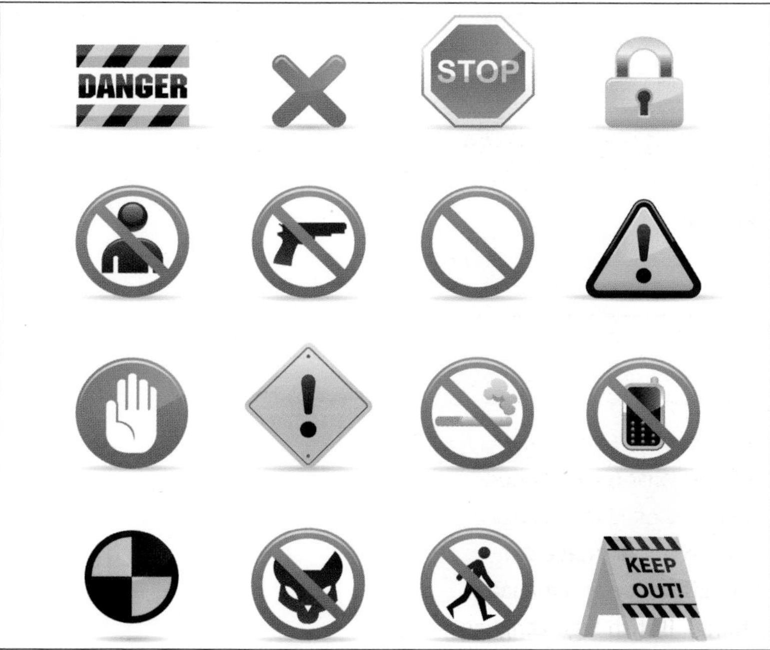

Figure 1.5 Health and safety symbols.

Communication passports

These are personalised booklets containing practical information about a person and their communication needs and preferences. A communication passport is designed to give people, such as care professionals, useful information about an individual so that they can adapt or adjust the way they communicate with the person. An individual's communication passport should indicate their likes, dislikes and preferred methods or styles of communication.

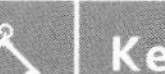

Key terms

Symbol: *an item or image that is used to represent something else*

Discuss

Do you recognise any of these symbols? What does each one mean or communicate to you?

Investigate

Find out about groups of service users who use communication passports.

P1 Human aids to communication

In situations where people speak different languages or prefer to use different communication systems – such as British Sign Language or Makaton – effective communication may only be possible if assistance is provided by a third party. Care organisations and agencies may use one or more of the following human aids to ensure that communication is effective in these circumstances:

- interpreters who act as a link or bridge between speakers of different languages. Interpreters usually listen to a person speak in one language and then communicate what they have said to a second person using a different language.
- translators who translate what is written in one language into a second language (English to Hindi, for example)
- signers who use forms of sign language to communicate what has been said or written into a sign language such as British Sign Language or Makaton, for example.

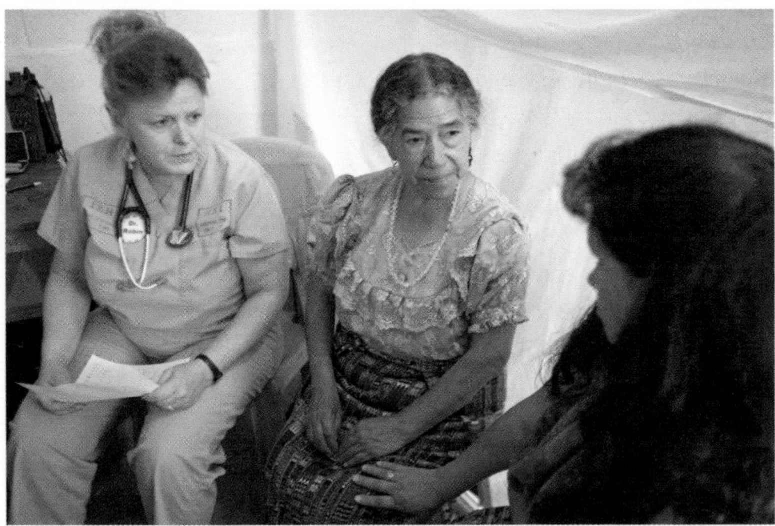

Interpreters can act as a communication bridge in care settings.

Cultural differences

Britain is a multicultural country. Care professionals need to have an awareness of and sensitivity to cultural differences when communicating with others. For example, people speak a range of languages, use different words, phrases and dialects in different regions of the UK and may use different forms of non-verbal behaviour to express themselves during interactions. If care professionals don't develop an awareness of cultural variations in communication and in interaction styles and preferences, communications may be misunderstood or may make no sense at all.

Your assessment criteria:

P1 Explain the role of effective communication and interpersonal interaction in a health and social care context

Reflect

What different languages are spoken by people living in your local area? Have you seen any non-English information leaflets or signs at your local health centre, hospital or library designed with these communities in mind?

Expressive activities, objects and technology

As we have seen, care professionals use a variety of different forms of communication in their day-to-day work. However, there are some care-related situations where a person's ability to express their thoughts or feelings is impaired or limited. This might occur if a person has a learning disability, a brain injury or a condition (such as dementia) that limits their ability to use or understand language. Some people who are experiencing mental health problems also struggle to talk about experiences or to express thoughts and feelings that are distressing and painful. In situations like these, a care professional may make use of:

- expressive activities based on music and drama to enable a person to express their emotions in a non-verbal way
- **objects of reference**, for example toys, clothes, jewellery or photographs, that have a special meaning for the individual and which are used to reassure, comfort and remind them of happier times
- arts and crafts activities that allow the person to produce images or objects which express feelings they cannot verbalise.

Care professionals may also encourage some people to make use of technological aids, such as electronic communicators, hearing aids and videophones, to overcome specific communication problems. These kinds of technological aids are specifically designed to help individuals who have difficulty sending or receiving the messages that form their communication with others (see page 52).

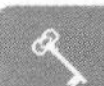

Key terms

Objects of reference: *objects that have a particular meaning for a person (such as a special ring or ornament)*

Reflect

Do you or members of your family have any objects of reference that carry special meaning?

What do you know?

1. Identify two reasons why care professionals need to be able to adapt their communication approach to the needs and preferences of people who use care services.
2. Describe how a signed language works.
3. What characteristics does a sign or symbol need to have to communicate information effectively?
4. What is a communication passport and how can it help to make communication more effective?
5. Explain why care professionals need to be aware of the way cultural differences affect communication and interaction.
6. Describe an example of an object of reference and explain how it could play a part in communication between people.

Theories of communication: the one-to-one situation

A theory is a set of ideas that can be used to understand, explain and make predictions about something. Theories of communication provide ways of analysing communication between people and give care practitioners an insight into what works and why.

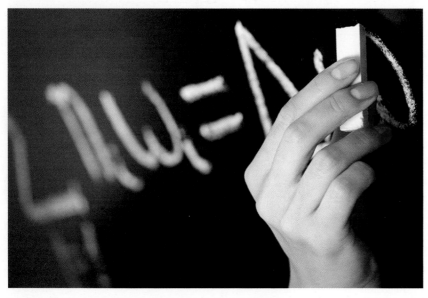

Figure 1.6 The theoretical notation symbolising a theory.

Your assessment criteria:

P2 Discuss theories of communication

M1 Assess the role of effective communication and interpersonal interaction in health and social care with reference to theories of communication

P2 The communication cycle

Michael Argyle (1925–2002) was a **social psychologist** who researched and developed theories about human communication and interpersonal interaction. He focused on both verbal and non-verbal communication, carrying out **experimental research** to test and develop his theoretical ideas (see Argyle, 1967, 1969 and 1975). Argyle's 'communication cycle' theory sets out to understand, explain and predict how communication occurs between people in one-to-one situations.

In *The Psychology of Interpersonal Behaviour* (1967), Argyle proposed that communication is a skill that needs to be learnt and practised like any other skill. Argyle's (1967) claim was that human communication is essentially a two-way process that involves people sending, receiving and responding to each other's verbal and non-verbal messages.

Key terms

Experimental research: *research that investigates cause and effect relationships*

Social psychologist: *a psychologist who studies the relations between people and groups*

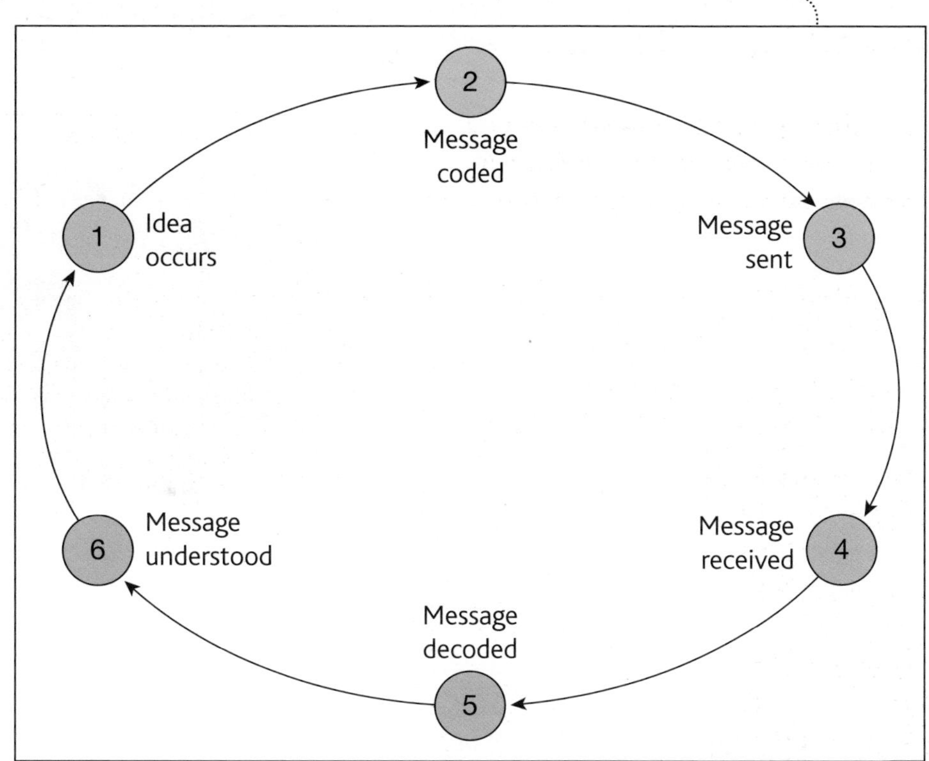

Figure 1.7 The communication cycle.

Figure 1.7 illustrates the way in which the communication cycle works. There are six main stages:

1. an idea occurs
2. a message is coded (by choosing words, using **NVC** or sign language, for example)
3. a message is sent (via speech, writing, signing or use of NVC)
4. the message is received
5. the message is decoded (the recipient has to interpret the message using their knowledge of language, NVC, signs or symbols, for example)
6. the message is understood (the recipient correctly interprets the message or understands the information sent).

The receiver of the message keeps the communication going by responding to or by giving feedback to the original message. This process then repeats and builds into a communication cycle.

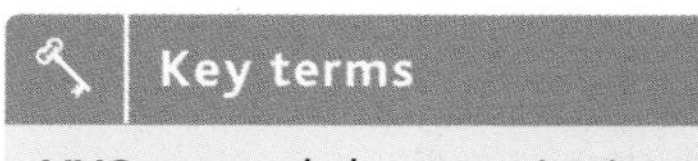

Key terms

***NVC:** non-verbal communication*

M1 Making one-to-one communication effective

The concept of a 'communication cycle' makes it clear that effective communication is a two-way process. As well as getting their messages across to others in a clear and unambiguous way, care professionals need to understand and respond to the verbal and non-verbal feedback of the people they communicate and interact with. According to Argyle's (1967) theory, care professionals can improve the effectiveness of their communication and interaction skills by adapting to verbal and non-verbal feedback from others.

So, effective communication involves effort from both the sender and recipient of a message. Getting your message across, and correctly interpreting the messages communicated to you, are vital to effective communication. However, communication isn't always effective as the receiver can easily misinterpret messages. Problems can occur at every stage of the communication cycle (see Figure 1.8). Care professionals can minimise these problems with clear, concise and well-planned communications and through the effective use of their interaction skills.

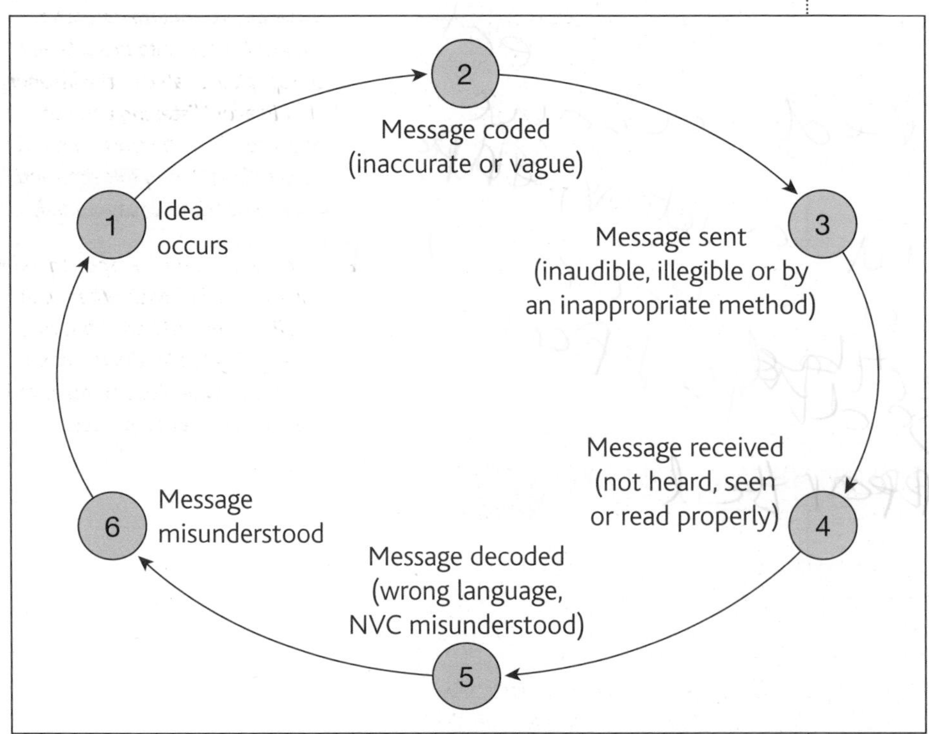

Figure 1.8 Problems in the communication cycle.

Your assessment criteria:

P2 Discuss theories of communication

M1 Assess the role of effective communication and interpersonal interaction in health and social care with reference to theories of communication

The turn-taking pattern of speaking and listening is one of the factors that allow the communication cycle to work effectively. Interrupting people who are speaking – or not listening to what they are saying – disrupts the sending and receiving process of the communication cycle. Additionally, communication is most effective when the message is clear and unambiguous; the person receiving the message will have few difficulties in interpreting its meaning. However, communication is only effective when both the sender and receiver understand the same information as a result of communication. A variety of factors, including cultural differences, background noise and language problems, can disrupt the smooth flow of the communication cycle (see Figure 1.8) and act as barriers to effective communication (see page 40).

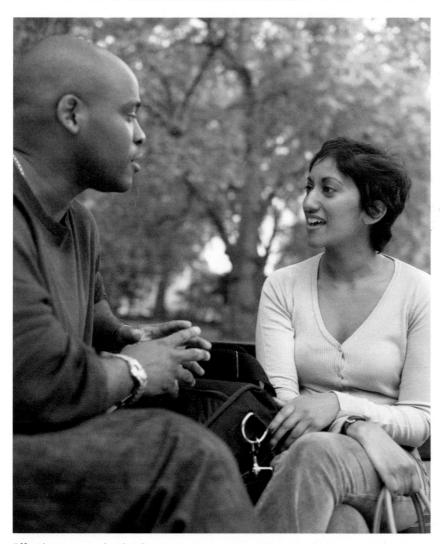

Effective communication is a two-way process.

Discuss

What happens when the communication cycle doesn't work as effectively as it should? Try the following activity with a partner:

1. *Take it in turns to talk to each other about a health-related subject for a minute or so. While the speaker is talking, the listener should avoid listening and not pay attention. The speaker should keep talking during this time and the listener should stay seated.*
2. *After each person has spoken, take it in turns to tell each other what you liked and disliked about the activity. Try to identify the main factors that inhibited or disrupted the communication process.*

Theories of communication: the group situation

Care practitioners need to have an understanding of group processes and patterns of group behaviour in order to interact and communicate well in the various group situations that they experience. Understanding how groups form and then develop is an important part of this.

Your assessment criteria:

P2 Discuss theories of communication

M1 Assess the role of effective communication and interpersonal interaction in health and social care with reference to theories of communication

P2 Tuckman's group formation theory

Bruce Tuckman (1965) outlined a model of group development based around a number of stages, or a sequence, of group activity. Tuckman's (1965) theory suggests that groups must go through these stages to be effective and that the pattern of communication in each of the four stages is different (see Figure 1.9):

1. **Forming** involves group members coming together and asking basic questions about the purpose and aims of the group, each member's role within it and commitment to it. In this first stage of group development, members tend to feel quite anxious, often prioritise their own interests and may feel 'disorientated' in their interactions with others. A leader usually emerges in this early stage.
2. **Storming**, the second stage, is a period of conflict within the group. Members may argue over the purpose of the group, may contest its aims and sometimes resist the authority and role of the leader. In this stage, power and control are the main issues. Eventually, the purpose of the group and the roles within it become clearer as power and control battles are won and lost. Without tolerance and patience at this stage, the team will fail. Co-operation between members should begin to develop towards the end of this phase.
3. **Norming** is the stage when the group's identity develops. A strong set of shared values, norms of behaviour and a group 'culture' emerge. The group arrives at one goal and agrees a shared plan to achieve it. The group becomes more cohesive and group members tend to work together to resolve conflicts.
4. **Performing** is the stage when the group finally matures and gets down to working effectively. Members tend to focus more on the overall goal rather than on relationships between themselves. Relationships have, by this stage, become more comfortable and are based on trust and mutual support.

Key terms

Forming, Storming, Norming, Performing: *stages in group formation theory*

Reflect

Think about your friendship group or class at school or college. Can you see how Tuckman's theory applies to the formation of this group? Which stage is the group currently at?

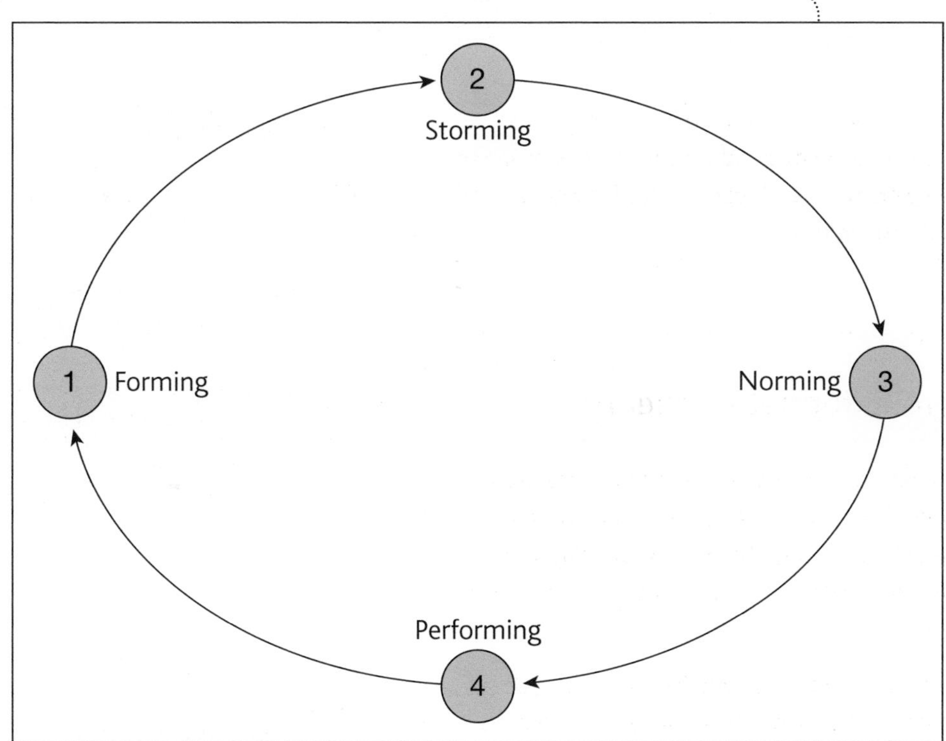

Figure 1.9 The process of group formation.

A group may or may not reach the performing stage: effective, high performing teams do but other less effective groups may get stuck at one of the earlier stages, particularly if they are unable to resolve the challenges or crises associated with that stage of group development. Effective communication within a group situation is a key influence on whether a group reaches the performing stage.

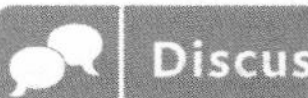

Discuss

How might high staff turnover affect the performance of a team of care practitioners? How does Tuckman's theory help to explain this?

M1 Group communication is different!

People often interact and communicate differently in group situations compared with when they are interacting in one-to-one situations. Typically, people are more restrained and formal in group interactions than in one-to-one situations. Philip Burnard (1992) partly explains this by pointing out that people have to make compromises in the way they communicate within group situations because there is always a tension between the needs of the group and those of the individual. The interests, ideas and needs of the individual are secondary to the goals and shared work of the group as a whole. Despite this, observations of group communication in action can show that some people do not, in fact, put the needs of the group first. Instead they may behave in challenging, competitive and negative ways when in other circumstances they are supportive, co-operative and productive.

M1 Communication strategies in groups

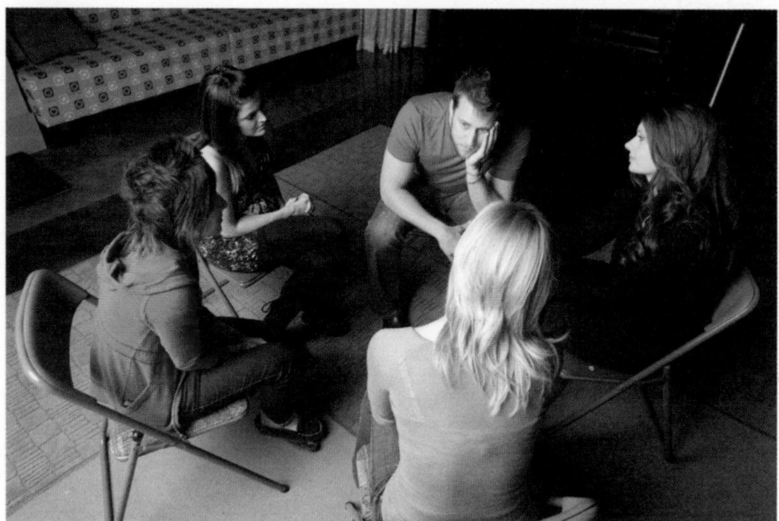

Group communication follows different patterns to one-to-one communication.

R.F. Bales (1970) and his colleagues at the Harvard University social relations laboratory identified and studied a number of different communication **strategies** that are used in groups. These include:

- **proposing** strategies where new ideas, suggestions or plans of action are put forward in a positive and constructive way
- **building** strategies in which a group member extends or develops ideas and proposals offered by other group members; these tend to be positive, constructive interactions
- **supporting** strategies where group members communicate active support for, or agreement with, the contributions of one or more other group members, making the group more cohesive and co-operative
- **dominating** behaviours where an individual or clique monopolises communication opportunities to gain and use power in their interactions with other group members
- **disagreeing** where a difference of opinion or disapproval of the contributions or behaviour of other group members is expressed; disagreements can be made in a constructive way or in a negative, critical way
- **defensive** strategies in which group members put up a defence of their own position, ideas or views when other group members question, disagree with or attack them

Your assessment criteria:

M1 Assess the role of effective communication and interpersonal interaction in health and social care with reference to theories of communication

 **Key terms**

Strategies: *plans of action. Different types of communication strategy are covered in this section*

 **Reflect**

Do you use any of the communication strategies identified by Bales (1970) either at school or college, or in your family? What about other people you know – which strategies do they tend to use? Reflect on the positive and negative effects these strategies can have on your opportunities to communicate with others.

- **attacking** strategies that challenge other group members' ideas or behaviour; these may be met by defensive responses
- **blocking** strategies which are used to place obstacles or difficulties in the way of other group members' proposals or contributions – these tend to be negative manoeuvres, designed to frustrate other group members' efforts
- **summarising**, a communication strategy that seeks to support and maintain the work of group members; it involves a member restating or summing up the contributions and previous discussions of the group
- **pairing** which occurs where a couple of group members talk to each other 'off task', distracting attention from the main focus or work of the group
- **inclusive** behaviours which aim to bring less powerful or more isolated group members into discussions; these strategies usually involve seeking the views, ideas and thoughts of these group members to encourage interaction within the wider group
- **exclusive** communications have the opposite intention and effect to inclusive behaviours – they aim to block other people's communication and frustrate interaction.

Some of the strategies listed above are designed to promote and support effective communication in groups. However, others are clearly more negative in their intent and effects. Sometimes negative behaviours are inadvertent and do accidental damage to communication within a group. At other times, activities such as irrelevant talking, changing the subject and using complicated language are used deliberately to disrupt communication, exclude group members or as a way of gaining control of the group communication process.

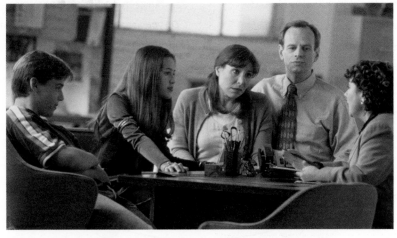

Group communication strategies are often used in families.

M1 Group structures and communication patterns

Patterns of communication in a group are strongly influenced by the group's structure. This is because the structure of a group determines the possible relationships and communication opportunities that group members can have.

Communication in a group or team is fed downwards based on a **hierarchy** (see Figure 1.10). People at the bottom and top have few opportunities to interact with one another. Hierarchical relationships were a common feature of health and social care settings in the recent past. The main criticism of this kind of group is that it limits communication opportunities and leads to 'top down' decision-making. Increasingly, care practitioners and service users are demanding the right to make a contribution to care and treatment decisions. As a result, the power of medical and other care professionals is increasingly being challenged by a rejection of hierarchical group relationships.

A circular group structure provides more opportunities for members to interact with one another; relationships are also on a more equal footing. Circle-type structures are often a feature of community-based health and social care teams where leadership rotates between members, communication with the people who use services is more direct and decision-making is a shared activity.

Your assessment criteria:

M1 Assess the role of effective communication and interpersonal interaction in health and social care with reference to theories of communication

Key terms

Hierarchy: *a system of people or things arranged in a graded order*

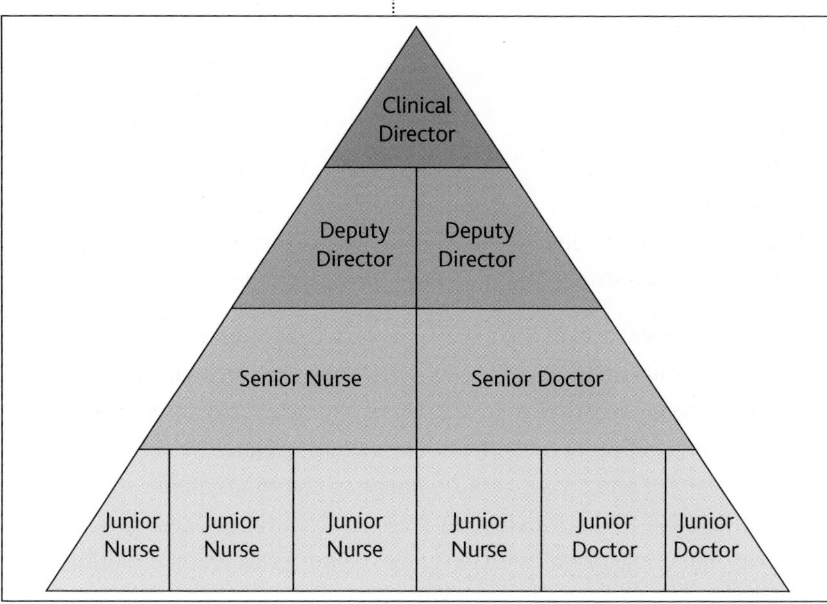

Figure 1.10 Hierarchical group relationships.

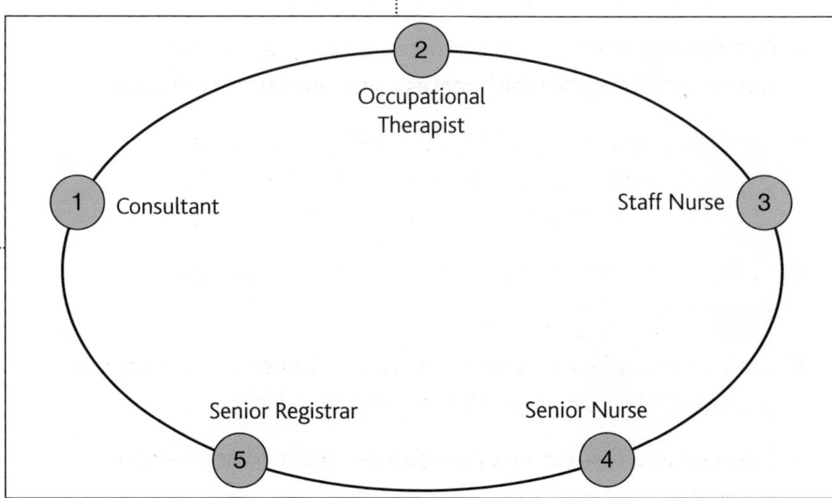

Figure 1.11 Circular group structure.

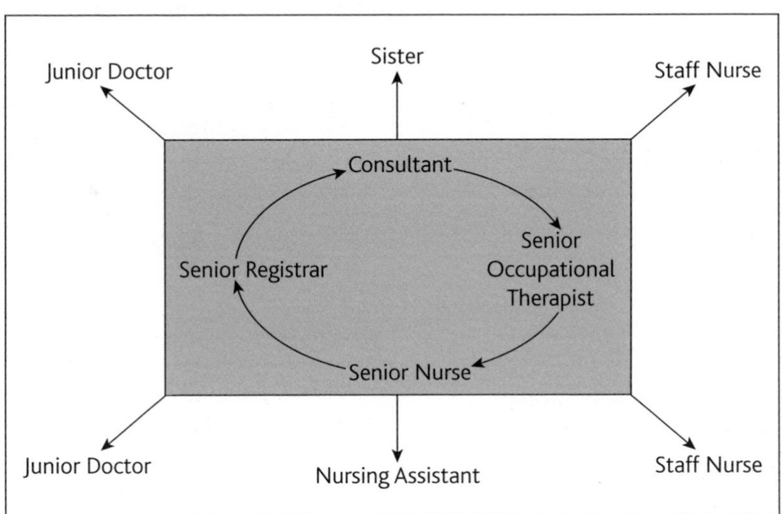

Figure 1.12 Clique structure.

The **clique** is a complex type of group. The people who belong to the 'inner' group tend to be in close contact and to communicate well with each other. The other members of the group are more isolated and find it harder to communicate and interact with the group as a whole. Communication can be fragmented and may not flow freely in groups with clique-style structures.

In real health and social care situations, work teams can be based around a combination of different group structures. For example, multidisciplinary teams are, ideally, based around circular structures but they may also incorporate an internal clique (see Figures 1.11 and 1.12).

Reflect

Think about the teams that you have been part of (on work placement, at school or college, or in your personal life, for example a care team or a sports team). What type of group structure did these teams have? How did this affect your ability to communicate with other team members?

Key terms

Clique: *an exclusive group of people with a shared purpose or interest*

What do you know?

1. Can you list the six stages of the communication cycle?
2. Describe one problem that can occur at each stage of the communication cycle which makes communication ineffective.
3. How could a knowledge of Argyle's (1967) theory of the communication cycle help to make a care professional's communication and interaction more effective?
4. Name the four stages of Tuckman's (1965) theory of group interaction.
5. Describe two differences between communication in a one-to-one situation and communication in a group situation.
6. Explain how the structure of a group can affect communication within it.

Factors influencing communication and interpersonal interaction

A range of environmental factors influence communication and interaction in health and social care settings. These factors are typically so familiar in our everyday and working lives that people tend to take them for granted.

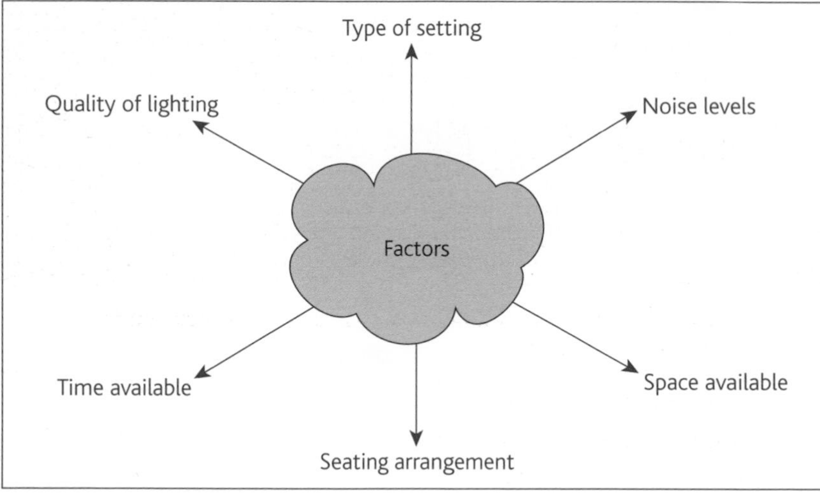

Figure 1.13 Factors affecting communication.

Your assessment criteria:

P3 Explain factors that may influence communication and interpersonal interactions in health and social care environments

P3 Positive and negative influences on communication

The effectiveness, or success, of communication and interaction in health and social care settings is influenced by a number of factors (see Figure 1.13). Some of these factors promote interaction and effective communication, while others can limit interaction and be a **barrier** to effective communication. Care professionals can often overcome 'barriers' to effective communication by:

- being aware of possible problems and solutions
- adapting their interaction approach and communication skills to take account of likely 'barriers'
- making simple modifications to the physical environment of a care setting.

Environmental factors

Aspects of the physical environment can affect the quality of communication between people and may even deter individuals from making an effort to communicate with one another in the first place.

Key terms

Barrier: *something that blocks or prevents communication from being effective because it disrupts the flow of messages*

In particular, the nature of the setting in which communication takes place, noise levels, the arrangement of seating, the quality of lighting, and the amount of available space and time can all impact on the effectiveness of interaction and communication.

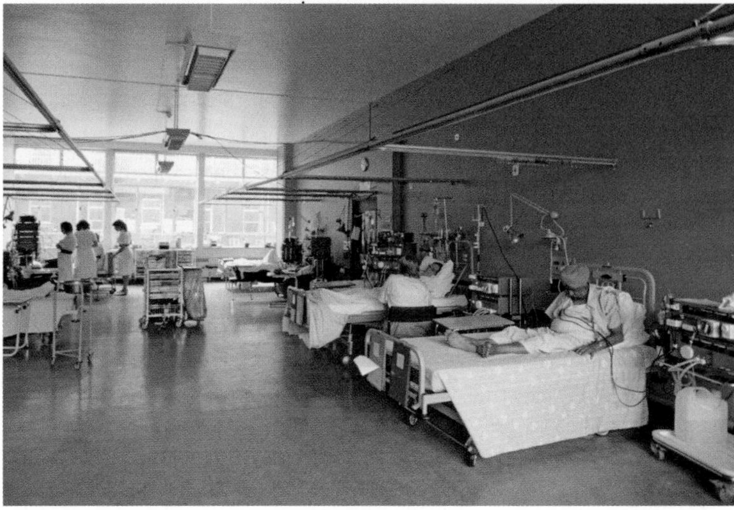

Care environments can be a barrier to communication for some service users.

Considering the setting

People who use care services may interact and communicate with care professionals in their own homes, in community facilities, such as GP practices or day centres, in residential care settings or in institutional settings like hospitals. Where a setting is very busy and there is little privacy, communication may be inhibited. An individual may not feel comfortable talking about themselves or aspects of their life or personal situation in a public environment, for example. However, where efforts are made to ensure the person can talk in private without being overheard, interaction and communication is likely to be more effective. Similarly, people may become isolated and have few opportunities to interact and communicate socially in domestic, community or residential settings that lack comfortable, well-organised **communal** spaces. It is important to ensure that care settings have private spaces, as well as areas where people can meet and talk more publicly.

Key terms

Communal: *shared*

Noise

An environment where there is a lot of noise, either from within or outside of the building, can be a barrier to effective communication. Background noise from a television or radio, from people talking close by or from traffic passing outside a window can make communication very difficult for someone with a hearing impairment, for example. This can be a problem for people who use hearing aids as the background noise is amplified to the same level as the voice of the person speaking to them.

Investigate

Find out how loop systems for hearing aid users work. How do they help people with hearing impairment to communicate more effectively?

Seating

The way that the seats are organised in a room can have a big impact on interaction and communication. Seating that is organised in rows or a line around the outside of the room is less likely to promote interaction than seating organised into small clusters, for example. The seating in a room should be organised in a way that brings people into relatively close proximity, promoting eye contact. While people need to be close enough to interact and talk, seating arrangements shouldn't cause the room to feel cramped or oppressive.

P3 Lighting

The quality of lighting in a person's home or in an institutional care setting may affect communication. Dark and gloomy rooms, for example, make it difficult for care workers to pick up the details of another person's facial expression or body language. The glare of a light, sunshine on a window or shiny surface, or standing in front of a light source can also obscure the speaker's face.

People who have a hearing impairment find that their ability to communicate with others is particularly affected by poor lighting. This is because it reduces their ability to lip read, as well as to pick up the non-verbal features of communication.

Space

The way in which the physical space of a care setting is used can have an impact on communication. For example, in residential and nursing home settings there are often rooms where residents can meet to talk, watch television or join in other shared activities. The extent to which people can communicate can be restricted by poor use of space. With careful thought and planning, the physical space of a care setting can be used to encourage communication to take place. The layout of a room, the careful use of light, and considered selection of furniture and decor can all promote more effective communication.

Time

Interpersonal interaction and communication can be affected by time issues in a number of ways. For example, it is sometimes necessary to book meeting rooms in large care settings. Having a time limit on a meeting can restrict the quality of communication; members of a group or team may have to get through an **agenda** quickly or the meeting may be curtailed by the next group arriving. Similarly, where a care practitioner, such as a GP or a practice nurse, has a lot of people to see, they may need to impose strict time limits on each consultation. If the care practitioner is preoccupied with keeping to their appointment schedule, this again can limit the quality of interaction.

Reflect

Have a look around the classroom where you spend most of your time. Does the space and the way it is organised affect people's ability to communicate? Has anything been done to promote more effective interaction and communication in the room?

Your assessment criteria:

P3 Explain factors that may influence communication and interpersonal interactions in health and social care environments

Discuss

Try having a one-to-one interaction with a friend or colleague after dimming the lights in a room so that they are only just on, or while wearing sunglasses.

1. *Which aspects of communication were affected by changing the lighting conditions?*
2. *How did the lack of good lighting make you feel while communicating with the other person?*
3. *What could the person you were interacting with have done to make communication more effective, despite the poor lighting conditions?*

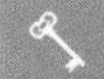

Key terms

Agenda: *an organised plan or list of items to be discussed*

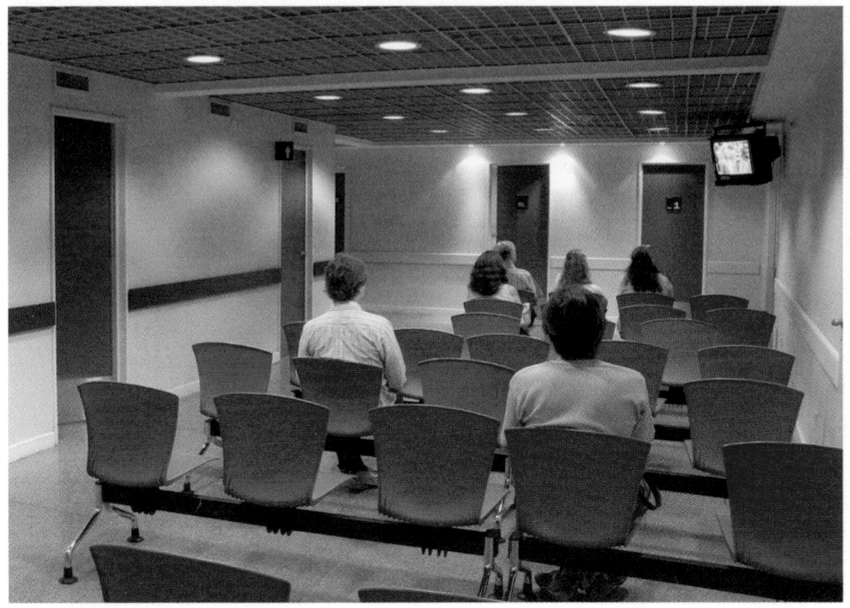

Reflect

Design a room in a health and social care context that would promote interpersonal interaction and effective communication. Your room could be communal with the purpose of promoting group interaction or could be a room where a practitioner communicates one-to-one with a service user.

What do you know?

1. Identify five different environmental factors that can influence the effectiveness of communication in health and social care settings.
2. Describe the possible impact of poor lighting on communication and interaction in a residential care setting.
3. Identify three sources of noise that could impact on communication within a care setting.
4. What is communal space and why is it important to have this in a residential care setting?
5. How can the seating in a communal room be used to promote more effective group communication and interaction?
6. Identify two ways in which time can influence the effectiveness of communication and interaction in a care setting.

Barriers to effective communication

There is a range of barriers to effective communication and interaction in health and social care environments; care practitioners must consider ways of overcoming these barriers. A communication barrier is something that disrupts or stops the flow of messages in the communication cycle (see pags 26-29).

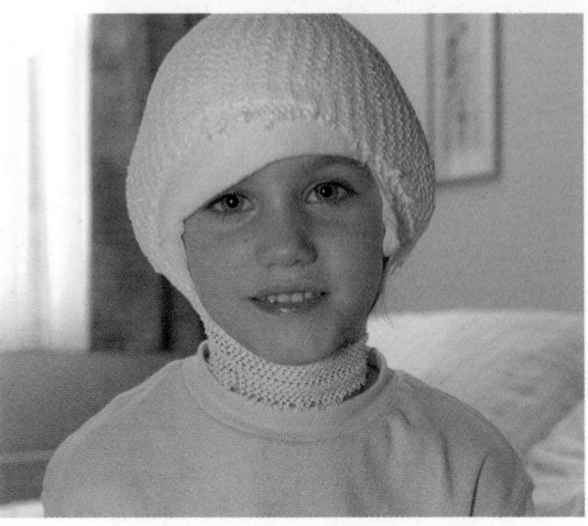

This little girl may be having trouble hearing but could also be experiencing barriers to communication that are not obvious from her appearance in the photo.

Your assessment criteria:

P4 Explain strategies used in health and social care environments to overcome barriers to effective communication and interpersonal interactions

P4 Barriers associated with difficult, complex or sensitive issues

Communication barriers can occur for a number of reasons (see Figure 1.14). Care practitioners need to have flexible and effective communication skills in order to deal with the many different situations that can arise in a care setting. For example, they may be asked to explain difficult and complex information about a person's health problems, treatment or the medication that has been prescribed. The sensitive nature and complexity of the information a care practitioner

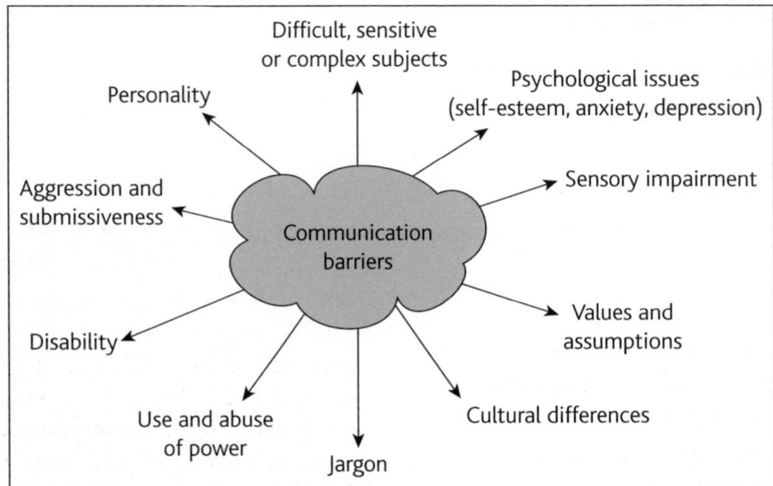

Figure 1.14 Examples of barriers affecting communication in care settings.

has to give can sometimes be a barrier to effective communication, unless they are able to make it accessible and understandable. This is obviously important where the information relates to a person's care or treatment or has implications for their health and wellbeing.

Interpersonal interactions are most effective when people are able to communicate in a supportive atmosphere. People communicate best when they:

- feel relaxed
- are able to **empathise**
- experience and are able to express warmth, genuineness and sincerity
- give and receive respect.

Key terms

Empathise: *Putting oneself in another person's position to appreciate how they feel or what they think about something*

Providing care for people can be an emotionally demanding and difficult task; sensitive issues and stressful incidents arise regularly in the course of care work. This is particularly the case where people receiving care have life-threatening or life-limiting conditions, where an individual is in a lot of pain or is experiencing mental distress. In circumstances like these, people who use care services may be reluctant to talk about their problems. This barrier to communication can have implications for a person's health and wellbeing as they may not receive appropriate support or access to the services they need.

Strategies for overcoming barriers associated with difficult, complex or sensitive issues include:

- using appropriate verbal and non-verbal communication skills to establish and maintain an emotionally supportive and reassuring relationship with the person
- using the person's preferred method of communication to provide information in a clear, unambiguous way that doesn't overload them with detail, use complex language or jargon
- providing reassurance that confidentiality will be maintained
- making sure that the environment is suitable for promoting effective interaction and communication (private, comfortable, quiet, with suitable lighting)
- using staff training and support services to reduce stress levels and develop effective counselling skills, so that care practitioners are able to listen and remain empathetic.

Often, the most effective way of communicating with people who are struggling to talk about or understand a sensitive issue is to reassure them non-verbally. Giving basic information, perhaps in written form, using empathy to understand the other person's feelings, being prepared to listen and spending time with someone are all ways of communicating acceptance and promoting understanding in these circumstances.

Discuss

What advice would you give to a male GP who is wondering how he can communicate more effectively with young women who make appointments about sexual health and contraception issues? Share your ideas and produce a list of key points.

P4 Barriers associated with values and beliefs

A person's values and beliefs encompass their ideas about what is important in life, how they should live and how others ought to behave, for example. Your own values and beliefs may be very similar to those of your friends and family members, but there may be areas where your values and beliefs differ. These areas of difference can sometimes lead to misunderstandings – we may assume that others see things in the same way that we do. A difference in values and beliefs can lead to a failure to understand what somebody is trying to communicate or to outright conflict.

Barriers associated with values and beliefs can be overcome by:

- learning about the values and beliefs of others to understand what they are communicating or why they may be taking a particular approach to an issue
- acknowledging and accepting diversity
- promoting and respecting the rights (to confidentiality, respect, effective communication) of each individual
- being aware of your own values and beliefs and the ways they affect your communication and interpersonal interactions.

Barriers associated with language needs and preferences

Most people have a preferred language or method of communication. Being aware of people's preference and adapting communication to suit will improve interaction with them. However, the way a person uses language may also become a barrier to effective communication. For example, a strong accent, use of a dialect, technical jargon or slang can all make apparently 'plain English' very difficult to understand. Messages can be misunderstood as a result. Additionally, care practitioners who assume that all service users can understand English are making cultural assumptions that may limit some users' communication opportunities.

Barriers associated with language needs and preferences can be overcome by:

- finding out about an individual's preferred language and communication method
- using your own verbal and non-verbal skills in a clear, unambiguous way
- checking your understanding of the other person's messages through summarising and paraphrasing
- clarifying the meaning of any words or phrases that you are not sure about

Your assessment criteria:

P4 Explain strategies used in health and social care environments to overcome barriers to effective communication and interpersonal interactions

Reflect

Do people in your local area use a dialect, slang terms or speak with a strong accent? How does this affect communication with people from outside the area?

- providing multi-lingual signposting within care settings and having letters and leaflets translated into the languages used by members of various local communities.

Where English is not a person's first or preferred language, and in situations where the person uses a different communication system (BSL or Makaton, for example), an appropriately skilled interpreter may be needed to ensure communication is effective.

Barriers associated with assumptions

Care practitioners need to take time to build effective relationships in order to understand the needs of the people who use care services. Making assumptions on the basis of stereotypes or prejudices is not a good way of understanding other people's needs, feelings or circumstances. Assuming almost always leads to misunderstandings that become a major barrier to effective communication; it is important to check your understanding with the other person. Assumptions are a barrier to communication because they prevent care practitioners from getting to know people and limit understanding of their real needs.

Investigate

Assumptions are often made about the needs, abilities and likely behaviour of groups who receive care services. Investigate some stereotypical assumptions associated with:

- *physically disabled people*
- *people with mental health problems*
- *homeless people*
- *teenage mothers.*

Case study

Kimberley, aged 26, tells student nurses a story about an incident that happened to her during her nurse training as a way of encouraging them not to make assumptions about people. Kimberley was on her first nightshift duty on a ward for older people with mental health problems. The shift was quite busy, but Kimberley liked having lots to do. She responded fast when she heard someone press the buzzer at the front door to the ward. Walking quickly, Kimberley wondered whether this might be somebody for admission or perhaps the senior nurse manager doing her rounds. When she looked through the small window in the door, Kimberley was very surprised to see an old man standing there; he had a shock of messy grey hair, looked half asleep and was wearing a scruffy old coat. As she opened the door, the man went to come in. Kimberley blocked his path and said, 'I'm sorry you can't come in. Relatives can visit after 9 in the morning.' The man looked at her and was about to speak when Kimberley said, 'If you need to see a doctor, you'll have to go to A and E – there is no doctor here.' The man replied, 'I *am* the duty doctor. Can I come in?'

1. What assumptions do you think Kimberley made as she looked through the ward door?
2. Were Kimberley's assumptions based on stereotypes and prejudice?
3. How did Kimberley's assumptions act as a barrier to communication?

P4 Barriers associated with cultural variation

Acknowledging and responding to the cultural aspects of a person's identity and care needs are strategies that are likely to enhance communication. While most care workers would agree with this, situations can occur when this doesn't happen. For example, if care practitioners make a general assumption that their beliefs about issues such as diet, personal care practices, sleeping arrangements and health are shared by all service users, they risk imposing their cultural beliefs on people who don't share them. The danger of imposing dominant cultural assumptions like this is that both the identities and care needs of service users who don't belong to the dominant culture are neglected. This obviously makes interaction and communication less effective. A person's cultural background and experience also influences their understanding of verbal and non-verbal communication. Failing to notice and respond to cultural variations in the use of verbal and non-verbal language can lead to misunderstandings.

Barriers to communication associated with cultural variation can be overcome by:

- developing knowledge and awareness of cultural differences, particularly with regard to communication behaviours (eye contact, touch and proximity, for example)
- monitoring and checking the cultural meaning of non-verbal messages that you receive
- being aware of the way you use verbal and non-verbal messages in your own communication
- ensuring you don't make inappropriate assumptions about the ability of other people to understand you.

Barriers associated with the use and abuse of power

Care practitioners are in a privileged, relatively powerful position in relation to people who use care services. They get to know a lot about the personal circumstances, problems and health issues of the people in their care. Additionally, people receiving care are often emotionally vulnerable and are sometimes physically dependent on care practitioners. The potential power imbalance in care relationships could be misused by an unscrupulous care practitioner to dominate, control, bully, abuse or exploit the people they provide care for. Bodies that regulate the conduct of care professionals, such as the Nursing and Midwifery Council (NMC) and the Health Professions Council (HPC), produce codes of practice and codes of conduct that aim to prevent

Your assessment criteria:

P4 Explain strategies used in health and social care environments to overcome barriers to effective communication and interpersonal interactions

Discuss

Why do some Muslim women wear a niqab or face veil? What impact might this have on their communication with health and social care practitioners?

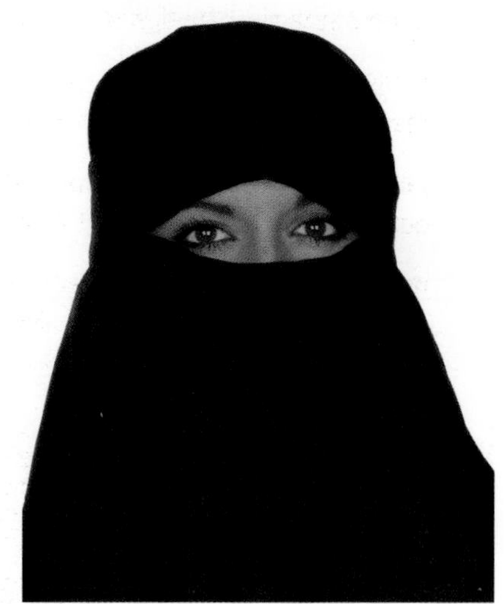

the misuse of power. Where power is misused in a care relationship, communication is likely to be ineffective because:

- the service user may feel frightened and intimidated by the care practitioner, becoming withdrawn and avoiding communication
- a service user's self-esteem may be damaged through being controlled and manipulated
- service users who are dominated or controlled by practitioners are unable to make their own choices or assert their rights.

Care practitioners can minimise the risk that the use and abuse of power could become a barrier to effective communication by:

- respecting each service user's individuality, rights and identity
- **empowering** service users to make choices and to control their own lives as much as they are able
- being aware of and always acting according to the code of conduct or code of practice produced by the body that regulates their profession
- using verbal and non-verbal communication appropriately and responding to service-user feedback
- gaining consent or asking permission before undertaking any task or activity that involves or will affect the service user
- maintaining confidentiality when discussing issues relating to the service user; people generally feel more confident about disclosing personal information if they are reassured about confidentiality.

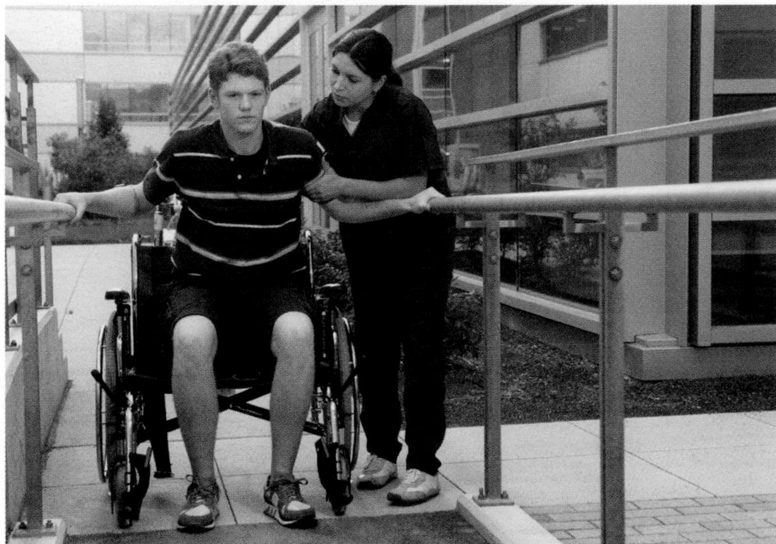

Effective communication can be used to empower service users.

Key terms

Empowering: *giving or delegating power or authority to another person*

P4 Barriers associated with drugs and alcohol

Alcohol and drugs impair a person's ability to communicate effectively. People who are under the influence of alcohol or drugs may not be able to receive or retain the messages that are communicated to them or may interpret the messages in a distorted way. This can lead to misunderstandings, frustration and aggression.

Care practitioners can overcome the impact that alcohol and drugs have on an individual's ability to interact and communicate effectively by:

- giving the individual affected by drugs or alcohol plenty of time to collect and express their thoughts and feelings
- using simple, direct and clear language when speaking
- using a calm tone and a relatively slow pace when talking to the person
- taking care to ensure that their non-verbal communication is unthreatening and consistent with what they are saying
- summarising and paraphrasing to clarify what the person is saying
- paying close attention to the person's non-verbal communication.

Barriers associated with personality, self-esteem, anxiety and depression

People who have low self-esteem or who are experiencing anxiety or depression often feel threatened by and incapable of dealing with the challenges that they face. Lack of confidence, negative thinking and low mood can all impair an individual's ability to communicate effectively. Care professionals can overcome barriers associated with personality, self-esteem, anxiety or depression issues by:

- building up an individual's self-esteem through a supportive relationship
- focusing on more positive aspects of the individual's thoughts and achievements to boost their self-esteem
- encouraging the person to set goals and to plan constructively for their future
- maintaining confidentiality in order to prompt and support the person's efforts to communicate and interact with others.

Your assessment criteria:

P4 Explain strategies used in health and social care environments to overcome barriers to effective communication and interpersonal interactions

Reflect

Have you ever had to help or support a person affected by drugs or alcohol? How did this affect their behaviour and communication skills?

Investigate

Find out about the role of care workers such as clinical psychologists, counsellors and mental health nurses. How do these care practitioners help people to rebuild their confidence and self-esteem?

Barriers associated with sensory impairment and disability

A person may have a hearing, visual or speech impairment that affects their ability to communicate effectively. In particular, people with hearing and visual impairments may not be able to receive messages that are conveyed verbally or non-verbally. To overcome barriers associated with sensory impairment and disability, care workers can:

- assess a person's communication needs and abilities (this may require specialist assessment from other practitioners)
- ask the person (verbally or in writing, for example) how they would prefer to communicate and what aids they may need
- adapt their own communication approach and skills to meet the particular needs of the person
- use a skilled interpreter or signer if the person's preferred system of communication is BSL, Makaton or another non-spoken language
- ensure that the environment is appropriate for the person's communication needs by checking that the lighting is sufficient, that background noise is low and that seating is appropriately organised, for example.

Investigate

You can find out more about the impact of sensory impairment on communication by exploring these websites:

- *The Royal National Institute for the Blind website at* www.rnib.org.uk
- *The Royal National Institute for the Deaf website at* www.rnid.org.uk

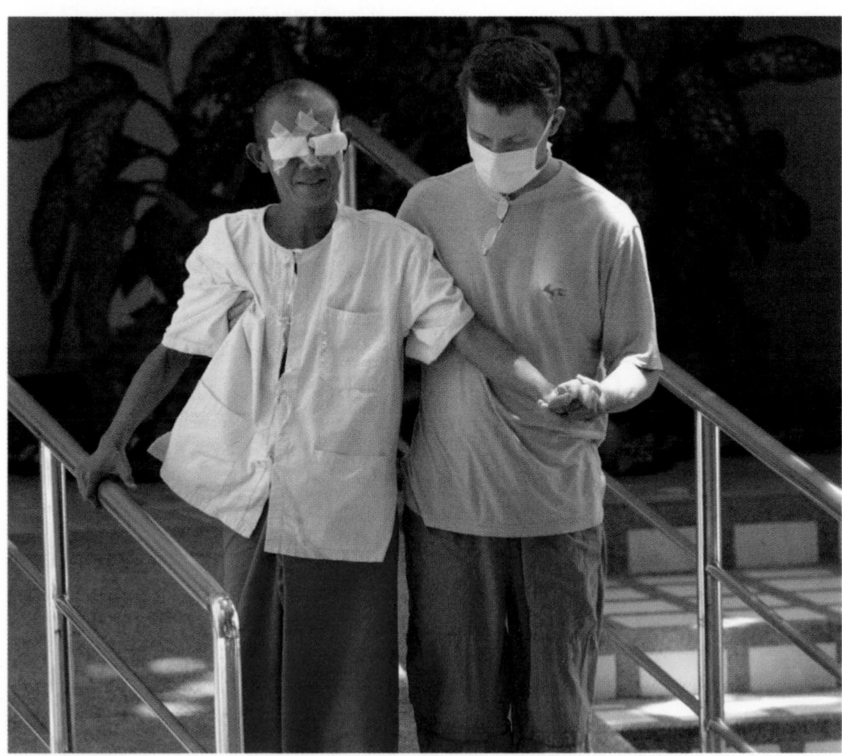

Adapting to the needs of others is necessary to overcome the communication barriers associated with sensory impairment.

P4 Barriers associated with aggression and submissiveness

Some people become aggressive when they are frightened or frustrated. In contrast, other people become withdrawn and submissive when they feel stressed or threatened. In both situations, an individual's ability to interact and communicate effectively is likely to be affected. Aggression can quickly escalate to a point where a person's hostility prevents them from engaging in or responding to two-way communication. Similarly, a person who is submissive may be unable to express their thoughts, assert their rights or gain the services or support they require.

Care practitioners can overcome the problems associated with aggression and submissiveness by:

- using their own verbal and non-verbal communication skills in a calm, non-threatening way
- being clear and assertive in the way that they communicate with people who are aggressive, and supportive towards those who are submissive
- ensuring that the environment (space, lighting and proximity) is used to defuse or de-escalate an aggressive situation
- empowering people to take control of situations that they find stressful
- avoiding physical contact or getting into arguments as a way of 'hitting back' at people who are being aggressive
- using reflective listening to clarify the source of any misunderstanding and to reassure the person that their perspective is valued and taken seriously.

Your assessment criteria:

P4 Explain strategies used in health and social care environments to overcome barriers to effective communication and interpersonal interactions

M2 Review strategies used in health and social care environments to overcome barriers to effective communication and interpersonal interaction

Reflect

Why do you think some people act aggressively or violently towards care practitioners at times?

M2 Reviewing the strategies used to overcome communication barriers

Health and social care organisations are keen to promote effective communication between care professionals and people who use care services. They may use a range of strategies to do this, all with the aim of prevent or removing barriers to effective communication. Figure 1.15 shows the questions that could be asked when reviewing the strategies an organisation uses to overcome barriers to communication.

Figure 1.15 Reviewing the strategies for overcoming communication barriers.

Stage of review	Question to ask
Find out about the range of strategies being used	What is being done?
Examine how the strategies are being put into practice	How are the strategies being put into practice?
Make a critical assessment of the effectiveness of the strategies	Are the strategies working?

The views and experiences of both the people who work in and the people who use a care organisation should be part of a review. The information gathered can then be combined with direct observations to assess the effectiveness of the strategies being used.

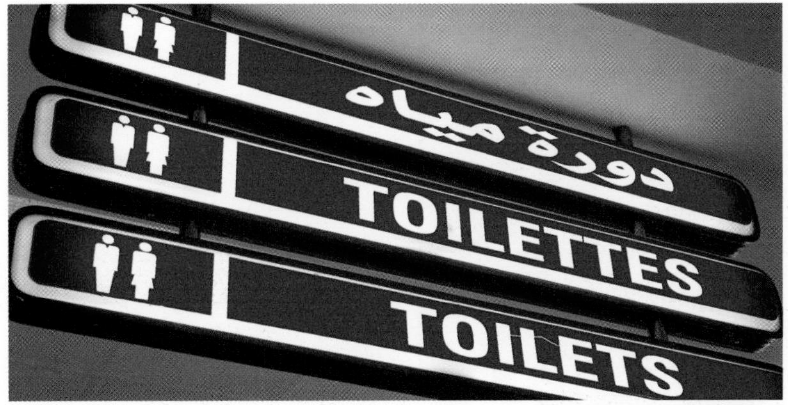

What do you know?

1. Identify four different barriers to effective communication.
2. Describe, using a practical example, how a care professional's values, beliefs or assumptions could become a barrier to effective communication.
3. Explain how communication barriers associated with cultural differences could be overcome by a care professional.
4. How can personality and self-esteem problems prevent effective communication?
5. What kinds of strategies could a care professional use to overcome the barriers to communication experienced by a deaf person?
6. Explain how aggression can act as a barrier to effective communication in a care setting.

Human aids to communication

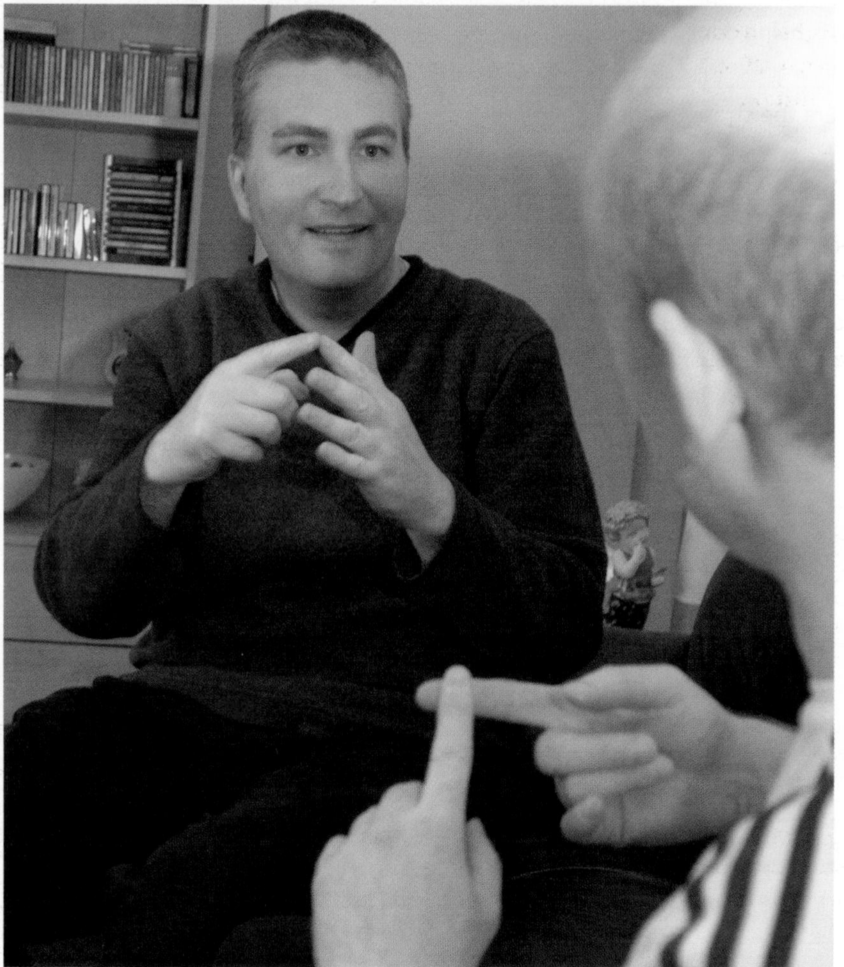
People like this specialist signer can be aids to communication.

Your assessment criteria:

P4 Explain strategies used in health and social care environments to overcome barriers to effective communication and interpersonal interactions

Key terms

Stroke: *a non-medical term for a cerebrovascular accident which results in a sudden loss of consciousness when the brain is starved of oxygen by a blockage in or rupture of an artery*

P4 Human aids can help overcome communication barriers

Specialist support is sometimes needed to improve the effectiveness of communication where individuals have specific communication problems or support needs. This can be the case where a person has a sensory impairment, a learning disability or where a health problem, such as a **stroke**, affects their ability to send or receive messages.

Advocates, interpreters, translators, signers, mentors and befrienders all play some part in promoting and supporting effective communication. Figure 1.16 describes how these professionals can help people overcome barriers to effective communication.

Figure 1.16 Examples of human aids to communication.

Work role	How this role helps overcome barriers to effective communication
Advocate	Advocates represent the views and interests of people who are unable to do this for themselves. An advocate may attend meetings or court to speak on behalf of the person or may discuss their everyday care needs with care practitioners. An advocate has to get to know a person very well to do this and should always be independent (not a staff or family member).
Interpreter/Signer	Interpreters and signers act as intermediaries in the communication cycle. They receive messages in one language (spoken or signed) and pass it on in another language, ensuring that people who speak or use different languages can communicate with each other.
Translator	A translator reads information in one language and then changes it into another language (French to English, for example).

Translators, interpreters and signers have to find ways of capturing the meaning of a message communicated in one language before passing it on as accurately as possible in another language. This can be quite complex as it is not always possible to find equivalent words or signs in each language.

Figure 1.17 Communication support roles.

Work role	How this role helps overcome barriers to effective communication
Mentor	Mentors provide support and guidance. Often a mentor will have a lot of experience in a particular area of care-related or support work. Mentors may support new and less experienced colleagues or may work with people who have low confidence or low self-esteem to boost their motivation and help them to achieve work or education-related goals.
Befriender	Befrienders are usually volunteers. They offer and maintain a supportive relationship with individuals who lack support and social contact. A befriender needs good listening and empathy skills, but is not expected to have or use professional care skills.

Technological aids to communication

P4 Technology can help overcome communication barriers

Hearing aids, textphones, minicoms, voice-activated software, relay systems and loop systems are all forms of technology that can help people overcome communication difficulties. Figure 1.18 describes the function of each of these technologies.

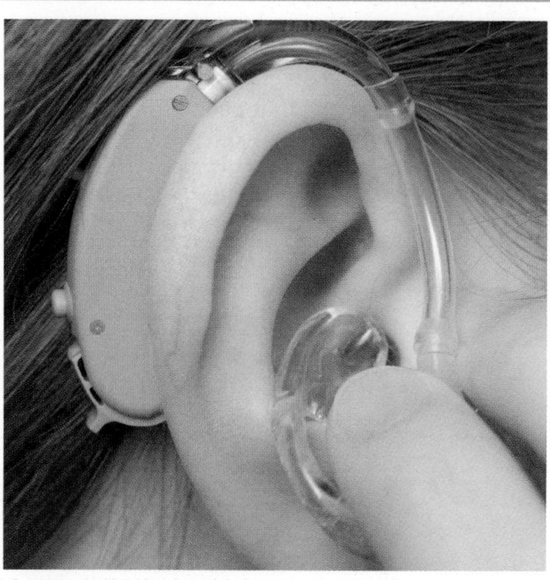

Hearing aids are an example of technological aids to communication.

Your assessment criteria:

P4 Explain strategies used in health and social care environments to overcome barriers to effective communication and interpersonal interactions

M2 Review strategies used in health and social care environments to overcome barriers to effective communication and interpersonal interaction

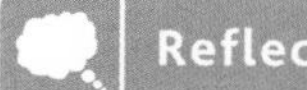

Reflect

Do you know anybody who uses a hearing aid? How does this affect the way they approach interactions with other people?

Figure 1.18 Technological aids to communication.

Technology	Function
Hearing aids	Hearing aids amplify sounds via small microphones. They can help a hearing impaired person to pick up verbal communication, but also amplify background noise. This can be problematic in a busy environment. Users must also remember to wear them and turn them on!
Textphones and minicoms	These devices have small keyboards and screens that allow users to type and read messages they wouldn't otherwise be able to send or receive.
Relay systems	The Royal National Institute for the Deaf (RNID) has a text relay system that allows deaf and hearing impaired people to text a message to an operator who then reads it to a hearing person (on the phone). The operator can then type the spoken reply so that the deaf or hearing impaired person can read it on their textphone or minicom device.
Loop systems	A loop system consists of wires and microphone sensors (usually hidden in a room) that boost sound and reduce background interference for people who use hearing aids. The person needs to switch their hearing aid to a special setting to receive the amplified sound from the loop system.
Voice-activated software	Voice-activated software programmes enable people to communicate directly with computerised devices simply by speaking. Computers with voice-activated software show a person's spoken words on the screen; there is no need to use a keyboard.

M2 Reviewing the use of human and technological aids to communication

Health and social care professionals need to be able to communicate effectively with people who use care services. Once they become aware that an individual needs assistance to communicate effectively, a care practitioner should ensure that suitable human or technological aids to communication are made available. Figure 1.19 shows the questions that could be asked when reviewing the effective use of communication aids.

The views and experiences of both the people who work in and the people who use a care organisation should be part of a review.

Investigate

How many different technological aids to communication do you know about? Find out about as many as you can.

Figure 1.19 Reviewing the use of human and technological aids to communication.

Stage of review	Question to ask
Find out about the availability of communication aids in a care setting	What is available?
Examine how care practitioners identify and obtain appropriate forms of support and assistance for people who need it	How is communication assistance provided?
Assess how effective the human and technological aids being used are at promoting communication	Do they work?

What do you know?

1. Identify three work roles that focus on promoting or supporting effective communication.
2. Describe the role of an interpreter, explaining how this is different to the role of a translator.
3. Explain why some users of care services need the support of an advocate to communicate effectively.
4. Describe how textphones and minicom systems can be used by hearing impaired people to communicate more effectively.
5. What is a 'loop system' and how does it improve the effectiveness of communication?
6. How might voice-activated software help a physically disabled person to communicate more effectively?

Assessment checklist

Your learning and level of understanding of this unit will be assessed through assignments given to you and marked by your teacher or tutor. Before you submit your assignment work for assessment you should make sure that you have produced sufficient evidence to achieve the grade you are aiming for.

To pass this unit you will need to present evidence for assessment which demonstrates that you can meet all of the pass criteria for the unit. The P5, P6, M3, D1 and D2 criteria relate to practical activities; you will need to participate in care-related tasks or undertake a work experience placement in a care setting to complete them. Your tutor will be able to explain how these criteria will be covered as part of your learning programme.

Assessment Criteria	Description	✓
P1	Explain the role of effective communication and interpersonal interaction in a health and social care context.	☐
P2	Discuss theories of communication.	☐
P3	Explain factors that may influence communication and interpersonal interactions in health and social care environments.	☐
P4	Explain strategies used in health and social care environments to overcome barriers to effective communication and interpersonal interactions.	☐
P5	Participate in a one-to-one interaction in a health and social care context.	☐
P6	Participate in a group interaction in a health and social care context.	☐

You can achieve a merit grade for the unit by presenting evidence that also meets all of the following merit criteria for the unit.

Assessment Criteria	Description	✓
M1	Assess the role of effective communication and interpersonal interaction in health and social care with reference to theories of communication.	☐
M2	Review strategies used in health and social care environments to overcome barriers to effective communication and interpersonal interaction.	☐
M3	Assess own communication and interpersonal skills in relation to each interaction.	☐

You can achieve a distinction grade for the unit by presenting evidence that also meets all of the following distinction criteria for the unit.

Assessment Criteria	Description	✓
D1	Evaluate strategies used in health and social care environments to overcome barriers to effective communication and interpersonal interactions.	☐
D2	Evaluate factors that influenced the effectiveness of each interaction.	☐

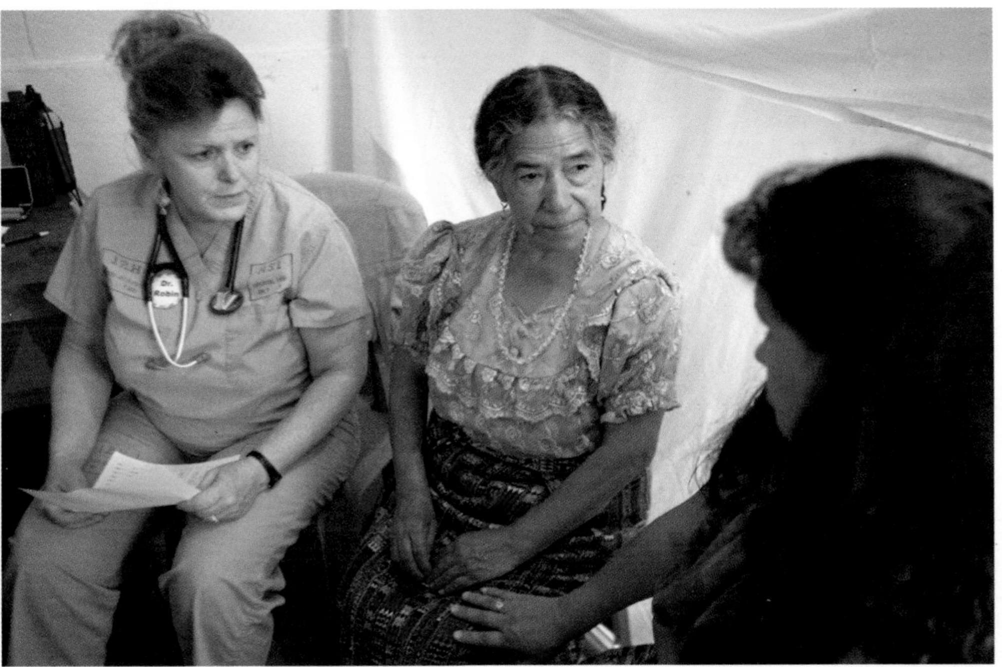

References

Argyle, M. (1967) *The Psychology of Interpersonal Behaviour,* Penguin, Harmondsworth

Bales, R.F. (1970) *Personality and Interpersonal Behaviour,* Holt, Rinehart and Winston, New York

Burnard, P. (1992) *Communicate!* Edward Arnold, London

Tuckman, B.W. (1965) 'Developmental sequences in small groups', *Psychological Bulletin,* 63, 384–99

2 Equality, diversity and rights in health and social care

LO1 Understand concepts of equality, diversity and rights in relation to health and social care

- benefits of diversity
- terminology
- settings
- active promotion of equality and individual rights in health and social care settings
- individual rights

LO2 Know discriminatory practices in health and social care

- bases of discrimination
- discriminatory practice
- effects
- loss of rights

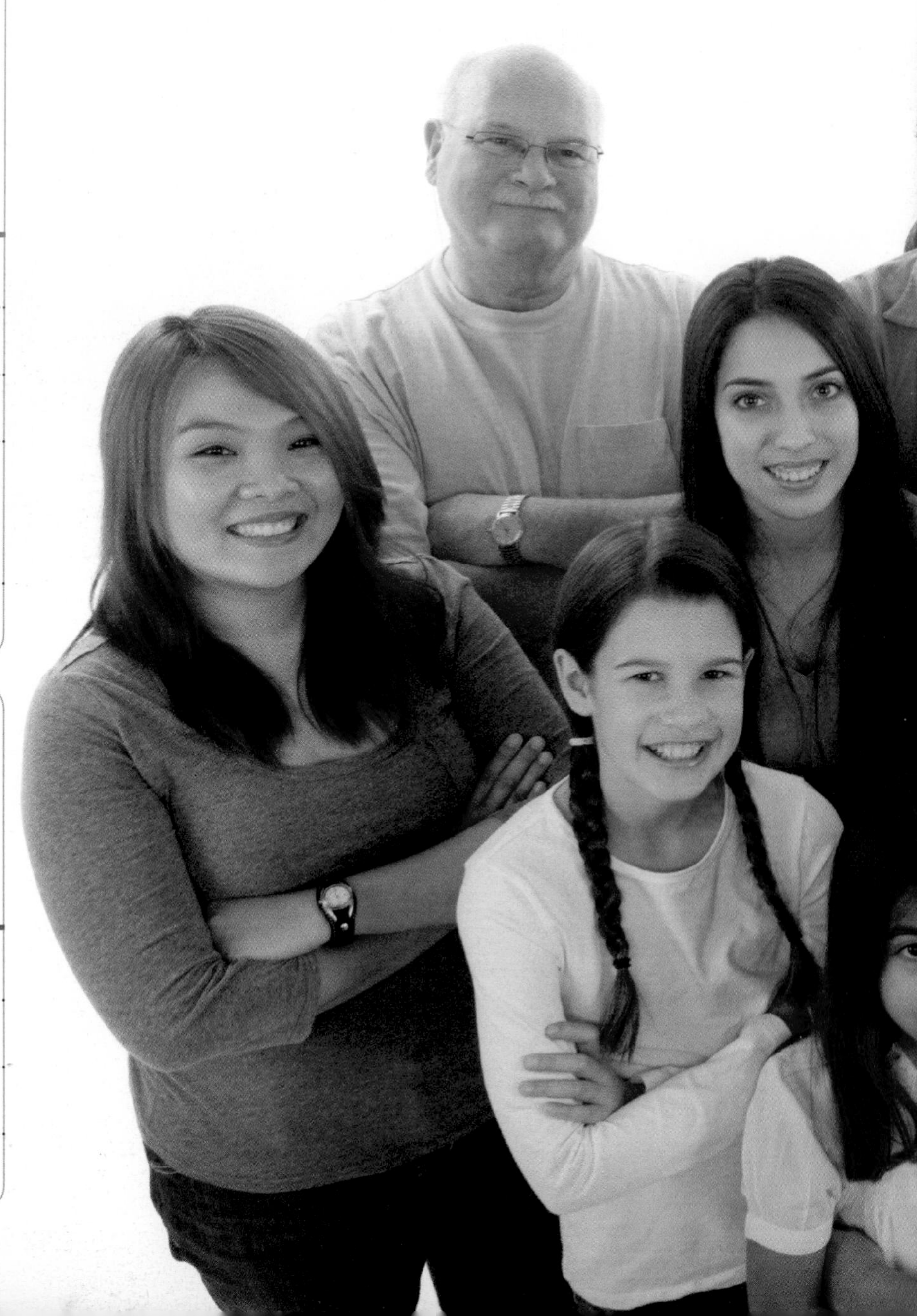

LO3 Understand how national initiatives promote anti-discriminatory practice

- conventions, legislation and regulations
- codes of practice and charters
- organisational policies and procedures

LO4 Know how anti-discriminatory practice is promoted in health and social care settings

- active promotion of anti-discriminatory practice
- personal beliefs and value systems

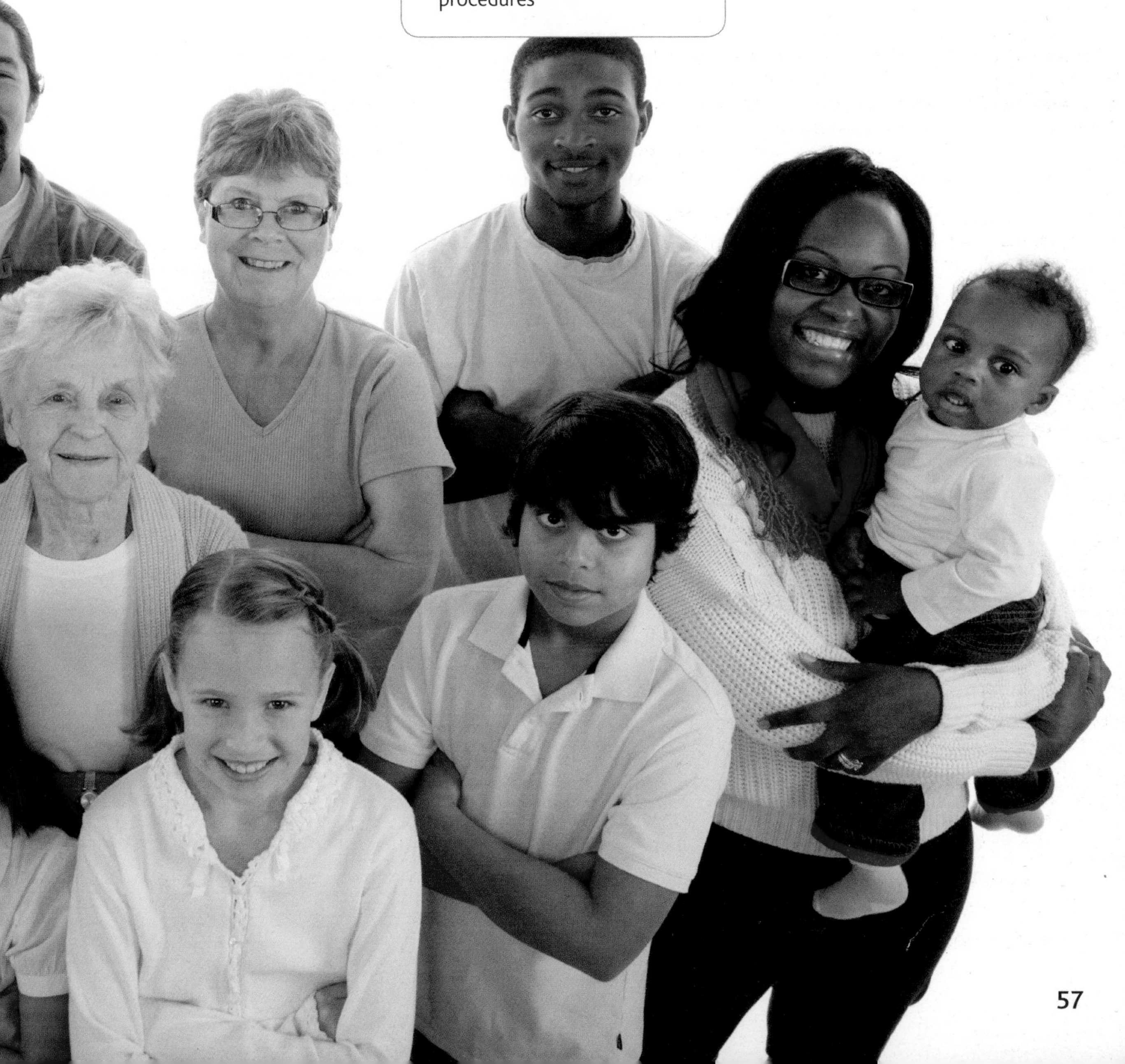

Understanding equality, diversity and rights

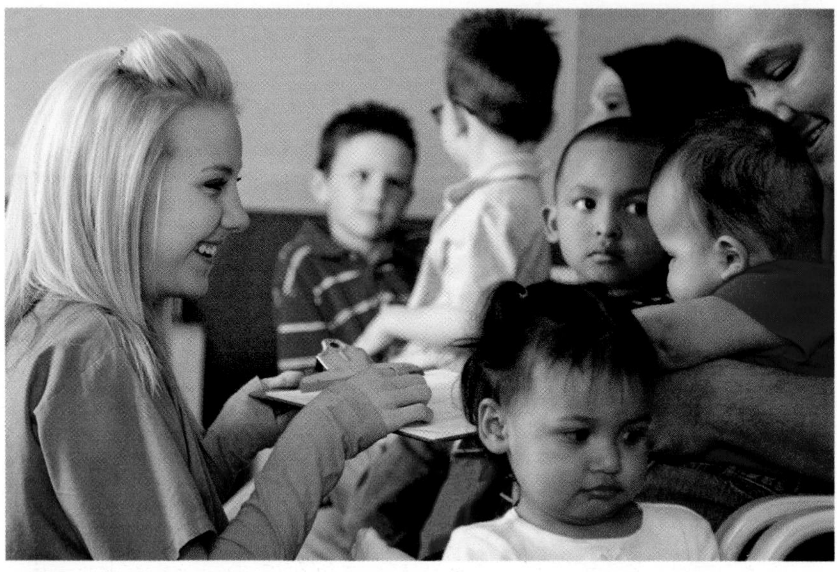

In what ways is this a diverse group of people?

Care practitioners work with a diverse range of individuals in contemporary British society. Health and social care practice should acknowledge, respect and accommodate this **diversity**. Promoting **inclusion** and **equality**, taking **rights** into account, is an important part of health and social care provision.

Your assessment criteria:

P1 Explain the concepts of equality, diversity and rights in relation to health and social care

Key terms

Diversity: *this refers to the social, cultural or ethnic differences within a population*

Equality: *treating people in an equivalent, fair way*

Inclusion: *the idea that all people, regardless of their background or characteristics, should be given fair and equal access to resources, services and opportunities*

Rights: *the legal freedoms or entitlements that people have*

P1 The language of diversity and equality

The United Kingdom has a population that is diverse in many ways. That is, the population consists of people who have a range of different characteristics and needs. Diversity within the UK population can be understood in terms of:

- ethnicity and culture
- gender
- social class
- sexuality
- disability
- age.

A central issue for care practitioners and care organisations is how best to respond to the needs of a diverse population, while also ensuring that every service user enjoys equality. For example, services have to meet the particular needs of people of different ages, different genders, people who have differing ethnic and cultural backgrounds and people with a broad range of abilities, disabilities, illnesses and impairments. Care practitioners need to appreciate the benefits of social and cultural diversity (see page 60) in order to provide appropriate care services in a fair and equal way.

Reflect

What do you think are the benefits of diversity for the UK?

The origins of diversity in the UK

The United Kingdom is now a diverse multicultural society. In part, this diversity is the result of a number of 'waves of immigration' that brought people from other countries to the UK in order to boost the economy.

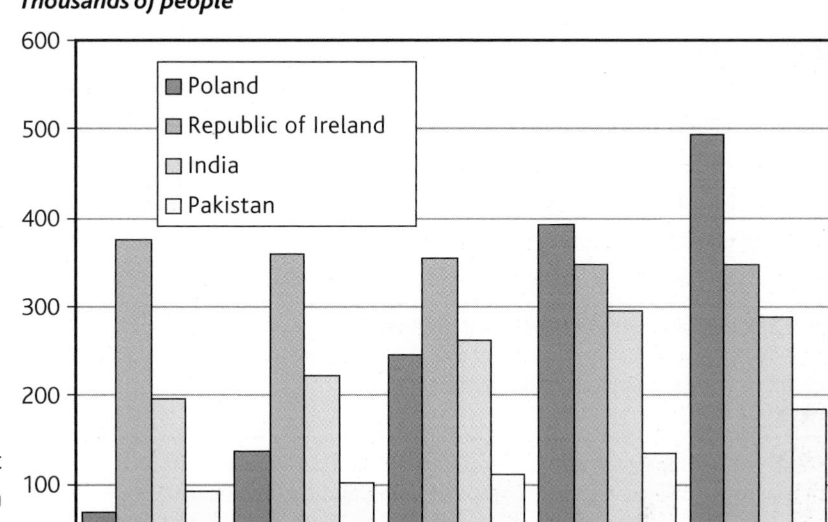

Figure 2.1 Number of non-UK nationals resident in the UK, 2004–2008.

Historically, immigration to the UK from Western Europe, the Caribbean, South Asia (India and Pakistan), Cambodia and Vietnam, and parts of Africa (e.g. Somalia and Nigeria), as well as more recent immigration from Eastern European countries, has made the UK more ethnically and culturally diverse. Despite this, minority ethnic groups still comprise only 7.9% of the overall UK population.

Figure 2.2 Ethnicity statistics are published by the Office for National Statistics.

Ethnic group	Population	Proportion of total UK population
White	54,153,898	92.1%
Mixed race	677,177	1.2%
Indian	1,053,144	1.8%
Pakistani	747,285	1.3%
Bangladeshi	283,063	0.5%
Other Asian (non-Chinese)	247,644	0.4%
Black Caribbean	565,876	1.0%
Black African	485,277	0.8%
Black (others)	97,585	0.2%
Chinese	247,403	0.4%
Others	230,615	0.4%

Employees and users of health and social care services may now come from a diverse range of cultural backgrounds, and will have differing beliefs and values.

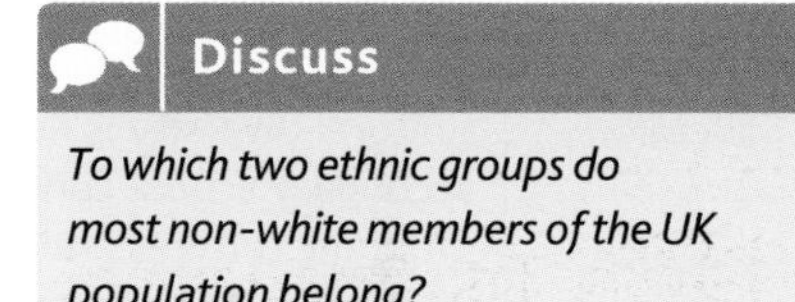

To which two ethnic groups do most non-white members of the UK population belong?

Diversity and types of discrimination

P1 The benefits of diversity

Arguably, diversity is beneficial for UK society as it brings together people from different backgrounds and cultures to share their knowledge, experiences and skills. Figure 2.3 outlines some of the benefits of diversity, including economic benefits, for the country as a whole.

Your assessment criteria:

P1 Explain the concepts of equality, diversity and rights in relation to health and social care

Figure 2.3 Social and cultural benefits of diversity.

Area of benefit	**Explanation and examples**
Cultural enrichment	Books, theatre, art and film productions give insight into different cultures, ways of living and the perspectives of different people. Knowledge from these sources can promote and develop understanding of diversity and enrich wider UK culture, improving quality of life for everyone.
Diet	A diverse population brings dietary diversity through knowledge of foods from different ethnic groups. Knowledge of these foods is needed when planning care and meeting individual's nutritional needs. For example, a knowledge of Halal and kosher food rules is important when planning care and meals for Muslim and Jewish service users.
Education	Cultural diversity is now explored in the primary and secondary school curriculum. Knowledge and understanding of different cultures and of diversity in the UK population enables young people to be more inclusive and non-discriminatory. Education and training courses are also a way of challenging **prejudice** and of preventing **unfair discrimination**.
Language skills	Employment practices that acknowledge and promote diversity in the workplace enable organisations to recruit staff who speak the languages (and dialects) of their local community. This enables care organisations to be more responsive to the needs of the local population.
Tolerance and social cohesion	A socially diverse population promotes and provides opportunities to practise tolerance of others. This is an important quality in health and social care practice. Minority ethnic groups may also bring social cohesion (at least within their own community) and supportive relationships. Health and social care team members need to promote and can benefit from this type of cohesion.
Labour force skills and national income	Immigration boosts the UK economy. It brings people with important work skills to the UK to fill vacant posts. These workers produce goods and provide services, and pay tax, leading to a more productive and stronger economy. Migrant workers bring new ideas, techniques and skills that can increase productivity and improve the quality of life for everyone.

Key terms

Prejudice: *an unreasonable or unfair dislike or preference towards an individual or social group*

Unfair discrimination: *treating some people less favourably than others*

Types of discrimination

Diversity is not celebrated by everyone in the UK, and is a source of fear and resentment for some people who believe they are being 'pushed out' or 'taken over' by 'outsiders'. This can lead to unfair treatment or unfair discrimination against those who are different from the majority (see Figure 2.4). Unfair discrimination that is obvious and deliberate is known as **overt discrimination**. Unfair discrimination that happens inadvertently or which is carried out in a secretive, hidden way is known as **covert discrimination**. Acknowledging diversity, and challenging prejudice and all forms of unfair discrimination are important elements of anti-discriminatory practice in care work.

Key terms

Covert discrimination: *unintentional unfair treatment or deliberately disguised unfair treatment*

Overt discrimination: *obvious and deliberate unfair treatment*

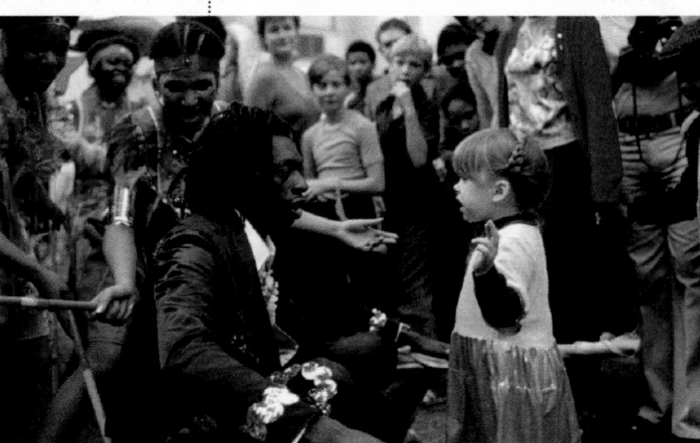

Children are not born with prejudiced attitudes - they have to learn these from others.

Figure 2.4 Examples of unfair discrimination.

Type of discrimination	What does this involve?
Racism	Unfair discrimination against people because of their ethnic background. It can be expressed as: • institutional racism where an organisation inadvertently disadvantages or deliberately treats people of one particular ethnic group less favourably • directly as overt racism • indirectly as covert or inadvertent racism. Minority ethnic groups are more likely to experience racism than members of the white majority group in the UK.
Sexism	Unfair discrimination against people because of their sex or gender. Sexism may: • occur at institutional, group or individual level • be direct and overt or indirect, inadvertent and covert. Women are more likely to experience sexism in the UK. The consequences can be fewer opportunities, lack of recognition and unequal pay compared to men, for example.
Homophobia	This is the fear and hatred of people who are homosexual and of their homosexuality. Homophobia is a prejudice that can lead to: • hostility and unfair discrimination • hate crimes • physical threats and violence. People who are homophobic often feel that heterosexuality is 'normal' and that homosexuality somehow presents a threat to normal social order.

Diversity, equality and rights issues in care settings

P1 Promoting equality in care settings

Equality, diversity and rights are sensitive issues – personally and professionally – for many people working in and using health and social care services. As a result, it is important to use terms relating to equality and diversity issues in appropriate ways. This will enable you to:

- communicate more effectively with service users
- communicate and interact appropriately with colleagues
- avoid treating or responding to people from a different background to your own in an inappropriate or insensitive way.

Your assessment criteria:

P1 Explain the concepts of equality, diversity and rights in relation to health and social care

Fairness in access to care

In health and social care contexts, ***equality*** involves treating everyone who uses care services (or who works within them) in a fair and equal way. People generally expect to receive fair access to treatment or services – they expect *equality of opportunity* or *equal rights*. The slightly different idea that all people are entitled to an *equal share* of health and social care resources (such as a practitioner's time or a particular drug treatment) is summed up by the concept of **equity**. Where treatment is provided equitably, every service user will receive their fair share of resources.

Key terms

Equity: *this refers to the idea of fairness, justice or a fair share of resources*

Case study

George Danver has pancreatic cancer. His GP wishes to prescribe a drug that will extend his life by up to 2 years. George's local Primary Care Trust will not fund this drug. George is angry about this as he knows that if he lived in the next county, 3 miles away, he would receive this drug.

1. Talk about George's situation in a small group or with a partner.
2. What kind of equality (equality of opportunity or equity) is George seeking?

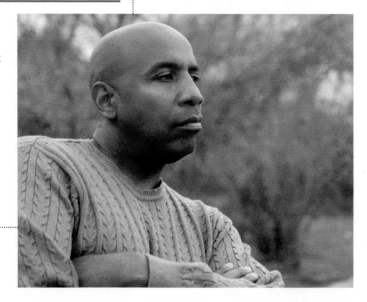

Social inequality

The various forms of social inequality that exist in UK society can lead some people to experience social exclusion and the health effects of **social disadvantage**, prejudice and unfair discrimination. These effects can be seen in the higher rates of illness, disease and premature death that people in the lower social classes and those in **marginalised** groups experience (see page 80).

It is important to note that social inequality is not a consequence of the physical, social or cultural differences that exist in the population. It is the unequal distribution of economic and social resources, prejudice and unfair discrimination and the inability, or reluctance, of governments, organisations and individuals to tackle sources of privilege and social advantage that have the effect of creating and maintaining social inequalities.

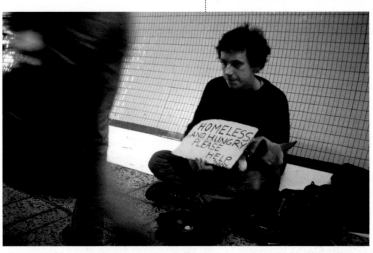

Homeless people are an example of a marginalised group.

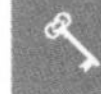

Key terms

Marginalised: *pushed out of mainstream society or the local community*

Social disadvantage: *the result of having fewer opportunities or resources in comparison to others*

Case study

Duncan left the Army 2 years ago. Almost immediately, he experienced a range of personal and financial problems. Duncan's efforts to start a small gardening business caused him a lot of stress and he used up all his savings. He began drinking to cope with the pressure, affecting his relationship with his wife and children. Duncan's wife asked him to move out of the house when his temper began frightening his daughters. Duncan stayed with a friend for a few weeks but soon found himself sleeping in the park.

Duncan got into the habit of using alcohol and drugs to get through each day (and night). He now feels hopeless and can't see a way out of this situation. He has applied for many jobs but is never successful. Most of all, he would like a safe place to live and enough money to eat properly each day.

1. How can the concept of social exclusion be used to explain Duncan's situation?
2. In what ways is Duncan socially disadvantaged?
3. Why is fair access to care services particularly important for people like Duncan?

Reflect

Are there any socially disadvantaged groups living in your local area? In what ways are members of these groups marginalised, socially disadvantaged or discriminated against?

Prejudice, stereotyping and labelling

The assumptions that a person makes about another individual or group of people is likely to affect the way they deal with them. Prejudice, **labelling** and **stereotyping** all involve making assumptions about what other people are like.

P1 Prejudice and stereotyping

A stereotype is a simplified or standardised view about a type of person or thing. Stereotypes can help us to make sense of the world, when we are looking for patterns and want to classify people or objects. However, they are unhelpful when used insensitively because they can lead us to jump to conclusions about people; we may become prejudiced against them. Assuming that all older people are frail, hard of hearing and have memory problems is an example of using a stereotype that isn't, in fact, true to life. Health and social care professionals who are influenced by this stereotype are likely to communicate less effectively with older service users than care practitioners who can see past these negative assumptions about older people.

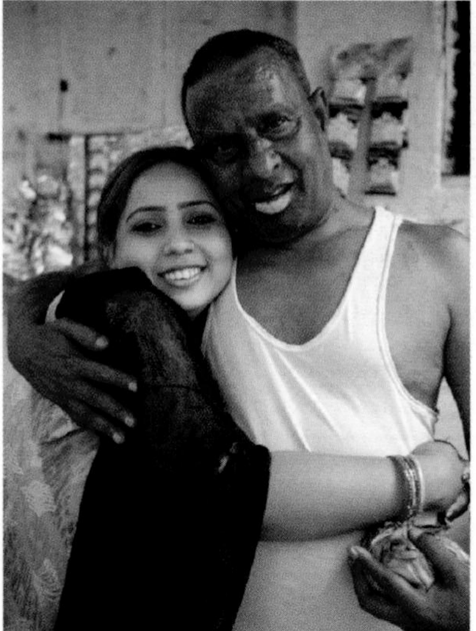

Prejudices and stereotypes prevent us from seeing the real person behind the label.

Labelling

The process of labelling people with diagnoses or other terms (for example, 'personality disordered', 'geriatric', 'manipulative') that carry a very negative social status is strongly discouraged and should be avoided in contemporary health and social care practice. Labelling and stereotyping are barriers to effective interaction because they restrict communication and prevent care practitioners from identifying each person's individual needs.

Beliefs and values

When a person becomes involved in stereotyping others they are applying their own **beliefs** and **values** to others in an inappropriate, often insensitive and usually ill-informed way. A person's beliefs refer to their ideas about the world and their place within it. Our beliefs influence our

Your assessment criteria:

P1 Explain the concepts of equality, diversity and rights in relation to health and social care

Key terms

Labelling: *describing someone in terms of a word or short phrase ('schizophrenic' or 'Down's child', for example)*

Stereotyping: *the process of applying simplified labels or standardised views to individuals or groups*

Discuss

In a small group, identify examples of medical 'labels' that you don't like and discuss the reasons why you think they are stigmatising.

Key terms

Beliefs: *things that a person accepts are true*

Values: *ideals that a person believes are important*

behaviour and lifestyle in a very broad way. For example, an individual's beliefs about health may affect the extent to which they exercise, eat a healthy diet and use or avoid potentially damaging substances like alcohol, tobacco or other drugs.

Beliefs are principles that are accepted as true, often without proof. Values are principles too, but they guide behaviour by giving us a sense of what is right and wrong. For example, a person's health beliefs may lead them to eat a healthy, balanced diet. However, their values in relation to animals may mean that they choose a vegetarian or even a vegan diet.

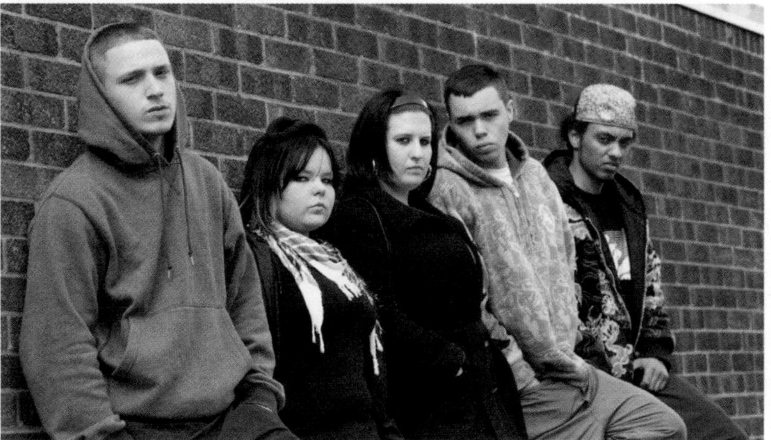

What stereotypical ideas can people have about teenagers like these?

Reflect

What stereotypical ideas are associated with teenagers?
Can you think of any ways in which the labelling of teenagers has a negative effect on their opportunities or treatment by other people?

Case study

Roseen, aged 22, had a breakdown 3 years ago following a very distressing bereavement. After taking an overdose, she was admitted to a psychiatric unit and treated for severe depression. Since then, she has received support from her GP and a community nurse; she has now stopped taking all medication and feels well.

Despite the success of her treatment and the positive way in which she has overcome her problems, Roseen has been unable to find work as a nanny or nursery nurse. Roseen believes that her past history of mental health problems, especially her admission to a psychiatric unit, puts off potential employers. This is frustrating her and is starting to get her down again.

1. How have Roseen's past problems caused her to be labelled?
2. What kind of stereotypical ideas do you think employers might have about people with Roseen's past health problems?
3. Would you be concerned about working with or employing Roseen in a childcare setting? How would you feel as a parent of a child that Roseen might be caring for?

Empowering vulnerable people

P1 Supporting vulnerable people

Health and social care practitioners often work with people who are at a vulnerable point in their lives. That is, because of illness, disability or personal problems, people who use care services are often unable to meet their own needs or protect their own interests. Babies, children and young people and older frail people, as well as those who are ill or disabled, may be more at risk of **abuse** or neglect because of their vulnerability. Safeguarding the interests of **vulnerable** people is, therefore, an important part of a care practitioner's role.

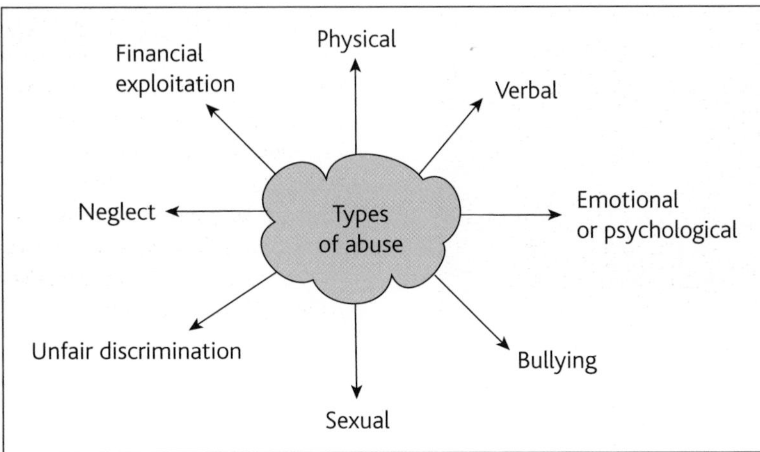

Figure 2. 5 Types of abuse.

Empowerment

Care practitioners often say that they work to *empower* people. **Empowerment** involves giving control or power to someone. Health and social care practitioners try to empower people to gain control over their own health and wellbeing, or over the life circumstances that are making them feel vulnerable.

Independence

The idea of promoting an individual's **independence** is very similar to empowerment. Typically, care practitioners try to work alongside an individual in a partnership, encouraging and supporting them to make decisions and choices that affect their life. This kind of supportive way of working empowers people to become more **autonomous** or self-determining. This is the essence of independence.

Your assessment criteria:

P1 Explain the concepts of equality, diversity and rights in relation to health and social care

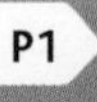

Key terms

Abuse: *the violation an individual's human or legal rights through some form of harm or neglect*

Empowerment: *giving an individual or group the power or ability to do something for themselves*

Vulnerable: *at risk of harm or exploitation*

Reflect

Identify as many reasons as you can to illustrate why a person with learning disabilities could be seen as being 'vulnerable' in a school or college setting.

Key terms

Autonomous: *freedom to make decisions and exercise choice*

Independence: *freedom from the control or influence of others*

Interdependence

It is debatable whether any individual is ever truly independent of others. In reality, people tend to be part of networks of personal and work contacts in which a number of people have **interdependent** relationships. For example, care practitioners typically work as part of a team and, outside of work, people are part of family and friendship groups. These different situations involve mutually supportive, interdependent relationships where people rely on each other and complement each other's skills, abilities and expertise.

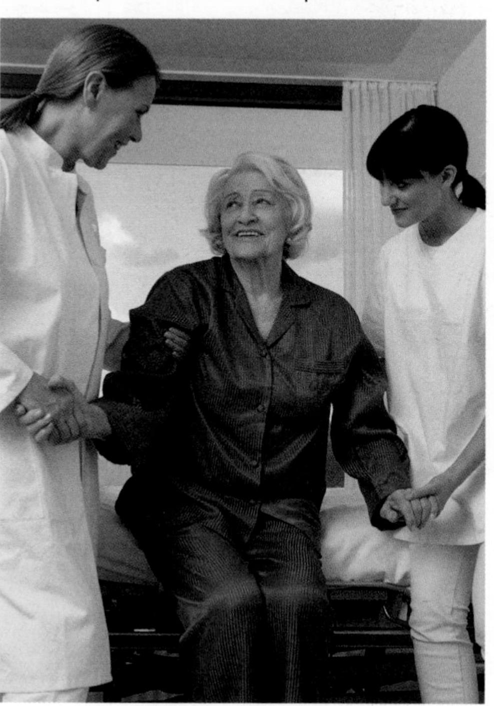

 Key terms

Interdependent: *depending on each other*

 Reflect

Think about your own relationships – in what ways are you part of an interdependent network of social support? Think about family relationships, friendships, work and peer group relationships, and the way in which support is given and received in these different contexts.

What do you know?

1. Identify four ways in which the UK population is socially diverse.
2. Describe two different forms of equality.
3. What is the difference between overt and covert racism?
4. Explain the concept of prejudice.
5. Describe an example of stereotyping that might occur in a health or social care setting.
6. Explain how and why care practitioners try to empower the people that use their services.

Promoting equality and individual rights

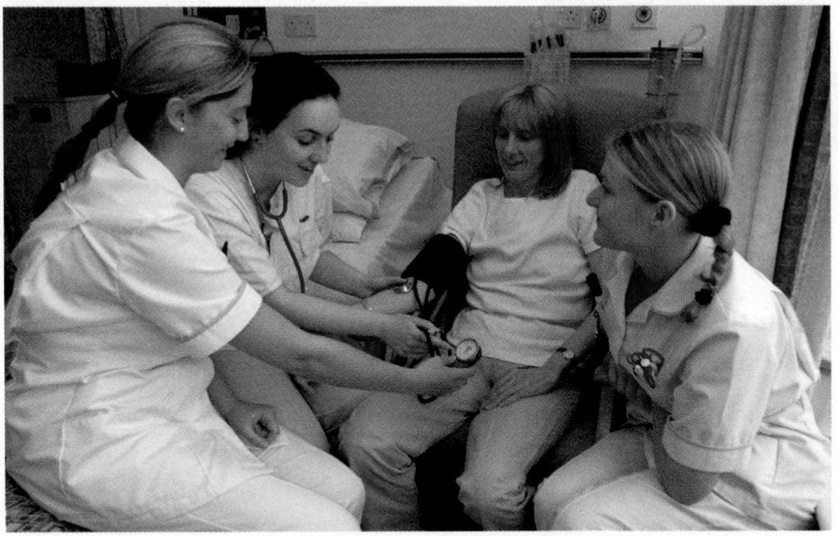

Care practitioners need to respect equality and rights issues when providing care for each individual.

Your assessment criteria:

P1 Explain the concepts of equality, diversity and rights in relation to health and social care

As we have seen, UK care practitioners work with a socially and culturally diverse population of service users and colleagues. Recognising how each individual's social and cultural background affects their personal and care needs, and their communication preferences (see page 24) is an important part of care practice. Care plans, treatment approaches and care relationships should all recognise and accommodate these aspects of an individual's identity, so that the person feels valued and respected.

P1 Care settings

Health and social care services are provided in a variety of different settings:

- Residential settings include hospitals and care homes; people live here either temporarily while receiving care or permanently because they have ongoing care needs.
- Some of these residential settings provide a high level of nursing care (sometimes specialist nursing care) to meet the physical and mental health care needs of residents.
- Other residential settings provide more practical help and day-to-day support for people who cannot live independently but who do not have specific health problems that require nursing care.

Investigate

Can you identify an example of each of the following types of health or social care setting in your local area?

- *a residential setting*
- *a day-care setting*
- *a setting providing nursing care*
- *a domiciliary care service.*

- Sometimes a person can live independently but requires some support or assistance; in this case they may receive **domiciliary** care at home. This is practical home-help care (assistance with meals, washing or dressing, for example).
- Day care, usually based around social activities, is available at day-care centres.

Promoting the individual's rights, choices and wellbeing

Whatever type of care setting a practitioner works in, they should actively promote the equality and rights of service users, of clients' relatives and of their own work colleagues. Care practitioners do this by using the principles of the **care value base** in their care practice. These principles include:

- promoting anti-discriminatory practice
- promoting **dignity**, independence and safety
- respecting and acknowledging personal beliefs and individual identity
- maintaining confidentiality
- protecting vulnerable people from abuse and harm
- promoting effective communication and relationships
- providing individualised care.

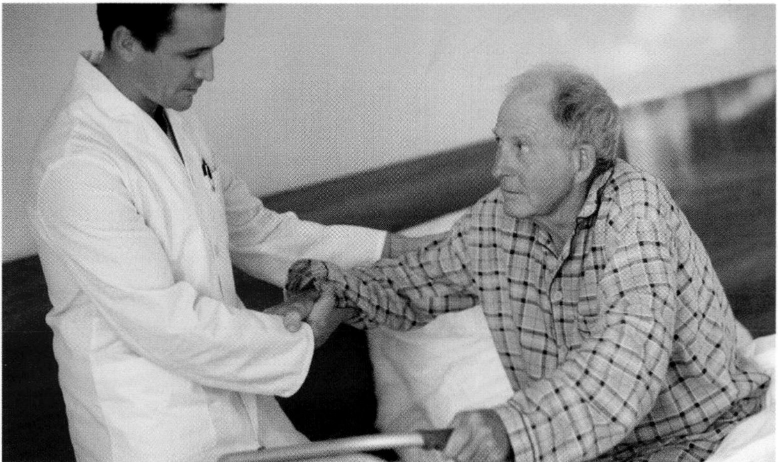

Care practitioners should always protect the dignity of vulnerable people.

Care practitioners who follow these principles will promote an individual's rights and choices, enabling the person to develop and experience a sense of wellbeing and control over their life. Putting the patient or service user at the heart of service provision is the key to this.

Key terms

Care value base: *a set of principles that guide care practice*

Dignity: *the right to be treated with respect*

Domiciliary: *home-based*

Reflect

Can you think of any occasions when a care worker has acted to promote your dignity, independence or safety?

Using an anti-discriminatory approach

P1 Anti-discriminatory practice

Anti-discriminatory practice is an approach to care work that explicitly seeks to tackle unfair discrimination as a way of promoting the rights and equality of each person using care services. Unfair discrimination occurs when individuals or groups of people are treated differently, unequally and unfairly in comparison to others. For example, an employer who refused to interview candidates under the age of 25 for a nursery manager post saying, 'In my experience, younger people are not good at accepting responsibility,' would be treating young people unfairly.

All users of care services should be treated fairly and equally. However, anti-discriminatory practice does not just mean treating everybody in the same way. It also means challenging and reducing any form of unfair discrimination that might be experienced by service users. Care practitioners who take an **anti-discriminatory approach** are:

- aware of the different forms of unfair discrimination that can occur in care settings
- sensitive to the ethnicity, social background and cultural needs of each individual service user
- prepared to actively challenge and try to reduce the unfair discrimination experienced by some service users.

Anti-discriminatory practice is a way of empowering patients and service users to take control of their own care, support or treatment needs. It can be difficult to challenge instances of unfair discrimination or prejudiced attitudes. However, not doing so can mean that you are reinforcing or supporting such discrimination. It is better to draw your manager's attention to situations that concern you.

Dealing with tensions and contradictions

Care practitioners sometimes have to deal with difficult situations where the rights of a service user clash with the legal or professional responsibilities of the care practitioner. For example, a doctor who is treating an obese person with weight-related health problems should advise them to lose weight. However, the doctor cannot refuse to treat the person if they refuse to change their diet or take exercise. Similarly, a social worker should support an individual with learning disabilities who wishes to try living an independent life, even where this involves some risk.

Your assessment criteria:

P1 Explain the concepts of equality, diversity and rights in relation to health and social care

Key terms

Anti-discriminatory approach: *an approach to care practice that challenges prejudice and unfair discrimination*

Reflect

Can you think of any instances where you have acted or worked in an anti-discriminatory way in a care setting? How could you adapt or develop your approach to care practice so that it became more anti-discriminatory?

Each practitioner has to manage the tension between the person's rights, the risks involved and their own professional responsibilities to monitor, support and provide care for the person.

Staff development and training

Continuous professional development is something that all health and social care practitioners are expected to undertake. To maintain a professional level of knowledge and skill, care practitioners need to keep up to date with the evidence, theory, new technology and practices in their area. Over time, care practitioners may need to update themselves on changes in legislation and policy, new care techniques and the use of new equipment, for example. There are a number of ways of doing this (see Figure 2.6).

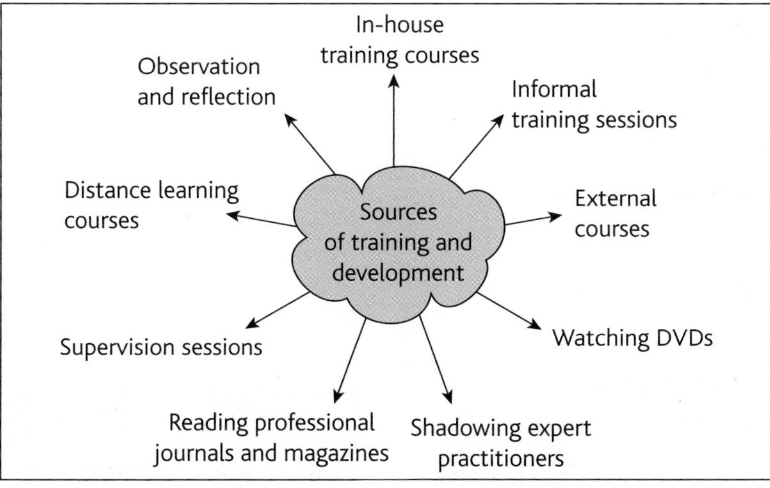

Figure 2.6 Sources of training and development.

Case study

Ian Berryman is a social worker who has just moved to a new post in the 'Older People' team. This is a new area of work for Ian who has spent the last 5 years in Child Protection. Ian is keen to develop his knowledge and skills relating to the older client group. He is about to discuss his learning and development needs with Barbara Korner, his new team manager.

1. Give two reasons why Ian should undertake some additional training as part of his new work role.
2. Describe two ways in which Ian could develop his professional knowledge and skills without taking time off work.
3. How might Ian benefit from shadowing a more experienced colleague for a few days when he starts his new job?

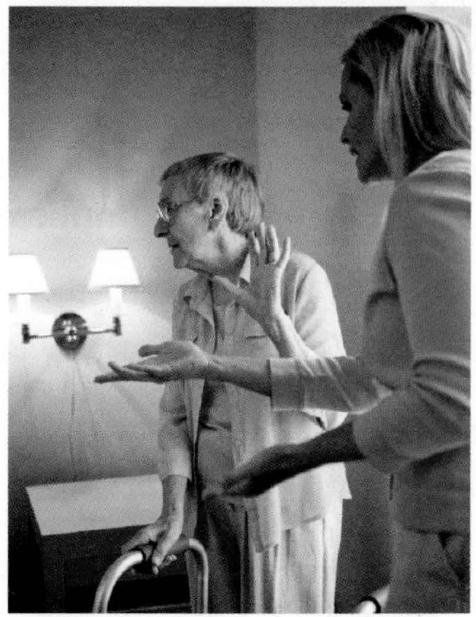

The tensions between rights, risks and responsibilities in care situations need careful handling.

Reflect

Have you ever been a situation where your own wishes, preferences or responsibilities (as a care worker perhaps) contradicted or were in tension with those of somebody else? How did you deal with this situation?

Key terms

Continuous professional development (CPD): *training or educational activity undertaken to maintain up-to-date professional knowledge and skills*

Rights and confidentiality

P1 Practical implications of confidentiality

Confidentiality is a very important care value. It involves recording, storing and sharing information about people in an appropriate way. Care practitioners have a professional and legal duty to maintain confidentiality at all times. Information must be handled carefully so that:

- an individual's wishes and privacy are respected
- the organisation's policies and procedures on confidentiality are followed
- the law is followed.

Care practitioners often obtain information when carrying out assessments or admitting people to a service for care or treatment. When doing this they should ensure that:

- they only collect information that is actually required
- the information they collect is used only for the intended purpose
- the individual's records are kept safe and secure
- all data protection guidelines are followed.

Your assessment criteria:

P1 Explain the concepts of equality, diversity and rights in relation to health and social care

Discuss

Why does confidentiality matter in care relationships? Share and discuss ideas about the importance of confidentiality in a small group. Think about the reasons why people value this important care principle.

Individual rights

As part of being anti-discriminatory, effective health and social care practitioners promote and protect individual's rights in relation to care. This includes the right to be:

- respected
- treated equally and fairly
- treated in a dignified way
- given privacy
- protected from danger and harm
- allowed access to information about themselves
- able to communicate using their preferred method and language
- cared for in a way that meets their needs
- protected and have their personal choices taken into account.

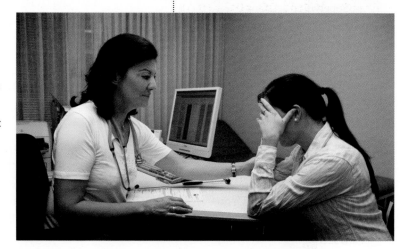

Confidentiality is the basis of trust in care relationships.

Figure 2.7 Ways of promoting an individual's rights.

Individual right	What do care practitioners need to do to protect this right?
The right to be respected	• use listening skills effectively • show patience and compassion • accept others' choices • use a non-judgemental approach • protect dignity and privacy • acknowledge others' beliefs
The right to be treated equally and fairly	• treat everyone equally and fairly • challenge instances of prejudice and discrimination • behave in a non-discriminatory way
The right to be treated in a dignified way	• preserve and promote the individual's dignity and self-esteem by explaining procedures and obtaining consent • ensure the individual has privacy when receiving personal care by closing curtains and doors as appropriate

Effective care practitioners express care values and promote people's rights in the way they provide care.

Discuss

How could a care practitioner promote an individual's right to each of the following?

- *privacy*
- *protection from danger and harm*
- *access to information about themselves*
- *communication using their preferred method and language*
- *care that meets their needs*
- *have their personal choices taken into account*

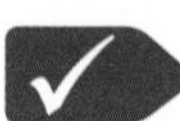

What do you know?

1. Identify four different types of care settings.
2. Name three principles of the care value base that are used to promote individual rights.
3. Explain what anti-discriminatory care practice involves.
4. What is the purpose of anti-discriminatory care practice?
5. Explain how staff development and training can help a care practitioner to promote an individual's rights.
6. What can a care practitioner do to protect confidentiality in the care setting?

Discrimination in society

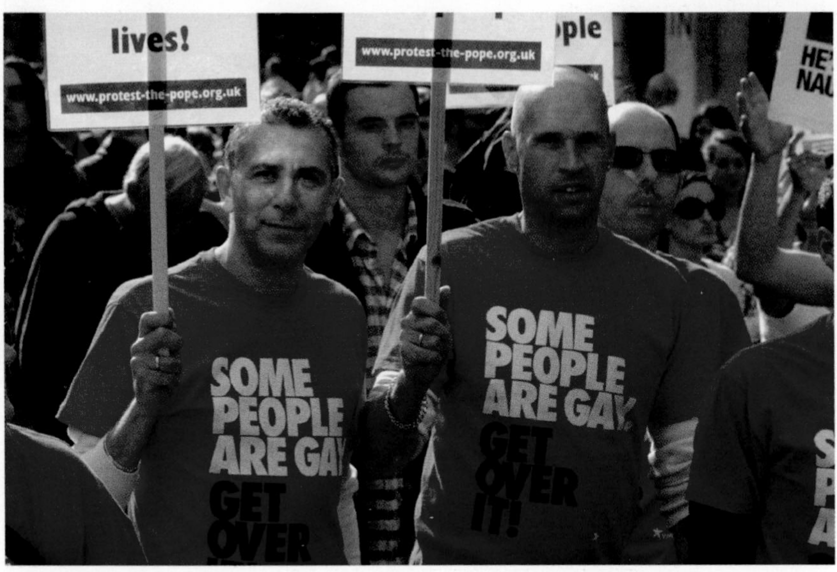

The legal rights of gay men and lesbian women have gradually improved in the UK.

Your assessment criteria:

P2 Describe discriminatory practice in health and social care

P2 Why does discrimination happen?

Care services that are based on equality of access and the fair and equal treatment of all service users are important features of any positive care environment. However, the persistence of various forms of inequality in British society means that some social groups are still struggling to achieve equal rights and equal treatment. Discriminatory practices may occur in health and social care settings with members of some groups being more vulnerable to this than others. These groups are frequently the focus of specific and powerful forms of prejudice and unfair discrimination in society generally.

The basis of discrimination

Unfair discrimination occurs when individuals or groups are treated unfairly, or less favourably, in comparison to others. The main bases of unfair discrimination in the UK are identified in Figure 2.8.

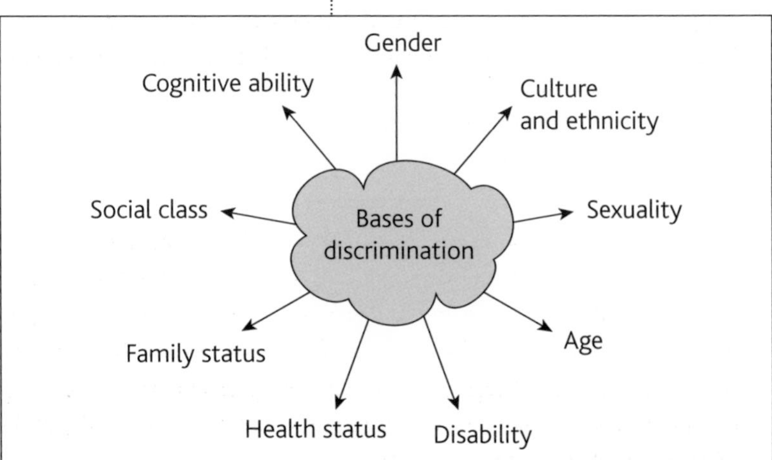

Figure 2.8 The bases of discrimination.

Culture

Government statistics regularly show that people from minority communities are discriminated against in a number of ways. For example, people from black and other minority ethnic groups are more likely to be unemployed than white people (see Figure 2.9).

Official labour force surveys regularly show that white people are less likely to be unemployed than members of black and other minority ethnic groups. Research carried out by Colin Brown and Pat Gay (1985) also found that when black, Asian and white people applied for the same jobs, there was a large difference between the positive responses that they received; 90% of white applicants gained positive responses while only 63% of Asian and 63% of Afro-Caribbean applicants received a positive response.

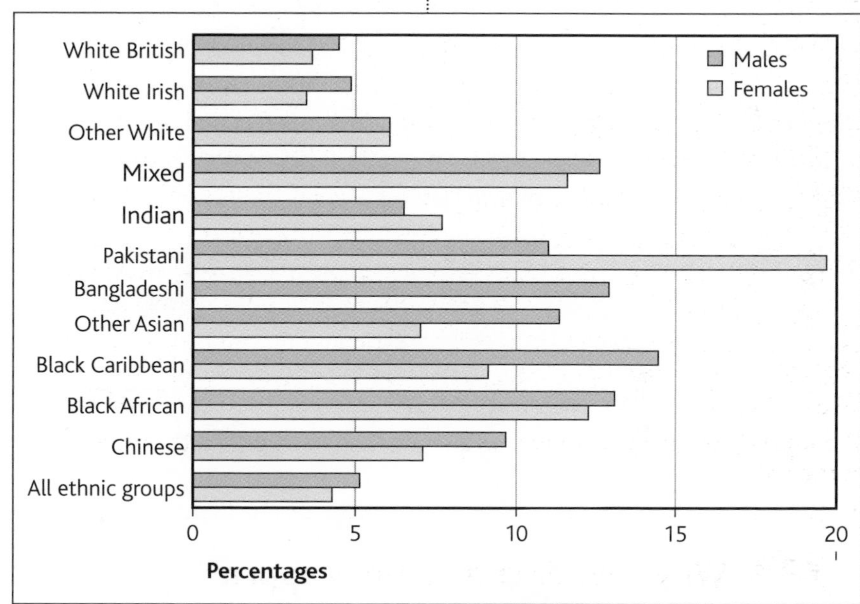

Figure 2.9 UK unemployment by ethnic group and sex, 2004.

Disability

A **disability** is a condition or problem that limits a person's mobility, hearing, vision, speech or mental function. A person may be born with a disabling condition or may acquire their disability as the result of an accident, illness or some form of trauma. Some people have more than one disability. A disabled person may be treated less favourably than an able bodied person because of deliberate prejudice against disabled people or because others don't understand their particular needs. Prejudice against disabled people is known as **disablism**. When people act on their disablist prejudices, disability discrimination may occur.

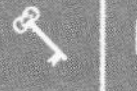

Key terms

Ageism: *prejudice relating to a person's age*

Disability: *a physical, intellectual or mental impairment that makes routine tasks or activities difficult or impossible*

Disablism: *prejudice relating to physical, sensory or learning disability*

Age

The UK population consists of a number of different age groupings; infants, children, adolescents, adults and older people are examples of age groupings. When an age group is given preference, an advantage or is more highly valued than others, **ageism** may occur. This kind of prejudice may lead to age discrimination if a person is treated unfairly purely because of their age. Assumptions about the needs and abilities of older people sometimes lead to this.

P2 Social class

A person's social class results from their occupation, income, education and their attitudes and values (or those of their parents). An individual's opportunities in life, and their health and wellbeing, are linked to social class.

People with a similar social class background tend to live similar lives. Discrimination can occur when people act on their class-based prejudices. For example, an employer with class-based prejudices may avoid interviewing job applicants from certain social classes because they favour people from their own class.

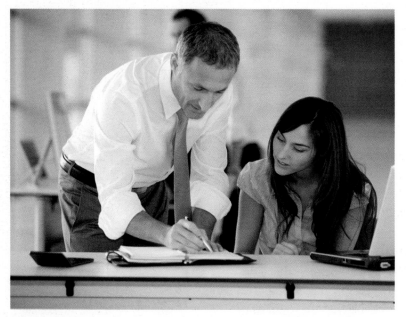

Do gender stereotypes and inequalities still exist in the modern workplace?

Gender

Sexism and unfair discrimination against the female **gender** has led to inequality of opportunity and under-representation of women in high status, higher paid jobs. Despite equal pay laws, women still earn, on average, only about 80% of what men earn per hour. This is due partly to their over-representation in lower status, lower paid jobs and partly to the fact that women are more likely to work part-time. However, despite the fact that more women than ever are now in employment outside the home, they still experience greater **vertical discrimination** and **horizontal discrimination** in the workplace.

Your assessment criteria:

P2 Describe discriminatory practice in health and social care

Discuss

Do you think that your own social class makes a difference to your life chances? Discuss this with a class colleague, identifying ways in which you think a person's class matters in life.

Key terms

Gender: *social characteristics and expectations that distinguish males from females*

Homophobia: *prejudice against (including fear and dislike of) people who are homosexual, and homosexuality*

Horizontal discrimination: *discrimination within the labour market generally that results in women being over-represented in low paid, low status service sector jobs, including care work*

Stigmatised: *to label someone or something as socially unacceptable*

Vertical discrimination: *discrimination that results in women being lower paid, having less status and being lower down the career ladder than men in the same profession*

Sexuality

A person's sexual orientation may be gay, lesbian, heterosexual or bisexual. People who identify themselves as gay, lesbian or bisexual have tended to experience prejudice (**homophobia**) and unfair discrimination because of their sexuality. In particular, some people judge non-heterosexual relationships as 'abnormal' and believe it is acceptable to deny gay and lesbian people the same basic rights as heterosexual people.

Reflect

What are the stereotypes of people who are diagnosed as 'mentally ill'? Why might these result in a person experiencing discrimination?

Health status

People who receive diagnoses that are socially **stigmatised** or feared, such as 'HIV positive' or 'mentally ill', may be discriminated against by those who misunderstand or are frightened by these health problems. This can occur where care practitioners avoid, stereotype or treat such people in a negative way.

Family status

There is a range of different family structures in the United Kingdom. These include nuclear families, extended families, lone parent families, blended families and foster families. In some families, parents are married while in others they cohabit and remain unmarried. If an individual makes judgements or holds prejudices about a person's family background, unfair discrimination can occur. For example, some people assume that it is better to come from a two-parent family and assume that lone parent families are less stable and less able to raise children successfully. Negative assumptions and prejudices about lone parent families sometimes lead to their labelling as 'problem families'.

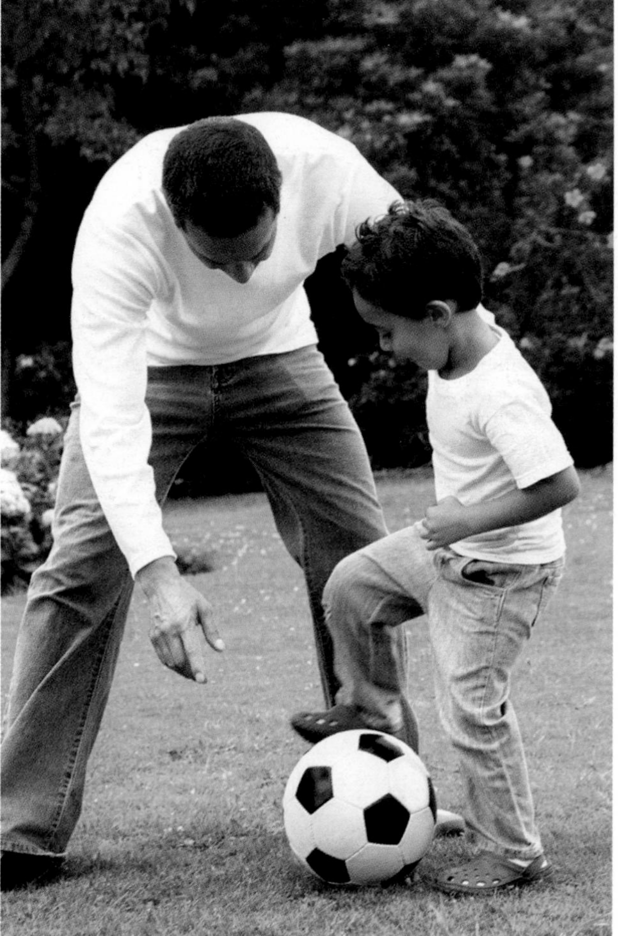

What are the stereotypes associated with lone parent families?

Cognitive ability

A person who has an inherited or acquired brain injury, a learning disability or a lack of education may be treated less favourably or unfairly because of their cognitive ability. People with learning disabilities are sometimes bullied, harassed or become the victims of hate crime because of prejudice about their cognitive abilities.

The effects of discrimination in health and social care practice

P2 Discriminatory practices

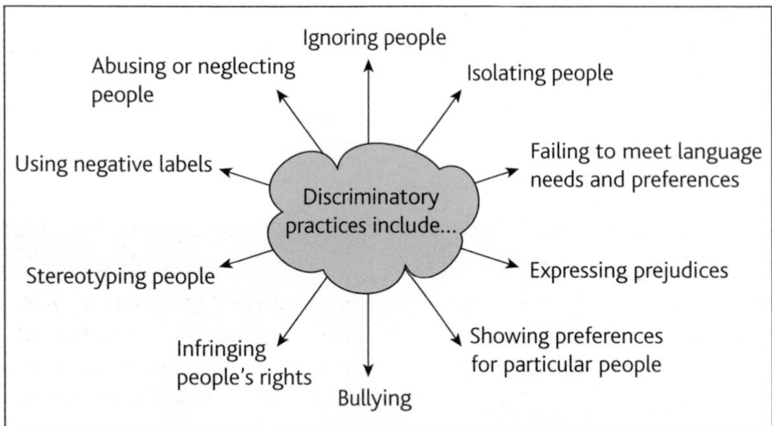

Figure 2.10 Examples of discriminatory practices.

Unfair discrimination can be expressed and experienced in a number of different ways. Direct discrimination involves deliberately treating one person less favourably than another and can be an overt abuse of power. The motive or intention behind such treatment is irrelevant. For example, unlawful direct discrimination would occur if a residential home refused to admit a disabled black person as a resident simply because she was black. It is also unlawful for residential homes to set quotas admitting people of different ethnic origins or to reserve places on a racial basis as this would lead to direct discrimination.

Unlawful discrimination isn't always overt and direct. Indirect discrimination, or the covert use of power, may also occur when a residential home sets a condition that, when applied equally, disadvantages some social groups because they are less able to satisfy it. Because the condition works to the detriment of some social groups (and to the advantage of others) it indirectly discriminates against them.

Your assessment criteria:

P2 Describe discriminatory practice in health and social care

P3 Describe the potential effects of discriminatory practice on those who use health or social care services

M1 Assess the effects on those using the service of three different discriminatory practices in health and social care settings

Case study

Pupinder Singh, aged 32, a baptised and practising Sikh police officer, was ordered by a senior officer to take off his turban during riot training. PC Singh refused, saying that this would be a violation of his dignity and was contrary to his religious beliefs. All officers undertaking riot training are required to wear a protective helmet. PC Singh could not because he was already wearing a turban. As a result, he was unable to complete riot training and has not been able to take up a new post in the Public Order Policing Unit. PC Singh claims that he has been subject to indirect discrimination and is now on sick leave with stress.

1. Is it reasonable for PC Singh to claim indirect discrimination in this situation?
2. Is this an example of indirect discrimination? Explain your answer.
3. What impact has the requirement to wear a specific type of helmet had on PC Singh's health and career opportunities?

Unfair discrimination doesn't just occur at an individual and interpersonal level. Institutions, including care organisations, have also been accused of operating in ways that discriminate unfairly. **Institutional discrimination** is usually associated with indirect forms of discrimination. This can occur, for example, where the policies or procedures of a care organisation disadvantage a particular social group with members who are less able to comply. Because care organisations are generally keen to promote open and equal access for everyone in their local communities, they now tend to take a positive approach towards identifying and tackling situations that may lead to institutional discrimination.

Key terms

Institutional discrimination: *unfair discrimination against an individual or group as a result of the way that an organisation operates or delivers services*

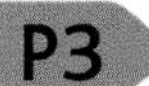

P3 M1 What is it like to experience discrimination?

Have you ever been bullied, treated differently to others or felt that you weren't given a fair chance to do something? If so, you will recognise that these kinds of 'less favourable' treatment can result in short-term distress and personal upset. But imagine how much worse it would be to be treated like that all of the time. How do you think that knowing others were prejudiced towards people like you would affect you when you were at work, when you were trying to make friends or when you were at home with your family?

The emotional and psychological effects of discrimination can be profound. A person's whole self-image and their sense of self-worth can be reshaped, almost always in a negative way, by the experience of prejudice and unfair discrimination. If an incident of discrimination is an isolated one, or if it is dealt with quickly, the person may only be affected temporarily. If the unfair discrimination is experienced over a long period, an individual's self-confidence and **self-esteem** can be damaged permanently. People can feel disempowered when they are devalued by unfair discrimination. As well as reducing people's work, education and lifestyle opportunities, unfair discrimination can lead to depression, negative behaviours (such as criminality and aggression) and long-term health problems.

Key terms

Self-esteem: *a feeling of pride in yourself*

P3 Social effects of discrimination

People who belong to social groups that are the target of prejudice and stereotyping experience forms of **social stigma**; they are marked out by prejudiced people as different, separate and of reduced social worth. The effect of this can be **marginalisation** and **social exclusion**. People who are marginalised are denied full access to society's resources and opportunities – they live on the edge of society and are unable to participate fully. Lack of effective access to education, employment and care services is experienced, for example, by many disabled and older people, by people with mental health problems, those who are homeless and by some members of black and minority ethnic groups – especially those who are recent refugees and asylum seekers. These and other social groups often live in poverty and lack both the economic resources and social influence to change their poor standard of living and circumstances. Health and social welfare services can be particularly important for such groups because poor living conditions eventually have negative effects on health and wellbeing.

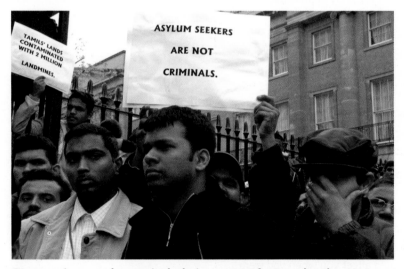

Care services can be particularly important for people who are marginalised and socially excluded.

Since the beginning of the **welfare state** in the late 1940s, governments have developed social policies and forms of health and welfare intervention to assist socially excluded and marginalised groups. However, as welfare groups and official statistics reveal, the problem of social inequality remains significant in the United Kingdom, with some social groups appearing unable to escape poverty. Various explanations are offered for this. Some politicians blame the socially excluded groups themselves for getting stuck in this position. Lack of personal responsibility, poor education, laziness and wasteful use of resources are cited as the reasons why individuals, families and whole social groups remain marginalised

Your assessment criteria:

P3 Describe the potential effects of discriminatory practice on those who use health or social care services

Key terms

Marginalisation: *being excluded or left out*

Social exclusion: *a process that results in certain social groups being pushed to the margins of society (e.g. because of poverty or discrimination), so that they are unable to participate fully*

Social stigma: *social disapproval of personal characteristics, behaviours (lifestyles) or beliefs that are felt to be beyond the cultural norm*

Welfare state: *an approach to government in which the state provides services to protect and promote the wellbeing of all citizens, but vulnerable people in particular*

and in poverty. Other explanations point to a more complex combination of social factors and processes that effectively oppress particular social groups and condemn them to marginalisation and social exclusion.

Key terms

Oppress: *to keep in a weak position through the use of force or power*

Loss of rights

In general, health and social care practitioners promote the individual rights of service users. However, there are some circumstances where an individual's rights can, and should, be overridden. For example, legislation such as the Mental Health Act (see page 84) allows care practitioners to detain a mentally unwell person in hospital – depriving them of their normal right to refuse treatment – if the person is a risk to themselves or others. Similarly, there are circumstances in which an individual's right to confidentiality can be overridden. For example, when:

- a court requires disclosure of information
- not disclosing information would put the person or others at risk of harm
- the care practitioner is aware that a crime has been, or may be, committed.

What do you know?

1. Identify four different bases of unfair discrimination.
2. Describe how cultural discrimination could occur in a health or social care setting.
3. Explain the term *ageism* and give an example of age discrimination relevant to health or social care work.
4. What does gender discrimination involve and how might it occur in a care setting?
5. Explain what institutional discrimination involves and how this could affect care service users.
6. Describe the impact that unfair discrimination may have on those who experience it.

Legal aspects of anti-discriminatory practice

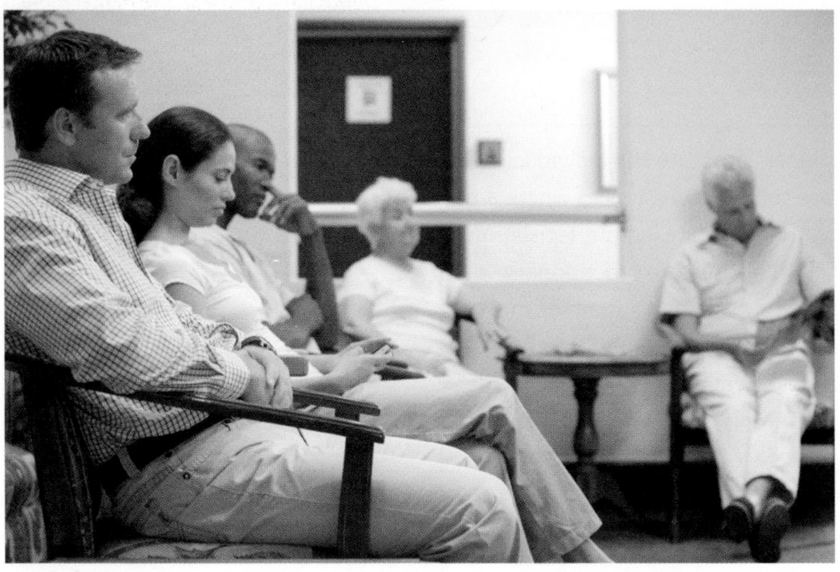

Every individual should be treated fairly and equally in health and social care settings.

Your assessment criteria:

P4 Explain how national initiatives promote anti-discriminatory practice

P4 Conventions, legislation and regulations

A range of equality and anti-discrimination **laws**, **regulations** and **policies** exists in the UK. This **legislation** provides the framework within which care practitioners must work. It also protects the rights of a variety of vulnerable groups to non-discriminatory treatment in many different areas. Examples of the **conventions**, laws and regulations that make up this framework include:

- The European Convention on Human Rights and Fundamental Freedoms (1950)
- The Human Rights Act (1998)
- The Sex Discrimination Acts (1975) and (1986)
- The Equal Pay Act (1970)
- The Mental Health Acts (1983) and (2007)
- The Mental Health (Northern Ireland) Order (1986)
- The Mental Health (Care and Protection) (Scotland) Act (2003)
- The Mental Capacity Act (2005)
- The Race Relations Act (1975)
- The Race Relations (Amendment) Act (2000)

Key terms

Conventions: *international agreements setting out generally accepted standards*

Laws: *rules imposed by Parliament, the Courts and other sources of authority*

Legislation: *Written laws, also known as* Statutes *and* Acts of Parliament

Policies: *written documents setting out an organisation's approach towards particular issues*

Regulations: *legal rules developed to implement legislation in specific ways or in relation to specific circumstances (e.g. moving and handling regulations)*

- The Convention on the Rights of the Child (1989)
- The Children Acts (1989) and (2004)
- The Disability Discrimination Acts (1995) and (2005)
- The Age Discrimination Act (2006)
- The Data Protection Act (1998)
- The Care Standards Act (2000)
- The Nursing and Residential Care Homes Regulations (1984) (amended 2002)

The European Convention on Human Rights and Fundamental Freedoms

This Convention established the European Court of Human Rights and provides the basis for the Human Rights Act (1998). It protects every individual's right:

- to life
- not to be tortured, punished or to receive degrading treatment
- not to be enslaved
- to freedom and a fair trial
- to freedom of thought, religion and expression
- to marry and join organisations
- not to be discriminated against.

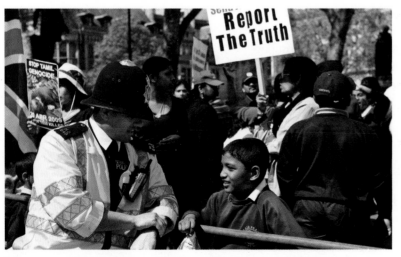

Demonstrations express a number of basic human rights and freedoms.

 **Reflect**

Each of these conventions, laws or regulations contains specific provisions that promote equality and protect the rights of individuals in particular circumstances.

Have you heard of or read about any of them before? What do you know about them?

 **Investigate**

Investigate the main provisions of the Human Rights Act (1998). Produce a table or a poster demonstrating the range of rights provided by this law and highlight those that are relevant to care practice.

P4 Sexual equality law

The Sex Discrimination Acts (1975) and (1986) promote sexual equality and make sexual discrimination illegal, the 1986 Act bringing Britain's sex equality laws into line with the rest of Europe. They define sexual discrimination as 'less favourable treatment on grounds of gender or marital status'. Although, the Acts apply to both men and women, women have benefited most as they face greater prejudice and experience more unfair discrimination on grounds of gender than men.

The inclusion of 'marital status' was an important feature of the 1975 Act. This prevents employers making assumptions that married women are more likely to have childcare responsibilities and are, therefore, 'less reliable' or 'less committed' employees than unmarried women. The original Sex Discrimination Act (1975) was amended in 1986 so that sex discrimination in employment in private households, in small firms, and in terms of retirement age was outlawed.

The Equal Pay Act (1970) is designed to prevent unfair discrimination between men and women with regard to the terms and conditions of employment. Where a woman is employed in similar work or in work that is of equal value to that of a man, she should be given equal pay. Equal pay has been the subject of a significant proportion of **Industrial Tribunal** cases.

Mental health law

The Mental Health Act (2007) updated the Mental Health Act (1983), the main piece of law affecting the treatment of adults with serious mental disorders in England and Wales. The Mental Health (Northern Ireland) Order (1986) is the main law relating to mental health issues in Northern Ireland. The Mental Health (Care and Protection) (Scotland) Act (2003) is the main law on mental health issues in Scotland. The Mental Health Act (2007) seeks to safeguard the interests of adults who are vulnerable because of their mental health problems by ensuring that they can be monitored in the community by care practitioners and admitted to hospital if they don't comply with treatment.

The Mental Health Acts (1983) and (2007) also protect the rights of people who use mental health services in a number of ways. Both Acts give individuals the right to appeal against their detention in hospital and give them some rights to refuse treatment; the 2007 Act gives individuals detained in hospital the right to refuse certain treatments, such as electroconvulsive therapy, and ensures that a person can be detained in hospital only if appropriate treatment is available for them.

The Mental Capacity Act (2005) provides a range of legal protections to people who are unable to make decisions about their own life because of their mental health problems. The Act supports each individual's right to

Your assessment criteria:

P4 Explain how national initiatives promote anti-discriminatory practice

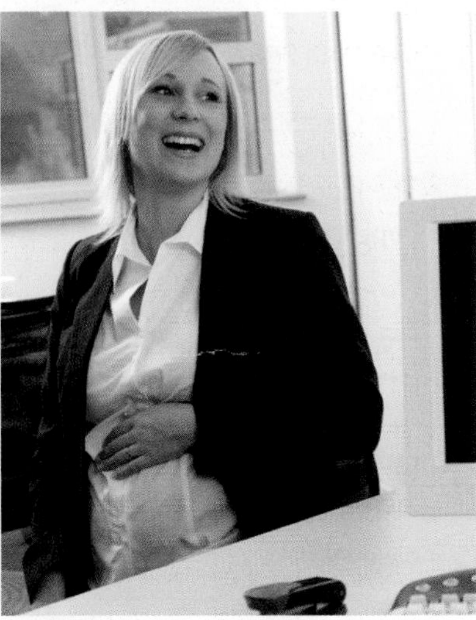

Pregnant women are protected by law from unfair dismissal at work.

Key terms

Industrial Tribunal: *a specialised form of court that hears employment-related cases*

Discuss

Why do people with mental health problems need the protection of laws and regulations? Discuss the reasons why people with these kinds of problems are seen as vulnerable and find out how they are protected in the UK by different mental health laws.

make decisions, ensuring that appropriate support is provided and that a proper process is followed which protects the individual's best interests.

The Race Relations Act (1976)

This is the key **statute** promoting racial equality and making racial discrimination illegal. It defines racial discrimination as 'less favourable treatment on racial grounds' and identifies several ways in which such treatment may occur. A person discriminates against another on the basis of race if:

a) 'he or she treats the person less favourably than they treat, or would treat another person on racial grounds; or

b) he or she applies a requirement, or condition to that other person:

   i. which is such that the proportion of the person's racial group who can comply with it is considerably smaller than the proportion of persons not of their racial group; and

   ii. which he or she cannot show to be justified irrespective of the colour, race, nationality or ethnic or national origins of the person to whom it is applied; and

   iii. which is to the detriment of certain people because they cannot comply with it.'

The Race Relations Act (1976) not only aims to eradicate racial discrimination but also promotes equal opportunities. Under the Act, it is unlawful for employers to unfairly discriminate in the selection of staff, the arrangements made for recruitment, promotion, training or transfer, and in the terms and conditions of employment and dismissal. The Race Relations (Amendment) Act (2000) extended the 1986 Act by placing a duty on public bodies, including health and social care organisations, to promote race equality and to show that procedures to prevent race discrimination are effective.

Key terms

Statute: *another term for an Act of Parliament or written law*

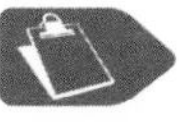

Case study

Jenny Lopez is a Health Visitor planning to return to work after a 3-year career break to have a child. She tells you that she is going to put an advertisement in the local paper and the newsagent's window for a 'young Spanish woman' to act as her childminder.

1. Is Jenny discriminating unfairly against any groups of people in her search for a childminder?
2. Will Jenny be breaking the law relating to race or sex discrimination?

P4 The Convention on the Rights of the Child (1989)

This convention introduced rights for children and young people under 18 years of age. It is based around the principles that:

- decisions about a child should be based on what is in the child's best interests
- children should not be discriminated against
- children should be free to express themselves
- children have the right to survive and develop.

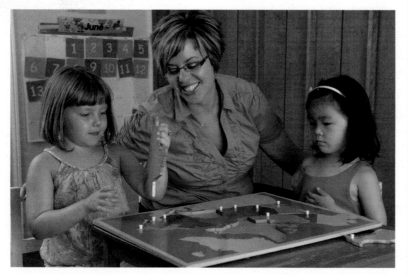

The rights of children in the UK are protected by a number of laws.

The Children Acts (1989) and (2004)

The Children Act (1989) established that care workers should see the needs of the child as **paramount** when making any decisions that affect their welfare. Under the 1989 Act local authorities are required to provide services that meet the needs of children who are identified as being 'at risk'. The 2004 piece of legislation updated the Children Act (1989) following an inquiry into the death of Victoria Climbié in 2000. The goal of the Children Act (2004) is to improve the lives of all children who receive informal or professional care. It covers all services that children might use, such as schools, day care and children's homes, as well as health care services. The Children Act (2004) now requires care services to work collaboratively so that they form a protective team around the child.

Your assessment criteria:

P4 Explain how national initiatives promote anti-discriminatory practice

M2 Assess the influence of a recent national policy initiative promoting anti-discriminatory practice

Key terms

Paramount: *most important*

The Children Act (2004) resulted from a report called *Every Child Matters* that led to significant change in the way services for children and young people are provided in the UK. The aim of *Every Child Matters* is that all children should:

- be healthy
- stay safe
- enjoy and achieve
- make a positive contribution
- achieve economic wellbeing.

M2 The national safeguarding initiative

The *Every Child Matters* programme of children's service development ensures that **safeguarding** remains the key priority for everyone who is part of the children's workforce. Anyone who works (or volunteers) with children, young people and vulnerable adults now has to submit to background checks by the Criminal Records Bureau (CRB). Since 2009, a Vetting and Barring Scheme that is administered by the Independent Safeguarding Authority and the Criminal Records Bureau has required all adults who work with children to register. Equivalent agencies called Disclosure Scotland and Access Northern Ireland operate in other parts of the UK.

Key terms

Safeguarding: *the process of providing protection*

P4 The Disability Discrimination Acts (1995) and (2005)

These Acts safeguard the rights of disabled people; 'less favourable treatment' of disabled people in employment, the provision of goods and services, education and transport is unlawful. The aim of the Acts is to ensure that disabled people receive equal opportunities and that employers, traders, transport and education providers make 'reasonable adjustments' to their premises and services to allow access.

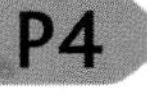

Investigate

Use the Equality and Human Rights Commission website (www.equalityhumanrights.com) to find out about the rights of disabled people and those with mental health problems.

The Age Discrimination Act (2006)

This Act makes discrimination against people on grounds of their age unlawful. All employment practices must now be based on skills and competencies, not on a person's age. A worker can sue their employer if they feel they have been harassed or victimised because of their age, for example. Also, employers are not allowed to recruit, promote, train or retire people on the basis of their age.

P4 The Data Protection Act (1998)

This Act established clear guidelines about service users' access to 'personal data': that anyone can ask to see their own records and how long it should take staff to prepare the records for viewing. **Data users**, such as NHS Trusts and local authority social services departments, are required to register their recording and use of service users' personal data with the Data Protection Registrar. They must then comply with the following Data Protection Act principles. Personal data must:

- be collected and processed fairly and lawfully
- only be held for specific, lawful registered purposes
- only be used for registered purposes or disclosed to registered recipients
- be adequate and relevant to the purpose for which it is held
- be accurate and, where necessary, kept up to date
- be held no longer than is necessary for the stated purpose
- be surrounded by appropriate security
- be subject to a right of access by the data subject (to records held about him or herself).

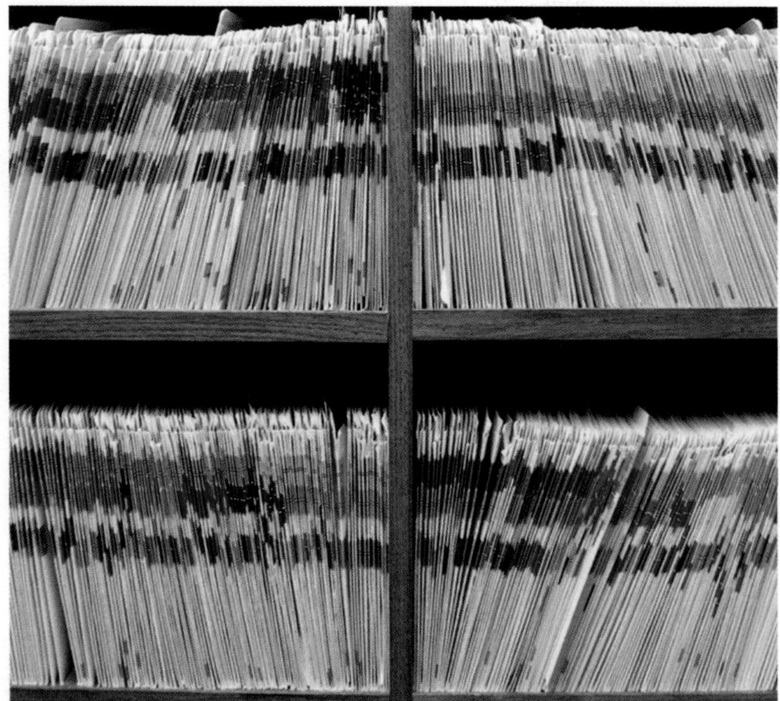

Care records: health and social care organisations have a duty to protect the information of service users.

Your assessment criteria:

P4 Explain how national initiatives promote anti-discriminatory practice

Key terms

Data users: *organisations who collect and make use of personal data*

Reflect

Who holds records or information about you? Think of three types of information – perhaps health, income, family matters. What might happen if the information held about you is incorrect or out of date?

Service users are entitled to know whether any information about them is being held by a care organisation. If it is, they have the right to apply for access to see it. Access to health records can be denied where the disclosure of the contents:

- would be likely to cause serious harm to the physical or mental health of the data subject
- would reveal the identify of others (not including care professionals) who have provided information in confidence and who have not then consented to it or their identity being disclosed.

Permission to see personal health records has to be sought from and given by the medical practitioner who is responsible for the service user's care. Applications must be made in writing and are also subject to the payment of a fee. Unless the exception principles given above apply, the applicant is entitled to a copy of the information contained in their records within 40 days of application. If this is not forthcoming, they can go to court to enforce their legal right or obtain enforcement from the Data Protection Registrar.

The Care Standards Act (2000)

The Care Standards Act (2000) established the legally required national minimum standards of care provision that health and social care organisations must achieve. The aim of this law is to ensure that everyone who uses care services receives fair and equal treatment. Care organisations are now inspected by the **Care Quality Commission** to check whether they meet the current national minimum standards of care.

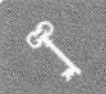

Key terms

Care Quality Commission: *the independent body that regulates and inspects health and social care services in England*

Nursing and Residential Care Homes Regulations (1984) (amended 2002)

These Regulations (1984) (amended 2002) affect the setting up and running of care homes. The regulations ensure that people who live in care homes have the right to be protected from danger and harm. Residential homes are inspected and must keep detailed information on residents and staff who work at the home. The 2002 amendments to these regulations set a range of legally enforceable minimum standards, such as room sizes, and access to bathroom facilities.

P4 Codes of practice and charters

Codes of practice and **charters** offer guidance to care practitioners and information to people who use services about expected standards and ways of approaching care provision. Codes of practice and charters have been developed by **regulatory bodies** and care organisations to guide the professional conduct and standards of performance of care practitioners. For example, the Nursing and Midwifery Council (NMC) and the General Social Care Council (GSCC) produce codes of practice for nurses and social workers respectively. These codes of practice set standards for good practice in care settings. Codes of practice establish the general principles and standards for care workers and should always refer to equality of opportunity. Examples of codes of practice and charters are now used in all care settings.

D1 Evaluating the success of anti-discrimination initiatives

The success of anti-discrimination initiatives may be evaluated by local and national government bodies, as well as by independent sector organisations that promote equality and diversity issues on behalf of a particular group of people. These organisations use a number of strategies to evaluate the extent to which initiatives have been successful, including:

- comparing from year to year the number of discrimination cases that go to court
- carrying out community surveys of attitudes towards equality and diversity issues
- reviewing and producing data on the diversity of the labour force or the patterns of admission to educational institutions
- carrying out audits and research studies to evaluate the effect that specific diversity or equality initiatives or laws have had on people's attitudes, behaviour or practices.

Data and reports on a range of equality and diversity initiatives and on the impact of anti-discrimination laws are usually published on the websites of government and independent sector organisations specialising in particular fields.

Your assessment criteria:

P4 Explain how national initiatives promote anti-discriminatory practice

D1 Evaluate the success of a recent initiative in promoting anti-discriminatory practice

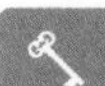

Key terms

Charters: *documents specifying rights and standards*

Codes of practice: *documents providing guidance on ethically appropriate and recommended ways of behaving or dealing with particular situations*

Ethics: *principles relating to right and wrong*

Regulatory bodies: *organisations that maintain registers of qualified practitioners in particular areas, give guidance on professional **ethics** and remove those unfit to practice*

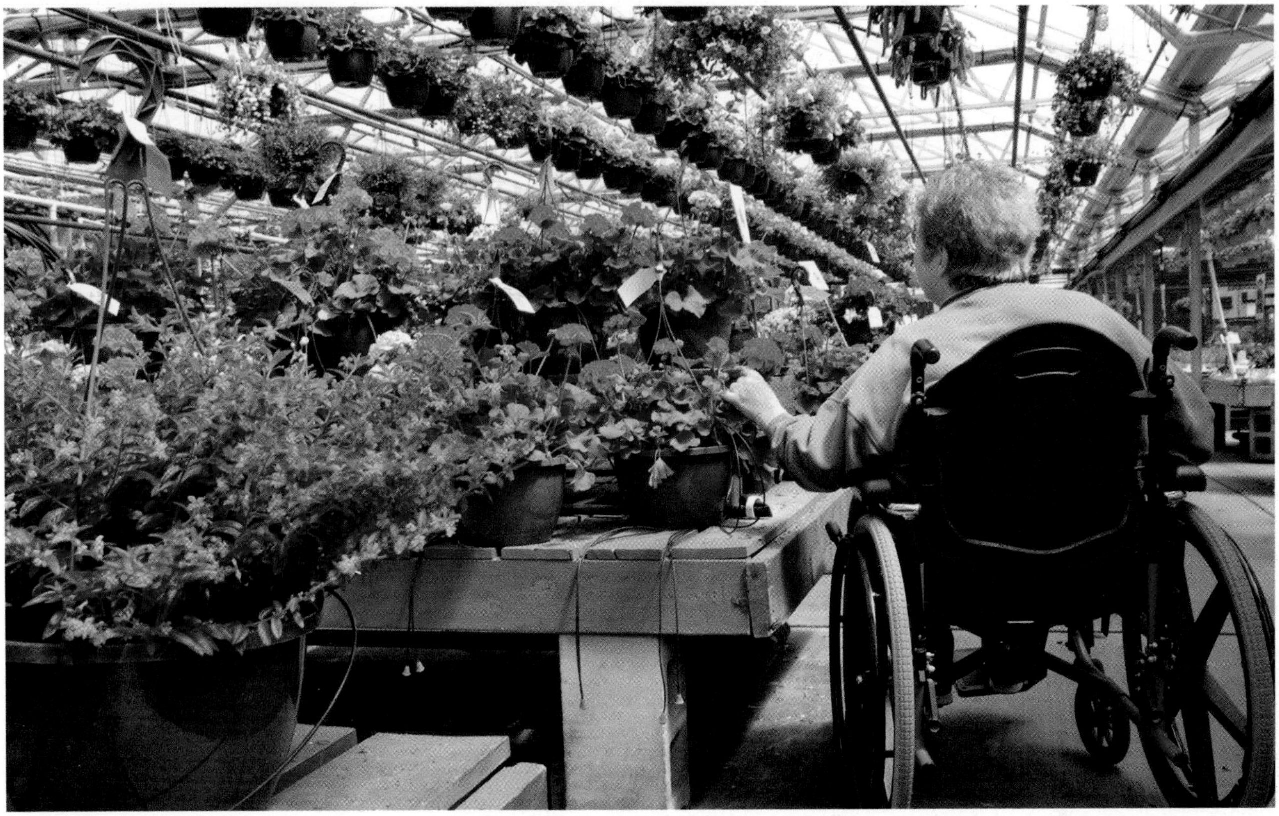

Has the Disability Discrimination Act reduced discrimination against disabled people?

What do you know?

1. Identify three client or service user groups whose rights are protected by specific anti-discrimination laws.
2. Describe the legal protection given to women by sexual equality laws.
3. Explain what racial discrimination involves and outline how legislation protects people from this.
4. Describe the purpose of the Children Acts (1989) and (2004).
5. Explain how the rights and interests of users of health and social care services are protected by data protection legislation.
6. Identify an example of a code of practice used in health and social care practice and explain how it helps to safeguard service users in health and social care settings.

Implementing anti-discriminatory practice in health and social care settings

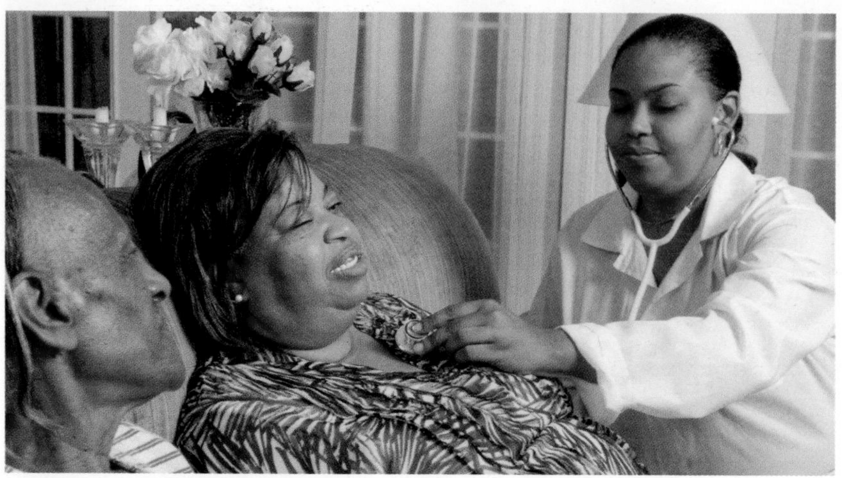

Anti-discriminatory practice is an important approach to care work in a diverse society.

Your assessment criteria:

P5 Describe how anti-discriminatory practice is promoted in health and social care settings

M3 Discuss difficulties that may arise when implementing anti-discriminatory practice in health and social care settings

Promoting equal opportunities and challenging unfair discrimination should be a real issue for all health, social care and early years practitioners. This is because care practitioners come face-to-face with people who experience health and social problems that are triggered by or made worse by unequal access to society's resources.

P5 Developing an anti-discriminatory approach to care practice

The best way of promoting equal opportunities is through anti-discriminatory practice. This means developing ways of working that:

- recognise the needs of people from diverse backgrounds including those who come from minority religious and cultural groups
- actively challenge the unfair discrimination that people experience
- counteract the effect that unfair discrimination has already had on people.

P5 M3 Responding to unfair discrimination in care

So, what can *you* do? Some suggestions include:

- Be **self-aware** and, within reason, self-critical.

Key terms

Self-aware: *a person's awareness of their individuality, ways of thinking and behaving*

- Question your own assumptions and be prepared to change your ideas and views about people.
- Continue developing yourself and reflecting on your ideas on equality.
- Adopt the view that people are different but of equal value, regardless of their physical, mental or cultural characteristics.
- Don't judge people.
- View people's physical, social and cultural differences as a positive and interesting feature of care work rather than something that is problematic.
- Read and become familiar with the **policies** and **procedures** of the care organisations in which you work.
- Ask questions about, and seek advice on, ways of implementing the equality and anti-discriminatory policies and procedures of the organisation.

Key terms

Policies: *written documents setting out an organisation's approach towards particular issues*

Procedures: *written documents that describe in detail the way in which tasks must be carried out or issues dealt with*

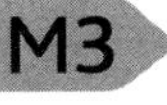

M3 Difficulties of implementing anti-discriminatory practice

As part of promoting equality in care settings, care practitioners need to address their own prejudices and tackle unfair discrimination when they see this occurring, a daunting and intimidating task. Challenging incidents of unfair discrimination or speaking out when people express prejudices can require a lot of courage and personal confidence. Not everyone feels able to do this on every occasion. As a result, anti-discriminatory practice can be difficult to implement, particularly in settings where basic equality issues have not been addressed and where there are weak complaints policies and **whistle-blowing** procedures.

Most care practitioners believe that they provide fair and equal treatment to all service users. However, some of the strategies that are commonly employed don't support equality of opportunity in the way that they're intended. For example, being 'blind' to the differences between individuals and to the particular characteristics of different social groups doesn't achieve the intended goal of valuing people equally. It is better to acknowledge and accept that people are different, but to value them equally. In this way cultural, religious and identity needs are clearly respected and can inform the way that care is provided.

Key terms

Whistle-blowing: *exposing wrongdoing in an organisation in the hope that it will stop*

Reflect

Do you have experience, through work or placement, of an organisation that has implemented an anti-discriminatory approach to care practice? If there was no such approach, do you think implementation would have improved practice in any way?

P5 Personal beliefs and value systems

Some care practitioners feel that they shouldn't impose their own **beliefs** and **value systems**, even if they believe in equality, on service users and work colleagues. They may also think that challenging prejudice and unfair discrimination is not their responsibility. However, acceptance, consideration for others and equality of opportunity are superior values to prejudice and unfair discrimination and they should prevail. Care practitioners should not remain silent or passive when prejudice is expressed or when unfair discrimination occurs. Failing to act could be seen as supporting the unequal and unacceptable treatment of an individual or group of people.

So, challenging prejudice and unfair discrimination is a part of the job of every care practitioner, not something that should be left to more senior colleagues or managers. Harm and distress must be minimised by swift action. Every health, social care and early years practitioner can help to promote equality of opportunity for care service users by developing their own awareness and knowledge of prejudice and unfair discrimination and by practising in ways that respect the diversity and rights of service users.

Your assessment criteria:

P5 Describe how anti-discriminatory practice is promoted in health and social care settings

D2 Justify ways of overcoming difficulties that may arise when implementing anti-discriminatory practices in health and social care settings

Key terms

Beliefs: *ideas that people accept are true, often without having any proof that this is the case*

Value systems: *sets of principles that guide thinking and behaviour*

P5 D2 Achieving change through anti-discriminatory practice

Anti-discriminatory practice aims to challenge social inequalities, prejudice and unfair discrimination and to address the effects of marginalisation and social exclusion that some social groups experience. Anti-discriminatory practice offers care practitioners an effective and powerful way of applying equal opportunities ideas in everyday work situations. As a brief recap, anti-discriminatory practice should:

- highlight and promote acceptance of **multiculturalism** and other forms of social diversity in society
- challenge forms of prejudice that affect service users in their lives, including racism, ageism, sexism, homophobia and disablism
- identify and work to rectify examples of stereotyping and unfair discrimination that deny people equality of opportunity and infringe their legal rights.

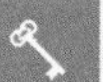

Key terms

Multiculturalism: *the peaceful and equal co-existence of different cultures within a society*

Anti-discriminatory care practice is achieved by:

- developing a personal awareness of how your own and other people's prejudices reveal themselves
- the development of greater self-awareness and tolerance of differences
- adopting a non-discriminatory approach to language (using non-sexist, non-racist and non-disablist words and phrases, for example)
- a commitment to the care value base
- working within the legal, ethical and policy guidelines set by legislation, professional bodies and employers.

Case study

Derek Bell is a 72-year-old patient on Green Ward at Oxford General Hospital. As a former Captain in the Royal Navy, he is used to giving orders and getting his own way. This morning Mr Bell shouted, 'Get your black hands off me!' at Jamilla, one of the nurses providing him with basic personal care. Jamilla was offended and upset by Mr Bell's attitude and by the language he used. Pauline, one of Jamilla's colleagues, thought the situation was funny and laughed. She then took over and provided care for Mr Bell herself.

1. In what way is Mr Bell being discriminatory?
2. Do you think that Pauline has helped or made this situation worse?
3. Explain what Pauline could do to practise in a more anti-discriminatory way.

What do you know?

1. Identify three things a care practitioner can do to develop an anti-discriminatory approach to care practice.
2. Why is self-awareness an important part of anti-discriminatory practice?
3. Describe some of the difficulties of implementing an anti-discriminatory approach in care settings.
4. How can an anti-discriminatory approach to practice improve the lives of the people who use care services?

Assessment checklist

Your learning and level of understanding of this unit will be assessed through assignments given to you and marked by your teacher or tutor. Before you submit your assignment work for assessment you should make sure that you have produced sufficient evidence to achieve the grade you are aiming for.

To pass this unit you will need to present evidence for assessment which demonstrates that you can meet all of the pass criteria for the unit.

Assessment Criteria	Description	✓
P1	Explain the concepts of equality, diversity and rights in relation to health and social care	☐
P2	Describe discriminatory practice in health and social care	☐
P3	Describe the potential effects of discriminatory practice on those who use health or social care services	☐
P4	Explain how national initiatives promote anti-discriminatory practice	☐
P5	Describe how anti-discriminatory practice is promoted in health and social care settings	☐

You can achieve a merit grade for the unit by presenting evidence that also meets all of the following merit criteria for the unit.

Assessment Criteria	Description	✓
M1	Assess the effects on those using the service of three different discriminatory practices in health and social care settings	☐
M2	Assess the influence of a recent national policy initiative promoting anti-discriminatory practice	☐
M3	Discuss difficulties that may arise when implementing anti-discriminatory practice in health and social care settings	☐

You can achieve a distinction grade for the unit by presenting evidence that also meets all of the following distinction criteria for the unit.

Assessment Criteria	Description	✓
D1	Evaluate the success of a recent initiative in promoting anti-discriminatory practice	☐
D2	Justify ways of overcoming difficulties that may arise when implementing anti-discriminatory practices in health and social care settings	☐

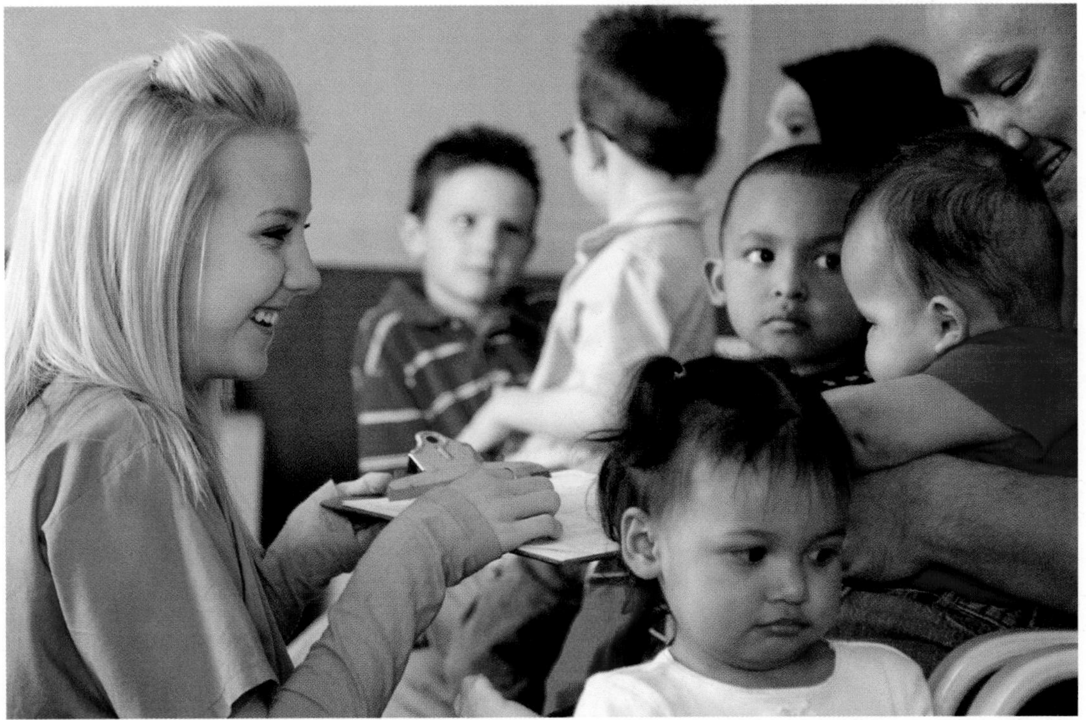

References

Brown, C. and Gay, P. (1985) *Racial Discrimination 17 years after the Act*, London, Policy Studies Institute

3 | Health, safety and security in health and social care

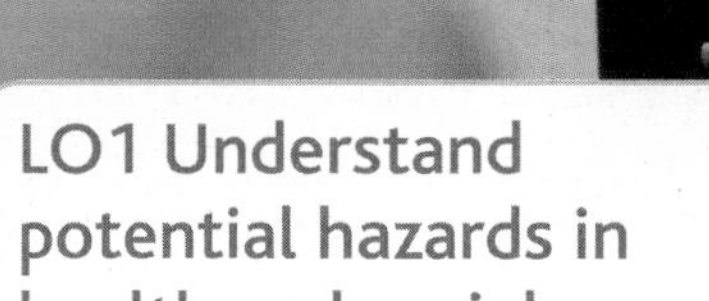

LO1 Understand potential hazards in health and social care

- hazards
- harm and abuse
- settings where hazards occur
- individuals who can be affected
- users of health and social care services

LO2 Know how legislation, policies and procedures promote health, safety and security in health and social care settings

- legislation and guidelines
- safeguarding
- influences
- policies and procedures
- roles
- responsibilities

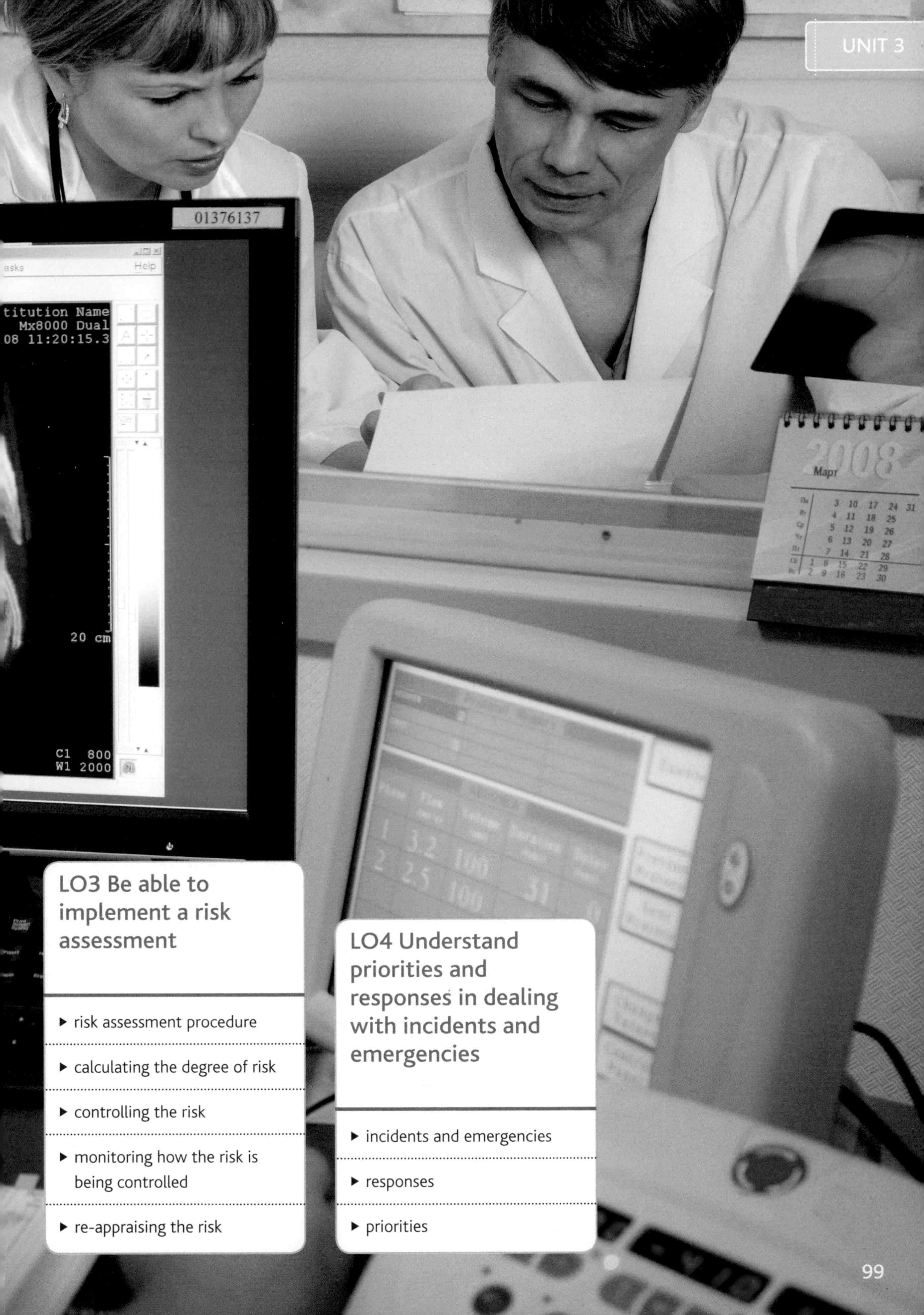

LO3 Be able to implement a risk assessment

- risk assessment procedure
- calculating the degree of risk
- controlling the risk
- monitoring how the risk is being controlled
- re-appraising the risk

LO4 Understand priorities and responses in dealing with incidents and emergencies

- incidents and emergencies
- responses
- priorities

Understanding hazards and risks

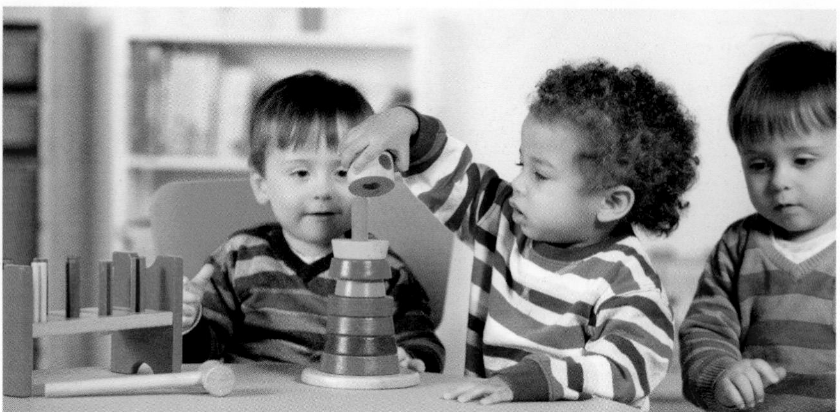

Identifying hazards is the first step to reducing risks in all care settings.

Your assessment criteria:

P1 Explain potential hazards and the harm that may arise from each in a health or social care setting

P1 Thinking about different settings

Health and social care services are provided in a range of settings that include:

- domestic homes (service users' homes and childminders' homes)
- residential and nursing homes
- day care centres
- pre-school nurseries
- infant schools
- community-based surgeries and health centres
- hospitals
- hospices.

Every care setting presents its own combination of physical characteristics and care facilities. These facilities should enable care practitioners to provide high quality care for individuals. However, care settings are also places that contain **hazards** and sources of potential health and safety **risk**.

Care practitioners may also work with people in public environments. Hazards and risks have to be assessed in relation to:

- retail areas
- swimming pools
- public parks

Key terms

Hazards: *things that can cause harm*

Risk: *the chance of harm being done by a hazard*

Reflect

Can you think of two different health and safety hazards that are present in a pre-school nursery or infant school setting?

- sports grounds
- beaches
- transport (cars, buses, trains and aeroplanes, for example).

Investigate

Can you think of reasons why care practitioners may find themselves working in each of the following public environments?

Public environment	Describe how this setting could be used in care development or support activities
Retail area (e.g. shopping street, supermarket, shopping mall, street market)	
Swimming pool	
Public park	
Sports ground (e.g. football stadium)	
Beach	
Public transport	

Case study

Jill is a childminder. Today she is looking after Elliot (4), Marley (3) and Olivia (3). Jill usually provides toys and organises games for the children to play at her home. However, it is a lovely bright sunny day – the first sunny day for a week. So, Jill and the children have decided they would like to go out somewhere. They have 2 hours to fill between 10 a.m. and midday, when they need to be back for lunch.

1. Suggest three public environments where Jill and the children could spend 2 hours.
2. Make a list of health and safety-related pros and cons for each type of environment you have chosen.
3. If you were in Jill's position and wanted to take the children out for 2 hours to a public environment near to where you live, where would you go?

In the same way that every care setting has its own hazards and risks, parts of the public environment are also associated with particular hazards and risks (see Figure 3.1).

Your assessment criteria:

P1 Explain potential hazards and the harm that may arise from each in a health or social care setting

Figure 3.1 Hazards in public environments can cause anxiety and other problems for vulnerable people.

Public environment	Possible hazards
Retail area	Modern retail developments often have good access and facilities for people with mobility problems. However, hazards include: • large crowds • tables and chairs outside cafés and restaurants • wet floors • delivery vehicles • boxes of goods and rubbish bags.
Swimming pool	• falling on wet floors • boisterous behaviour • diving in shallow end • crowded areas • overestimating own abilities.
Public park	• vehicles (tractors, grass cutters, refuse collection vehicles) • other users of the park (joggers, cyclists, people playing sports, people displaying anti-social behaviour) • poorly maintained play equipment, paths and grassy areas • overflowing rubbish pins, broken glass, needles • dog and other animal excrement.
Sports ground	In general, sports grounds are usually quite safe with plenty of fire safety measures and toilet facilities. However, hazards include: • large crowds • people pushing at the entrances and exits • lots of noise • hostility from opposing fans • getting lost.

Beach	• crowds, especially on hot days • fast or unpredictable tides, especially in bad weather.
	• vehicles and boats using the beach • strong sunshine • children and vulnerable people may get lost • inexperienced swimmers may get into difficulties.
Public transport	A significant number of pedestrians and drivers die in road traffic accidents each year. Other hazards associated with public transport include: • crossing the road too slowly or at an inappropriate place • not wearing a seat belt • standing too close to the edge of a railway platform • falling on the stairs or in the aisle of a bus • getting on the wrong bus or train.

Who is at risk?

Care service users tend to be more than usually vulnerable to harm, exploitation and abuse (see Figure 3.2). Professionals must be alert to the health and safety of service users, as well as to their own wellbeing and that of other staff. Health and safety, infection control, dealing with incidents and emergencies and following security procedures are all important issues in any care setting.

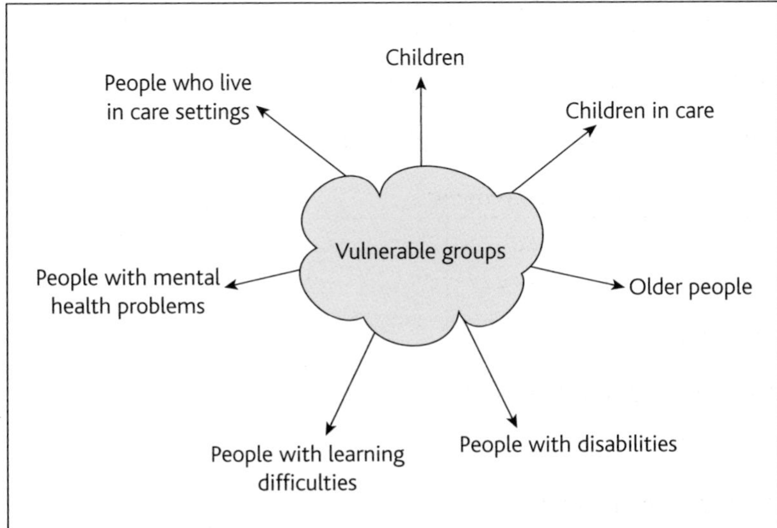

Figure 3.2 Vulnerable people tend to be more at risk from hazards.

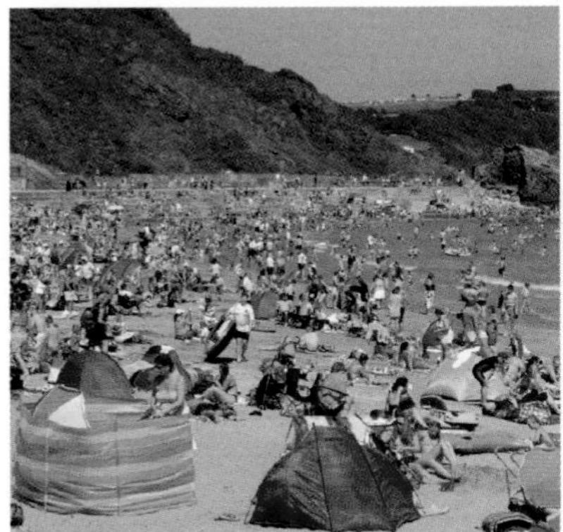

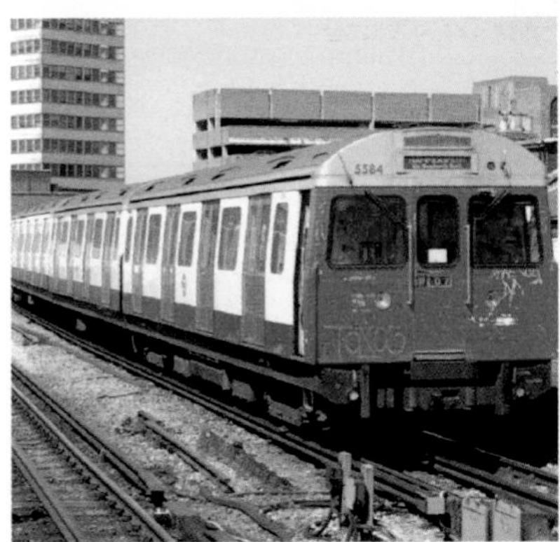

P1 Harm and abuse

Unfortunately, **abuse** and **neglect** are most commonly perpetrated by parents on children, by one partner on the other in a relationship, and by carers on vulnerable people who are unwell, frail or who have developmental problems. The different forms of abuse that members of vulnerable groups experience include:

- physical abuse
- sexual abuse
- emotional and psychological abuse
- financial exploitation
- neglect.

The abuse of vulnerable people in care settings is relatively rare but, regrettably, it still happens (see Figure 3.3). You may find this shocking and difficult to accept, especially because the vast majority of care practitioners, parents and partners in relationships never abuse or neglect those they care for. However, the perpetrators (people who carry out abuse, neglect or ill-treatment) are responsible for their actions and will not be allowed by their employers, the Police or the courts to make excuses for harming a vulnerable relative or service user.

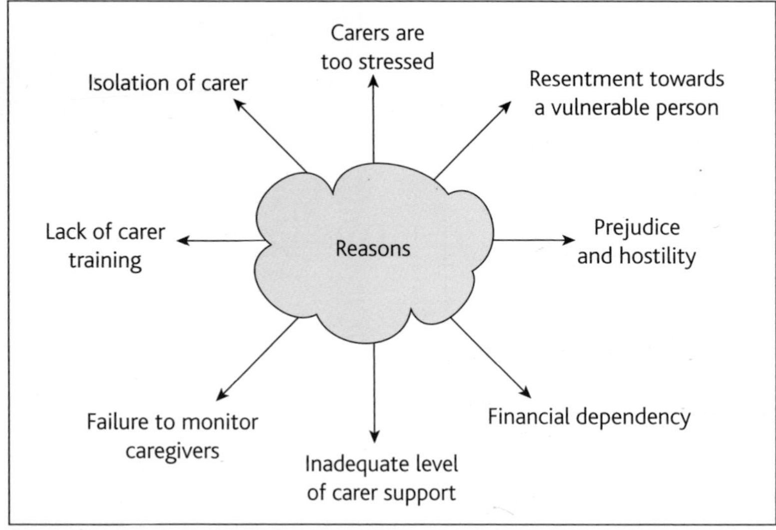

Figure 3.3 Reasons why abuse and ill treatment may happen.

Abuse or neglect of people who use care services can be deliberate, but is more likely to occur unintentionally. This could happen when, for example, care practitioners fail to follow correct infection control procedures or produce an inappropriate care plan for an individual who is then exposed to harm.

Your assessment criteria:

P1 Explain potential hazards and the harm that may arise from each in a health or social care setting

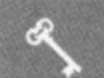

Key terms

Abuse: *any form of ill-treatment*

Neglect: *failure to provide appropriate care or take care of someone*

Figure 3.4 Harm can arise in a variety of ways, both intentional and unintentional.

Agent of abuse or harm	Possible consequences
Unintentionally exposure to harm by, for example: • failing to explain a physical procedure (e.g. lifting) • not demonstrating or supervising a task properly (e.g. chopping food) • failing to check the temperature of bath water.	Physical injury as a result of falling, cutting or scalding skin, for example.
Failure to follow infection control procedures, e.g. using unsterilised needles or not washing hands correctly.	An individual may acquire an infection such as HIV, *C. difficile* or hepatitis B.
Being verbally hostile towards or critical of an individual.	Psychological distress such as loss of self-esteem, loss of self-confidence, feeling anxious or upset.
Inaccurate assessment of an individual's needs or setting of inappropriate goals.	Inappropriate care planning can expose individuals to neglect and harm if they are unable to achieve care plan goals or their real care needs are overlooked.
Encouraging or allowing individuals to take inappropriate risks or expecting them to perform activities that are too difficult (e.g. walking long distances or getting in and out of the bath unsupported).	Inappropriate risk-taking can expose an individual to danger and physical harm – such as falling, getting lost or finding themselves in a situation where they are unable to cope.
Careless storage of an individual's property, failing to record accurately what they bring into a care setting or failing to follow security procedures.	Loss or damage to possessions may be emotionally upsetting, as well as causing financial loss.

What do you know?

1. Identify and describe a hazard that can be found in a care setting.
2. What does the term 'risk' refer to?
3. Describe three hazards that exist in public environments such as parks and retail areas.
4. Explain who the hazards you have described above present a risk to.
5. Identify three different forms of abuse that some vulnerable people experience.
6. Outline three reasons why abuse sometimes occurs in care settings and the impact this can have on victims.

Identifying hazards and risks in different care settings

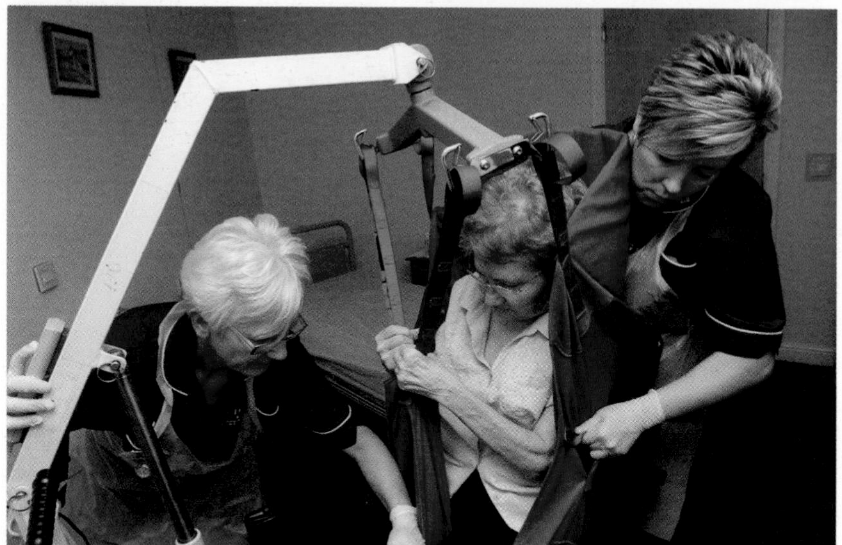
Care practitioners should always check risk assessments before carrying out care procedures.

Your assessment criteria:

P1 Explain potential hazards and the harm that may arise from each in a health or social care setting

P1 Potential hazards

Good health and safety in care settings is generally achieved through preventive measures such as **risk assessment**, safe care practice and the correct use of safety systems and procedures. Hazards and risks to health and safety can arise from several different sources (see Figure 3.5). Identifying the source of potential hazards to health, safety or security is the first step in a risk assessment.

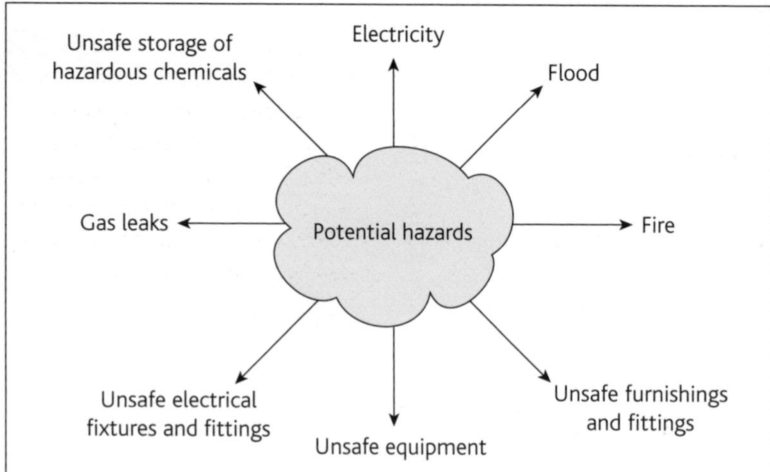

Figure 3.5 Potential hazards in care settings.

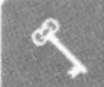 **Key terms**

Risk assessment: *the process of evaluating the likelihood of a hazard actually causing harm*

Examples of risks and hazards in care settings

Hazards in the physical environment of care settings include:

- Electricity – faulty electrical appliances and switches, overloaded sockets, frayed flexes and power surges can all lead to fires, burns and electrical shocks.
- Gas – faulty gas appliances and gas leaks can lead to fires, explosions, breathing difficulties, unconsciousness and asphyxiation.
- Water – leaks result in wet floors, walls and carpets, as well as rotten floorboards. All of these things cause accidents and injuries if people slip or trip. If there is contact between water and electricity, there is also a danger of electrocution.
- Kitchen – hazards include sharp knives, cooking appliances, overhanging pan handles, slippery floors and contaminated food.
- Living room and bedroom – hazards include worn or badly fitted carpets, loose rugs, poorly placed furniture, floor length curtains, clothes or bed linen left on the floor, trailing flexes, poor lighting, electrical appliances and fires without guards.
- Bathroom – hazards include hot water, slippery surfaces and floors, and electrical items near water.
- Stairs – can be hazardous if they lack hand rails, are steep or have poorly fitted, loose carpets.
- Work areas – these may present hazards if they are cramped, draughty or have poor lighting.

The areas in care settings that present the highest risks are:

- community rooms and lounges
- bedrooms
- kitchens
- community areas such as halls, entrance areas and stairs
- play areas (inside and outside)
- bathrooms.

Discuss

Think about your own experience of providing care on work placement. What kinds of health and safety hazards were you aware of in your placement setting? Share ideas with one or two class colleagues.

Investigate

Go to the website of the Royal Society for the Prevention of Accidents (www.rospa.com) and explore the information and guidance on home safety. Do the points made by ROSPA also apply to health and social care settings?

Reflect

Think about your own bedroom at home – what kinds of health and safety hazards are present there? How might a toddler or a physically infirm older person be at risk if they wandered into your bedroom?

Identifying hazards and risks in care practice

P1 Equipment hazards

Care practitioners use a range of equipment to make their work easier. For example, they use hoists, bath boards, wheelchairs and electronically operated beds in order to take some of the physical strain out of moving people. Personal protective equipment such as aprons, gloves and masks are also examples of health and safety equipment.

The equipment used by care practitioners must be in good condition and should only be used by people who have received appropriate training. Examples of equipment hazards that present health and safety risks to individuals and care practitioners include:

- mobility aids that are the wrong size or which do not work properly
- faulty or damaged lifting equipment
- brakes and hydraulics on beds that do not work properly
- computer display screens and keyboards that are badly located, poorly serviced or over-used
- blades and syringe needles that are stored or disposed of incorrectly
- unlabelled, incorrectly labelled or leaking bottles and containers
- old and faulty electrical and gas-fuelled appliances
- excessively full or faulty waste disposal equipment.

Care practitioners should always check the equipment they intend to use to ensure it is safe and free of hazards. They should not use equipment that is faulty or which they have not been trained to use. Faulty, unsafe equipment should be reported and removed from the care setting.

Infections

Preventing infection is one way of protecting people who use services. Care practitioners should follow basic measures to reduce the risk of the spread of infection in care settings. Many of the bacteria and viruses

Your assessment criteria:

P1 Explain potential hazards and the harm that may arise from each in a health or social care setting

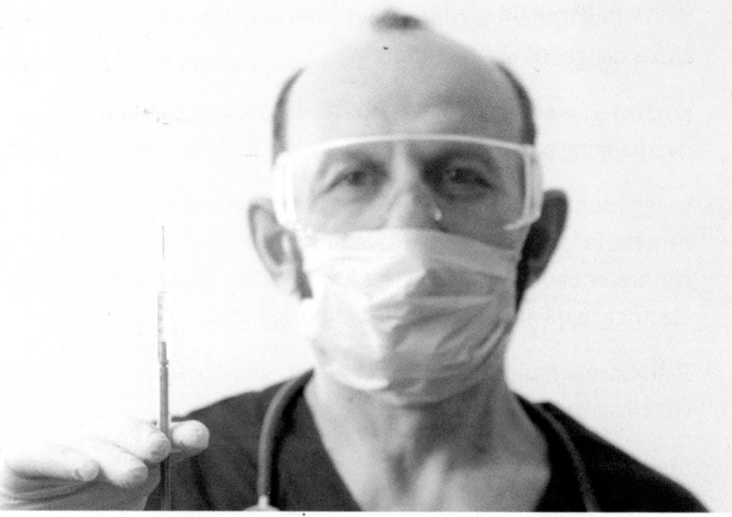

Needles and sharp blades are hazardous because they can cause injury and transmit infection.

Reflect

Why does each of these pose a health risk?

- *needle-stick injuries*
- *hours spent typing without a break*
- *unlabelled bottles in a kitchen area*

that cause infections are present in everyday life. However, new and more unusual infections may also be present and can be contracted in hospitals and residential care settings. People who are physically frail or who are suffering from significant health problems tend to be more vulnerable to common infections and rarer infections can be devastating.

Care workers should follow basic infection control procedures to minimise the risks of infection to themselves and others. These include:

- ensuring high standards of personal hygiene relating to dress, hair care, footwear and oral hygiene
- using personal protective clothing such as aprons, gloves and masks where appropriate
- following all health, safety and hygiene procedures in the workplace
- learning and using hand-washing procedures correctly (see Figure 3.6).

Discuss

Why do you think hospital-acquired infections have become more common over the last decade? Discuss the possible reasons for this and identify barriers to tackling this problem.

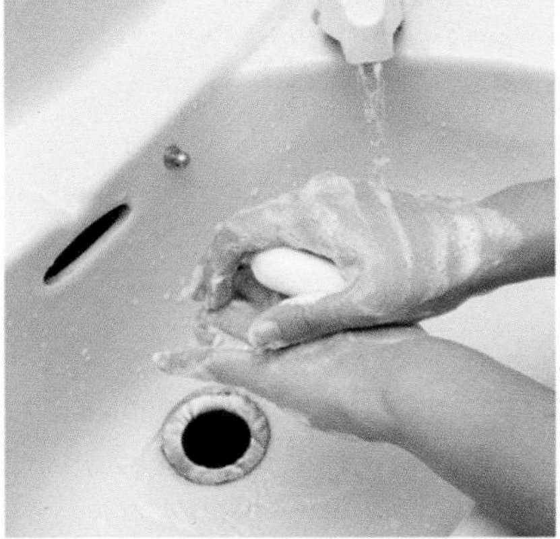

1. Lather hands with soap

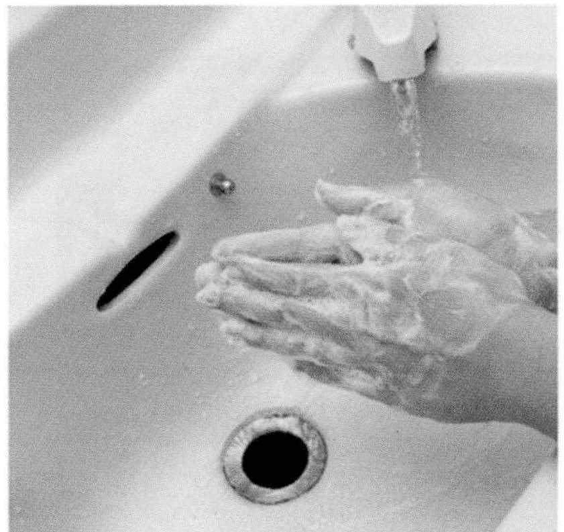

2. Rub both palms together

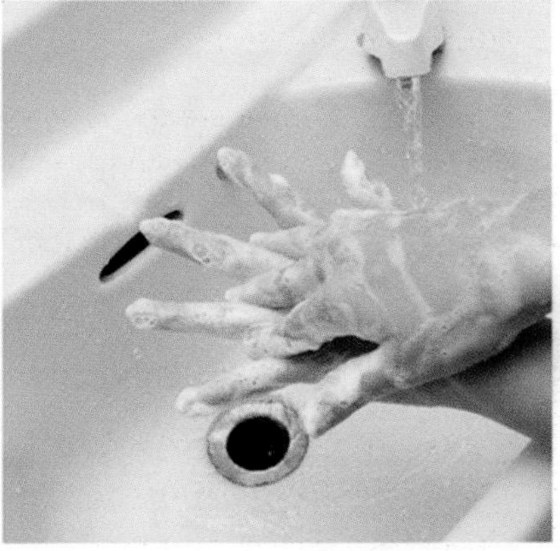

3. Rub each fingers and between fingers

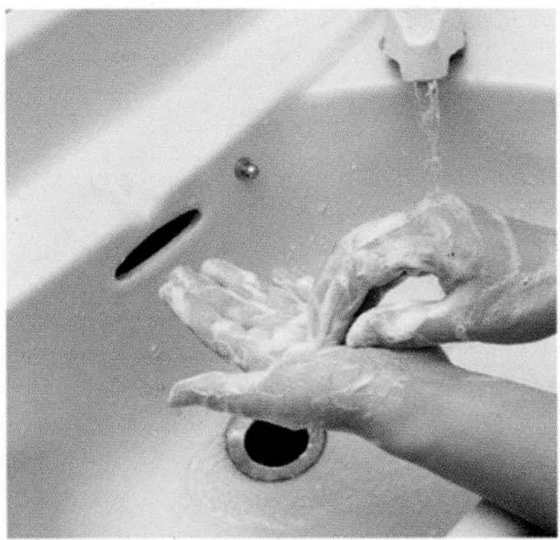

4. Rub palms with finger nails

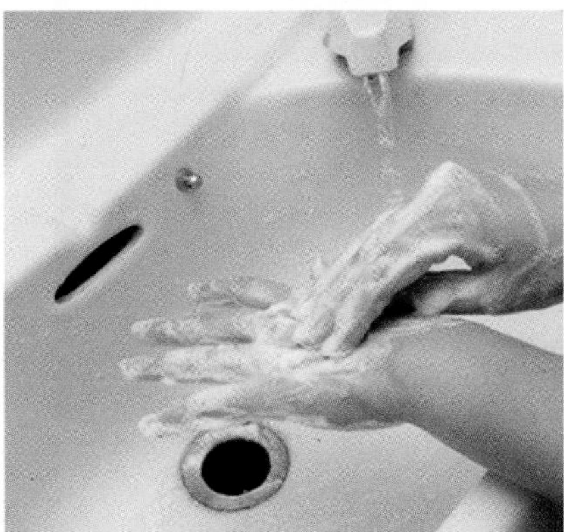

5. Rub back of hand with finger nails

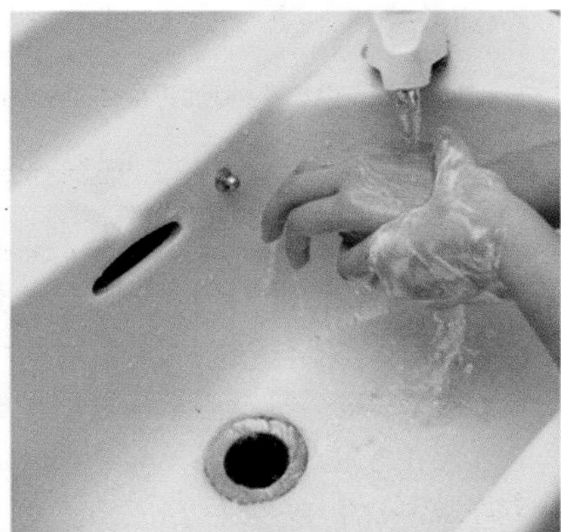

6. Wash thoroughly and towel dry

Figure 3.6 Correct hand-washing technique helps to prevent the spread of infection.

Correct use of systems and procedures

P1 Dealing with hazardous substances

A range of substances that are potentially hazardous to health are present in care settings. These include:

- cleaning agents, such as disinfectants and detergents
- sterilising fluids
- medicines
- art and craft materials (paints, glues and clay, for example).

Substances can be hazardous because they are **toxic**, **corrosive** or **irritant**. Hazard symbols (see Figure 3.7) should be printed on bottles, packets and canisters to indicate the kinds of dangers they pose.

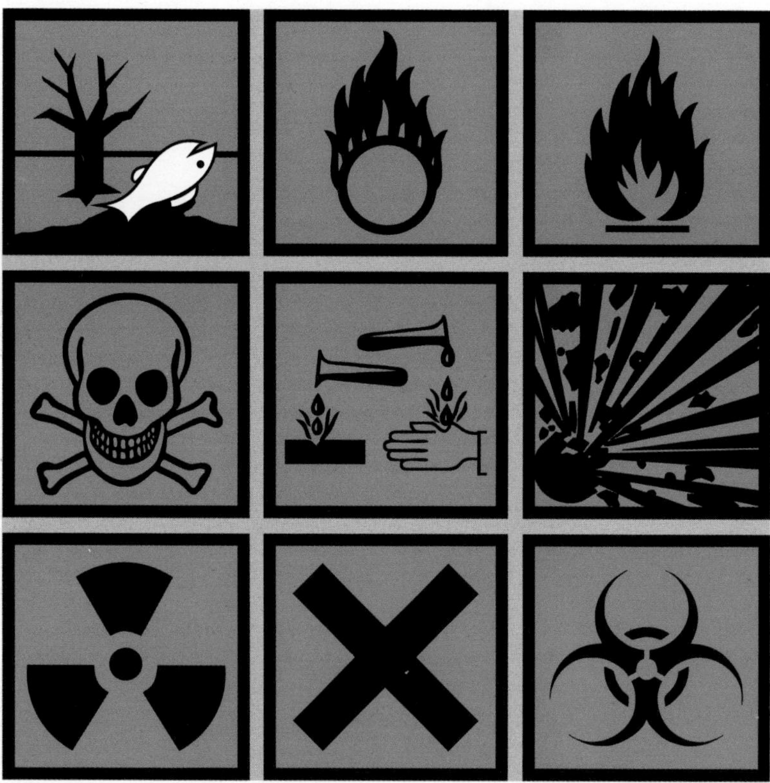

Figure 3.7 Hazard warning symbols.

COSHH Regulations (2005)

The Control of Substances Hazardous to Health (COSHH) Regulations (2005) state that all hazardous substances must be correctly handled

Your assessment criteria:

P1 Explain potential hazards and the harm that may arise from each in a health or social care setting

Key terms

Corrosive: *cause burns*

Irritant: *cause irritation*

Toxic: *poisonous*

Investigate

Are you familiar with any of these hazard symbols? If there are any you don't know, find out what they mean.

Investigate

When you are on work placement ask to look at the COSHH file. Find out about the procedures used to minimise risks from the hazardous substances stored in the care setting.

and stored to minimise the risks they present. The COSHH file that must be kept in each care setting provides details of:

- the hazardous substances that are present
- where they are stored
- how they should be handled
- how any spillage or accident involving a hazardous substance should be addressed.

Working conditions and practices

A care practitioner's working conditions are affected by factors such as:

- the number hours worked
- the amount of support received
- the quality of relationships between staff members
- whether there are sufficient members of staff on duty to provide the appropriate level of care.

A high turnover of staff and inadequate staffing levels can put care practitioners under a lot of pressure. This may cause staff to take short cuts or use risky working practices – such as lifting people alone – that increase the risk of injury and harm to themselves and the people they are caring for.

If care professionals have insufficient support, feel undervalued or are working under a lot of pressure, they may ignore important policies and procedures. Tired, unmotivated practitioners also make more mistakes, develop stress-related conditions and take more time off work through ill-health.

Discuss

What are the advantages and disadvantages of using temporary agency or 'bank' staff in a care setting when staffing levels would otherwise below due to sickness or high staff turnover?

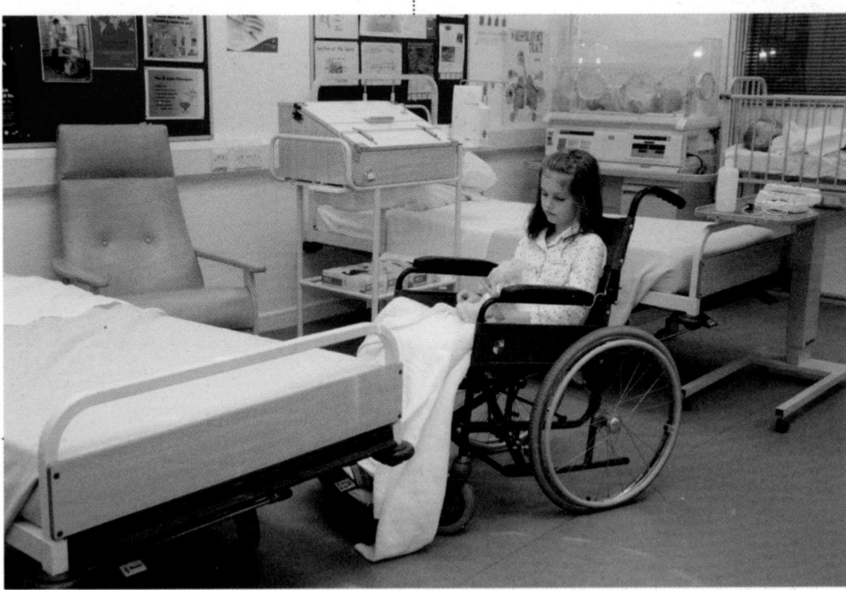

Inadequate staffing levels increase the risk of accidents and incidents occurring in care settings.

P1 Security systems

Increasingly, personal safety and security at work are becoming issues for care practitioners. Although, we may think of care settings as safe environments where people are cared for and not harmed, the threat from intruders and from increasing levels of violence and aggression towards care workers means that the security of buildings and personnel needs to be taken very seriously. In most care settings security provisions are designed to protect:

- personal safety
- property
- personal details and confidentiality
- service users who should not leave buildings unless it is safe for them to do so.

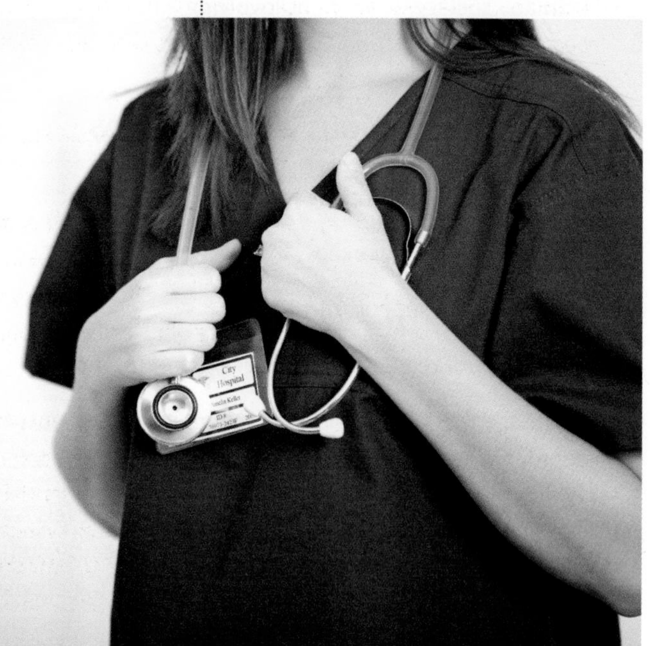

Identity badges are part of the security system used in many health care settings.

Internal and external security breaches

There are two different types of security breach in care settings – *external* and *internal* security breaches. External security is breached when an unauthorised person gets into a care setting. Care organisations use a variety of methods to minimise the risk of external security breaches including:

- developing security and incident policies and procedures, and training staff to follow and apply them
- having security staff or receptionists who check the identification of everybody entering the care setting
- using identity card systems
- fitting CCTV to monitor entrances, exits and corridors in care settings
- fitting electronic code pads on doors, window guards and high level door handles to combat unauthorised entry risks.

Care settings that do not use a range of security methods or where staff members fail to implement security procedures properly put the people in the setting at risk. Care practitioners can help to maintain high standards of security by:

- understanding the security and incident policies and procedures that apply in the care setting
- knowing how to operate any alarms or security systems that are provided

Your assessment criteria:

P1 Explain potential hazards and the harm that may arise from each in a health or social care setting

Reflect

What kind of security systems are in operation to prevent external breaches of security at your school or college?

- wearing an identification badge and carrying any alarms that are provided for security purposes
- asking visitors to identify themselves by showing some official identification badge or letter before letting them into the care setting
- locking doors and windows that are supposed to be locked for security purposes
- letting people know where they are and what they will be doing; this is especially important for care practitioners who work alone and those who visit service users at home
- signing in and out of work if the care setting uses a sign-in book or other logging system for employees.

Care practitioners should also remind service users living at home that they must never let unknown callers in. It is always important to check the identity of callers while using a security chain across the door. Bogus callers sometimes pretend to be police officers, council staff or maintenance people, for example.

Internal security breaches are more difficult to spot than external breaches. They tend to involve the theft of money or belongings from service users or staff members, or the theft of confidential information from files or from the care organisation's computer systems. Care organisations generally have internal procedures for checking, recording and storing money and valuables; service users' personal money should always be protected by a record-keeping system and large amounts of cash should not be held on the premises. Marking clothes and other possessions with their owner's name is also helpful.

Reflect

What would you tell an adult with learning disabilities or a frail older person living alone about the risk of letting unknown callers into their home? How could a person in this position protect their personal security?

What do you know?

1. Identify two types of hazard that can be found in the physical environment of a care setting.
2. Describe the kinds of hazards that exist in bathrooms in care settings.
3. Explain why care practitioners always need to carry out a risk assessment before using equipment to provide care.
4. Identify three ways of protecting people from hospital-acquired infections.
5. Describe examples of hazardous working conditions or risky practices that can occur in some care settings.
6. Explain how care practitioners can help to minimise the risk of external security breaches in care settings.

Legislation, policies and procedures

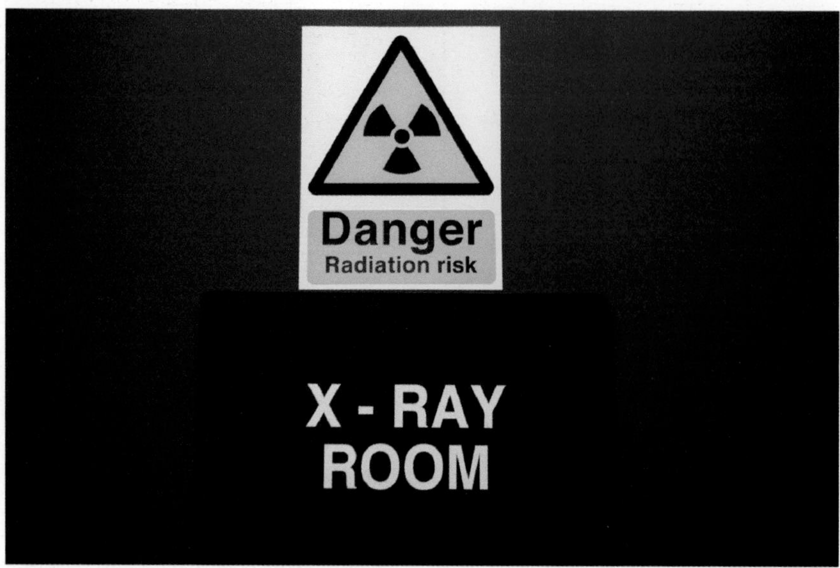

Your assessment criteria:

P2 Outline how legislation, policies and procedures relating to health, safety and security influence health and social care settings

Health and safety law affects many practices and procedures in health and social care settings.

The health and safety responsibilities of employers and employees result from the wide range of **legislation** that governs health and safety in all workplaces. A number of laws also exist covering health and safety issues that are specific to care settings. Legislation is necessary to ensure that safe working practices are followed when caring for individuals, to protect both service users and care practitioners.

Key terms

Legislation: *written laws made by an official law-making body such as Parliament*

Statute: *a form of written law also known as an Act of Parliament*

P2 The Health and Safety at Work Act (1974)

The Health and Safety at Work Act (1974) is the main piece of health and safety law in the UK. It affects both employers and employees. Under this **statute**, care practitioners share responsibility for health and safety in care settings with the care organisation that employs them. The care organisation is responsible for providing:

- a safe and secure work environment
- safe equipment
- information and training about health, safety and security.

In short, care organisations must provide a work environment that meets expected health and safety standards. They must make it possible for care practitioners to work safely. Care practitioners in turn have a responsibility to:

- work safely within the care setting
- monitor their work environment for health and safety problems that may develop
- report and respond appropriately to any health and safety risks.

To meet their legal responsibilities, care organisations must:

- carry out health and safety risk assessments
- develop health and safety **procedures**, such as fire evacuation procedures
- provide health and safety equipment, such as fire extinguishers, fire blankets and first aid boxes
- ensure that care settings have safety features, such as smoke alarms, fire exits and security fixtures (electronic pads on doors and window guards, for example)
- train their employees to follow health and safety **policies** and procedures, and to use health and safety equipment and safety features appropriately
- provide a range of health and safety information and warning signs to alert people to safety features such as fire exits and first aid equipment, and to warn them about prohibited areas and activities (no smoking, for example).

Care practitioners carry out their legal responsibilities by:

- developing an awareness of health and safety law
- following health and safety guidelines, policies and procedures
- monitoring the care environment for health and safety hazards
- where it is safe to do so, dealing directly with hazards that present a risk
- reporting health and safety hazards or the failure of safety systems and procedures to a supervisor or manager.

Key terms

***Policy:** a written document that sets out an organisation's approach towards a particular issue*

***Procedure:** a document that sets out in detail how a particular issue should be dealt with or how particular tasks should be carried out*

Reflect

Have you ever received any health and safety training relating to care work? How did you find out about health and safety procedures at your placement setting?

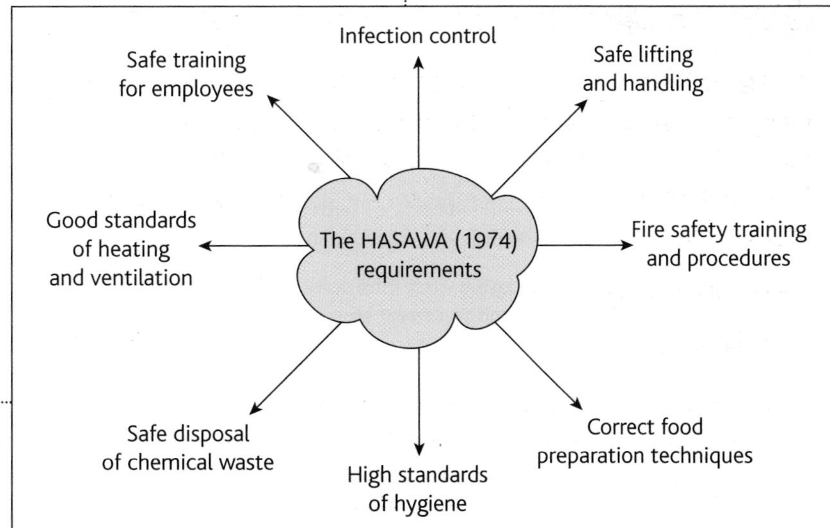

Figure 3.8 Requirements of the Health and Safety at Work Act (1974).

P2 Other health and safety legislation

Although the Health and Safety at Work Act (1974) enforces minimum standards of workplace health and safety and establishes a framework for safe working, in practice a range of regulations that apply to care settings extend and supplement this Act (see Figure 3.9).

Figure 3.9 Health and safety laws and regulations.

Regulations	Effects
Food Safety Act (1990)	This Act states that people working with food must practise good food hygiene in the workplace. Food must be safely stored and prepared, and must not be 'injurious to health'. Local authority environmental health officers enforce this law.
Food Safety (General Food Hygiene) Regulations (1995)	These regulations require people who prepare food in a care setting to identify possible food hygiene risks and to put controls in place that ensure any risk is reduced. The Food Safety Regulations also specify how premises that provide food should be equipped and organised.
The Manual Handling Operations Regulations (1992) (amended 2002)	These regulations cover all manual handling activities, such as lifting, lowering, pushing, pulling or carrying objects or people. A large proportion of workplace injuries are due to poor manual handling skills. Employers have a duty to assess the risks surrounding any activity that involves manual handling. They must put in place measures to reduce or avoid the risk. Employees must follow manual handling procedures and co-operate on all manual handling issues.
Reporting of Injuries, Diseases and Dangerous Occurrences Regulations (1995) (RIDDOR)	These require employers to notify a range of occupational injuries, diseases and dangerous events to the Health and Safety Executive or other relevant authorities.
Data Protection Act (1998)	This Act protects the individual's right to confidentiality of both paper and electronic records. An individual has the right to: • know what information is held about them and to correct this if it is inaccurate • refuse to provide information • have up-to-date and accurate data held about them

Your assessment criteria:

P2 Outline how legislation, policies and procedures relating to health, safety and security influence health and social care settings

Key terms

Regulations: *legal rules that are created using the authority of a statute*

Discuss

Do any of these health and safety laws affect the way people practise in your placement setting? With a couple of class colleagues, discuss the different ways in which they impact on the way care is provided where you work.

	• have data removed when it is no longer necessary for an organisation to hold it • have the confidentiality of their information protected.
Management of Health and Safety at Work Regulations (1999)	This places a responsibility on employers to train staff in relation to health and safety legislation, fire prevention, and moving and handling issues. Employers must also carry out risk assessments, remove or reduce any health and safety hazards that are identified and write safe working procedures based on their risk assessments.
Care Homes Regulations (2001)	These regulations aim to establish standards of good practice in care homes. Care homes must be registered and inspected by the Care Quality Commission (CQC). The manager of a home must have appropriate leadership and management qualifications and is responsible for health and safety at the home. This includes carrying out risk assessments and informing the CQC of any event that endangers the health, safety or wellbeing of people on the premises.
Control of Substances Hazardous to Health Regulations (2002) (COSHH)	These require employers to assess the risks from hazardous substances and take appropriate precautions to ensure that hazardous substances are correctly stored and used.
Civil Contingencies Act (2004)	The Act gives guidance on the responsibilities of public services in dealing with major public emergencies and accident hazards. Public services need to anticipate, prepare for, prevent, respond to and recover from major emergencies. Emergencies include extreme weather, terrorist attacks, industrial or other major accidents and pandemics (e.g. flu).
Care Minimum Standards	The Care Standards Act (2000) established National Minimum Standards for care services in 2003. Different standards exist for different types of care setting, but all have a health and safety focus. Each care setting should: • carry out a risk assessment on each individual service user • have relevant procedures and policies about security, abuse and neglect, bullying, and dealing with complaints, for example • carry out health and safety training of staff • have adequate security measures in place.

Key terms

Care Quality Commission: *the independent organisation that inspects and regulates all health and social care services in England*

Investigate

Go to the website of the Care Quality Commission (www.cqc.org.uk) and find a report on a health or social care organisation near to where you live. What does the report say about the standard of health and safety in the organisation?

Safeguarding vulnerable people

P2 Legislation for safeguarding

The recent development of a legal framework around **safeguarding** issues is designed to raise staff awareness of this important issue and to improve protection for vulnerable people. Procedures are now in place to identify abusers and sex offenders and, where appropriate, to bar them from working with children or vulnerable adults, whether in a paid post or as a volunteer.

The Independent Safeguarding Authority's (ISA) vetting and barring scheme aims to prevent unsuitable people from working with children and vulnerable adults. To achieve this, everyone who applies for such a post must be checked by the Criminal Records Bureau (CRB) , Disclosure Scotland or Access NI. Employers are responsible for ensuring checks are undertaken. People who work closely with children and vulnerable people require enhanced disclosure checks. This is a more detailed record check that identifies any previous cautions or offences (even if they are 'spent'). A 'barred' person who applies to work with or who is found to be working with children or vulnerable adults is committing a criminal offence and will be prosecuted. Employers who knowingly allow a 'barred' person access to vulnerable people are also committing a crime.

Factors affecting safeguarding

The legal framework surrounding health and social care influences a variety of issues in care organisations including:

- staff selection and staffing numbers, particularly the minimum staff–patient ratios needed to achieve acceptable standards of care
- inspection of premises by the Care Quality Commission (CQC)
- care practices.

M1 Using legislation, policies and procedures to promote safety

A care organisation's policies and procedures should incorporate the key points of health and safety law. This means that a care practitioner will be able to put health and safety laws into practice simply by

Your assessment criteria:

P2 Outline how legislation, policies and procedures relating to health, safety and security influence health and social care settings

M1 Describe how health and safety legislation, policies and procedures promote the safety of individuals in a health or social care setting

Key terms

Safeguarding: *the process of protecting children and vulnerable adults from abuse or neglect that may impair their health, development or wellbeing*

following their employer's policies and procedures. Care organisations need to develop a range of policies to ensure all aspects of the legal framework of care are covered. These will include policies on:

- health and safety
- safeguarding
- reporting of accidents
- waste disposal
- fire prevention and evacuation procedures
- security
- cleaning
- food safety
- dispensing and storing medicines
- lone working.

Implementation of health and safety-related policies and procedures should be monitored to check that employees are actually using them in practice. Employees are under a contractual obligation to implement their employers' policies and procedures and may face disciplinary action and possible dismissal for not doing so.

Case study

Christina is a health visitor based in a primary care health centre in a large city. She carries out checks on babies to ensure they are safe and developing normally. Christina also runs a number of child health clinics where she sees children up to the age of 8 years old. Christina works in an integrated care team with GPs, social workers, school nurses and staff from housing services, the police and the local children's centre.

1. How is Christina's work related to safeguarding?
2. What kind of safeguarding problems or issues relating to babies and younger children is Christina likely to be looking out for?
3. Give two reasons why it is better for Christina to work in a team of professionals who all have an interest in safeguarding children and vulnerable people.

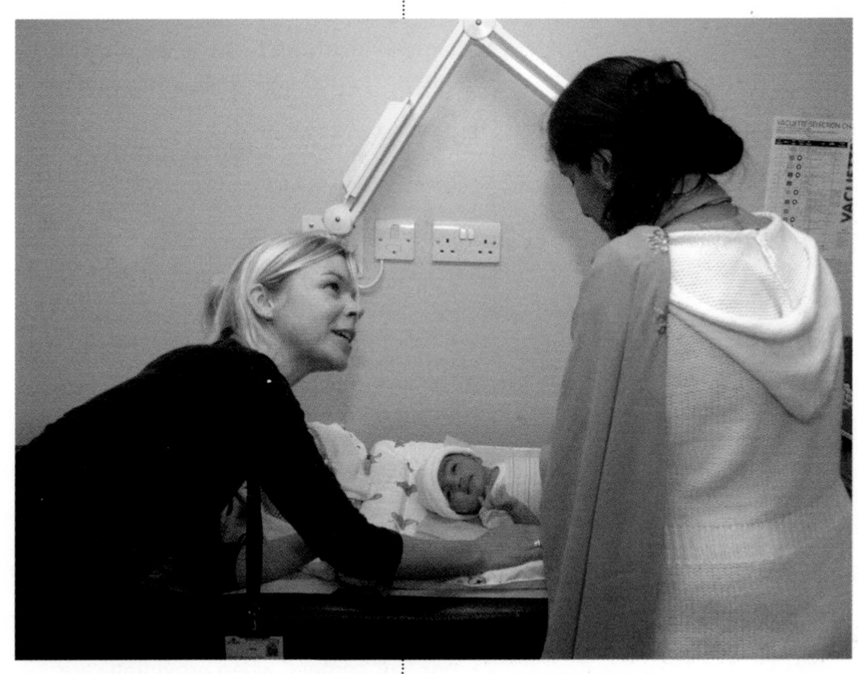

Roles and responsibilities

P2 Everyone has a role

Health, safety and security in a care setting are the responsibility of everyone involved in care provision, either directly or indirectly. The roles and responsibilities of the individuals and organisations involved in or affected by care provision are summarised in Figure 3.10.

Your assessment criteria:

P2 Outline how legislation, policies and procedures relating to health, safety and security influence health and social care settings

Figure 3.10 Different roles and responsibilities in care provision.

Participant	Role/responsibility
Employers	Legally, a care organisation takes on the employer's responsibilities for health and safety at work. In practice, managers are employed to oversee this aspect of the organisation's function. An employer's policies, procedures and practices are inspected and prosecution may result in the event of a breach of health and safety law. To be cleared of breaking the law, employers have to be able to show that suitable health, safety and security procedures were in place and were being followed correctly.
Health and safety representatives	Many care organisations delegate responsibility for health, safety and security issues to people who are specialist health and safety representatives. Ultimately, the care organisation is responsible for any breach of health and safety law but staff working as health and safety representatives undertake the day-to-day work needed to implement and monitor the organisation's policies and procedures. Health and safety representatives need to be well trained, experienced and committed to high standards to do this effectively.
Employees	All employees have to participate in health and safety training during their induction period and on an ongoing basis. Common induction standards cover: • moving and handling • fire safety • basic first aid • infection control • preventing abuse. An employee has a responsibility to always consider the health and safety of colleagues and the people they provide care for. In addition they must: • follow organisational safety and security procedures • make risk assessments and always minimise risks • report incidents and emergencies, and maintain adequate records • act within limits of their own ability and competence • not 'cut corners' when providing care.

Users of services	People receiving care are expected to behave in a responsible way and must not endanger the health, safety or security of others.
Visitors, relatives and volunteers	People who are visiting a care setting, or who have a volunteer role in a setting, are expected to follow all health and safety procedures, behave in a responsible way and be vigilant about possible health, safety and security hazards.
NHS Trust (see page 291)	National Health Service Trusts have a wide range of health and safety obligations. These range from fire safety and infection control, to protecting people within health care settings from violence and abuse.
Local authority (see page 289)	Local authorities provide advice and guidance to people employed in council-run and owned settings. They also employ community-based staff who provide health and safety advice to people receiving care at home. Many local authorities also provide aids and adaptations to people living in council-owned homes to improve and promote their health and safety.

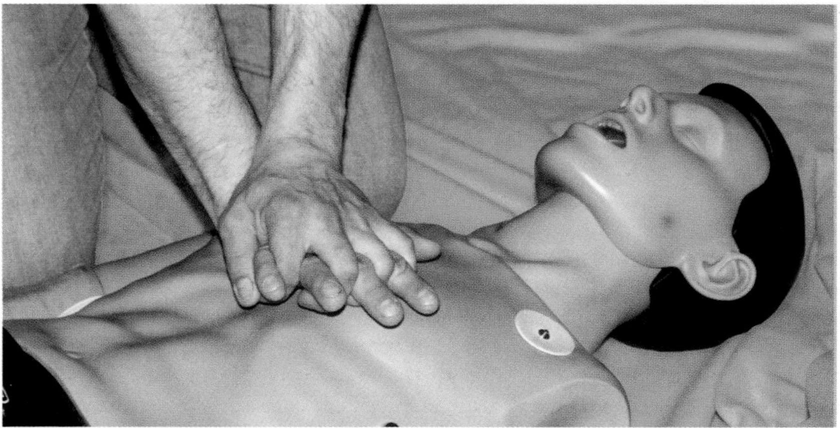

Basic first aid training forms part of the induction of most health and social care workers.

What do you know?

1. Identify the main piece of legislation covering health and safety in care settings.
2. Describe three ways in which care practitioners can ensure they meet their responsibilities under health and safety law.
3. What do COSHH and RIDDOR stand for and how does each affect care practice?
4. Explain how vulnerable people within the care system are protected by the Independent Safeguarding Authority.
5. Name four policies relating to health and safety that care organisations are expected to produce.
6. Explain the roles and responsibilities of employers and employees in care settings.

Risk assessment in care settings

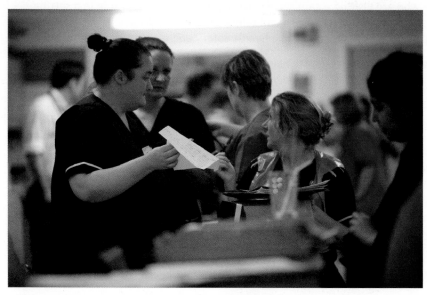

Risk assessment is usually a team-based activity in care settings.

Your assessment criteria:

P3 Carry out a risk assessment in a health or social care setting

P3 Why carry out risk assessments?

By law, care organisations are required to carry out formal risk assessments of their care settings. The process of **risk assessment** aims to identify potential risks to the health, safety and security of care practitioners, service users and visitors to a care setting. Risk assessment recognises that a range of care activities, equipment and even the way a care setting is organised can be hazardous, but that steps can be taken to minimise or remove the risk of people experiencing harm.

Care organisations employ and train care practitioners and specialist health and safety staff to carry out risk assessment procedures. Risk assessments in care settings tend to focus on areas of practice such as moving and handling, pressure area care, fire safety and food hygiene, for example.

Stages of risk assessment

The **Health and Safety Executive** has identified five stages of a risk assessment (see Figure 3.11).

Key terms

Health and Safety Executive: *the national, independent regulator of health and safety in the UK*

Risk assessment: *a process that aims to identify potential risks to the health, safety and security of all people at a specified location*

Figure 3.11 The stages of risk assessment.

Stage	Key questions	Purpose
1. Look for hazards	• What are the hazards?	• To identify all hazards
2. Assess who may be harmed	• Who is at risk?	• To evaluate the risk of hazards causing harm
3. Consider the risk – whether existing precautions are adequate	• What needs to be done? • Who needs to do what?	• To consider risk control measures • To identify risk control responsibilities
4. Document the findings	• Can you give a summary of the hazards and risks?	• To record all findings and the risk control plan
5. Review the assessment and revise if necessary	• Is the risk controlled? • Are further controls needed?	• To monitor and maintain an accurate and up-to-date risk control system

The Management of Health and Safety at Work Regulations (1999) place a legal duty on employers to carry out risk assessments in order to ensure a safe and healthy workplace. The risk assessments that are produced should clearly identify:

- the potential hazards and risks to the health and safety of employees and others in the workplace
- any preventive and protective measures that are needed to minimise risk and improve health and safety.

Care practitioners can also carry out their own ongoing risk assessments in their everyday work. Basically this involves:

- being alert to possible hazards
- understanding the risks associated with each hazard
- reporting any health and safety concerns that are identified.

Reflect

Do you know where the risk assessment documents relating to your work placement setting are kept? Ask to have a look at examples of risk assessments relating to practices or issues within the setting next time you are there.

M2 Assessing the severity of risk

Care practitioners should not only be able to identify hazards in their everyday work, but should be able to assess each hazard to consider the *degree* of risk posed. Risks may be associated with:

- moving and handling service users and equipment
- hazardous chemicals (such as cleaning and sterilising fluids, and disinfectants)
- medicines
- infection control
- personal security.

Your assessment criteria:

M2 Assess the hazards identified in the health or social care setting

D1 Make recommendations in relation to identified hazards to minimise the risks to the service user group

D1 Making recommendations to minimise risks

Risk assessment is an ongoing, cyclical process. This means that, once hazards are identified and risks are assessed, risk reduction strategies are put in place to minimise the likelihood of harm occurring. Risk reduction strategies must be monitored regularly to check that that they remain appropriate and that they are working. This is important because risk situations can change. For example, previously identified risks can diminish because of environmental changes or because people's behaviour changes; new equipment may make a particular task, such as lifting or moving patients, less risky. Alternatively, new hazards may be introduced into a care setting because new equipment is acquired or new procedures are introduced.

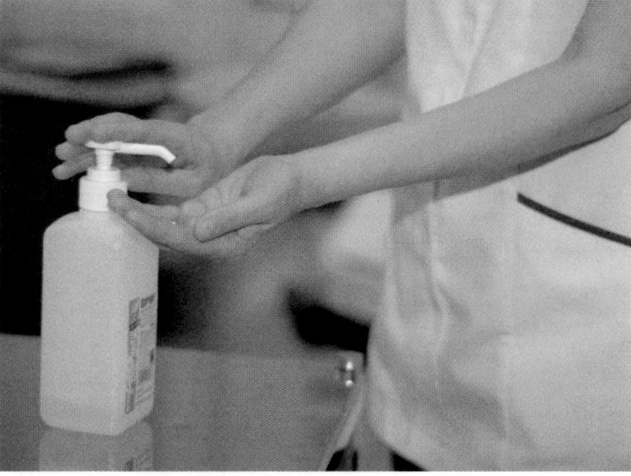

Effective hand-washing is the key to reducing infection rates in health care settings.

Regular reappraisal of hazards and risks is needed to ensure that safety remains the top priority. Where new hazards are identified or risk levels change, care practitioners, health and safety representatives or the managers of a care setting may need to make recommendations to minimise risks. Recommendations might focus on:

- changing aspects of the care environment (such as adding hand-gel dispensers or introducing hoists) to remove, exclude or minimise the potential impact of a hazard
- changing people's behaviour through additional training (for example in moving and handling) or information (perhaps about hand-washing) so that they can avoid hazards and reduce risk to themselves

- developing a new policy or procedure that recognises a hazard and delivers ways of avoiding potentially harmful effects.

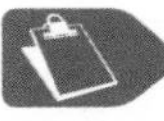

Case study

Using a scale of 1–5, where 1 is the highest risk and 5 is the lowest risk:

1. Identify the main hazard in each of the following scenarios.
2. Estimate the severity of the risk in each scenario.
3. Briefly describe how the risk could be minimised.

- Scenario A – at playgroup, the kitchen floor has just been washed and is still wet
- Scenario B – a half-full laundry bag of dirty linen has been left at the top of the stairs outside a hospital ward for older people
- Scenario C – in a nursing home, an elderly resident's window has been left wide open to air her room
- Scenario D – at a learning disability day centre, scissors have been left out on the craft-room table
- Scenario E – a workman fitting a new security pad to the front door of a nursery has left the door wide open and unattended while he goes to his van for some tools.

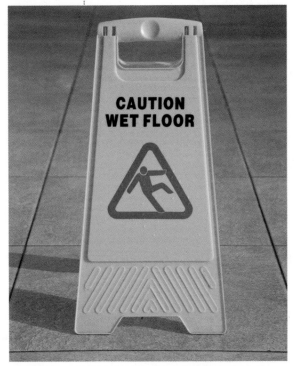

Scenario A – at playgroup, the kitchen floor has just been washed and is still wet.

What do you know?

1. What is the purpose of a risk assessment?
2. Identify the five stages of a risk assessment.
3. What should happen in the risk assessment process once hazards have been identified and risks have been assessed?
4. Identify three areas of care practice that should be risk assessed in a care setting.
5. Describe three ways in which care practitioners can incorporate risk assessment into their care practice.
6. Describe three things a care practitioner could recommend to minimise risks to service users in a care setting.

Accidents and first aid

Care practitioners work in a variety of different health and social care settings with a diverse range of people. Many people receiving care are vulnerable because of ill-health or other problems. As a result, care practitioners need to be able to respond effectively to different **incidents**, **accidents** and other emergencies that may occur.

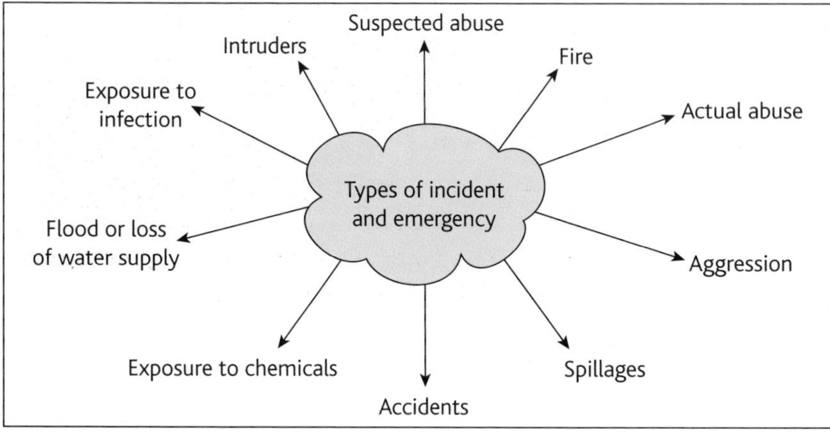

Figure 3.12 Different types of incident and emergency.

Your assessment criteria:

P4 Explain possible priorities and responses when dealing with two particular incidents or emergencies in a health or social care setting

Key terms

Accident: *an event that happens suddenly and unexpectedly or by chance*

Incident: *an event that may cause disruption or a crisis*

P4 Dealing with accidents

Accidents sometimes happen in care settings, even when care practitioners assess the risks in situations and are careful in the way they provide care. When an accident does occur, an effective response is needed to minimise any harm caused and to ensure that the situation does not get any worse. As a care practitioner you would use an *emergency response procedure* to deal with an accident. This could involve the following steps:

1. STOP and ASSESS – stop what you are doing to assess the situation
2. CHECK for any continuing danger
3. AVOID RISK – if the situation remains dangerous, avoid putting yourself or others at further risk
4. CALL for help by activating alarms, shouting to others or calling emergency services, for example
5. if it safe to do so, INTERVENE – establish whether the people affected by the accident have injuries and prioritise those needing most help.

Care practitioners and others who respond to accidents and emergency situations should always try to respect the dignity of people who need assistance. Discouraging onlookers from crowding the scene and staring, talking

Reflect

Think about two or three situations in which first aid would be needed. Have you ever experienced any of these situations or helped out when a person required first aid? What skills and personal qualities do you think a first aider needs to deal with accidents and unexpected health problems?

to casualties in a professional, reassuring way and covering people with blankets or coats are all ways of showing respect and protecting an individual's dignity.

The principles of first aid

A person who is injured in an accident or who suddenly develops unexpected health problems may need first aid treatment. The aims of first aid are to:

- preserve the casualty's life
- prevent further harm occurring to the casualty
- promote or support the process of recovery.

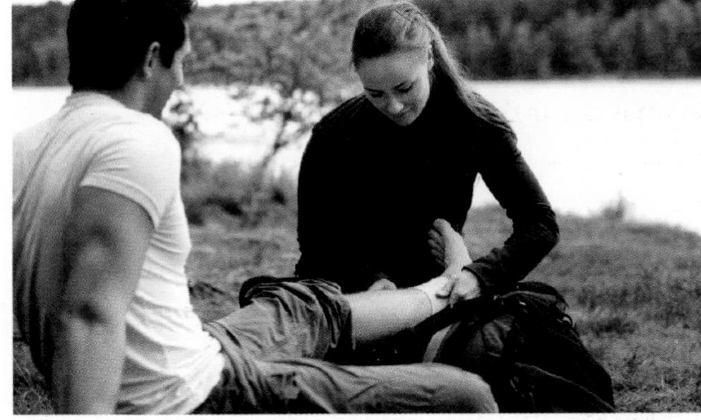

Accidents occur unexpectedly and may require prompt treatment to minimise injury.

The basic responsibility of a first aider is to provide a prompt response to injured casualties. Effective first aid is most likely to result if the responder has a calm, logical approach and prioritises the most seriously injured and physically unwell casualties. When managing casualties, first aiders should:

- observe the casualties to establish priorities
- respond to any unconscious casualties first
- check any unconscious casualty's airway, breathing and circulation (abc); the person will die if any of these vital body functions are absent
- help conscious casualties who are unable to walk or move themselves as the next priority; a conscious casualty may be suffering from serious fractures, head injuries or have bleeding wounds that need immediate attention
- not move or lift an immobile casualty unless the person is in danger of experiencing further harm (such as being run over); moving a person who is conscious but immobile can be dangerous if the person has unseen spinal injuries, fractures or open wounds
- do all they can to minimise the risk of cross-infection between themselves and a bleeding casualty; where possible a first aider would wear gloves, avoiding direct contact with open wounds and the casualty's blood and covering cuts and wounds with appropriate dressings and bandages
- arrange for casualties with minor injuries or distress to be taken to hospital for further examination and possible treatment
- always remain with casualties until help arrives, ensuring the safety of each casualty, providing comfort and reassurance, and monitoring each individual's condition in case this deteriorates.

Care practitioners are specifically trained to protect themselves and others, as well as to look after casualties, when they intervene in accident situations. This is important if blood or body fluids are involved or where there is continuing danger.

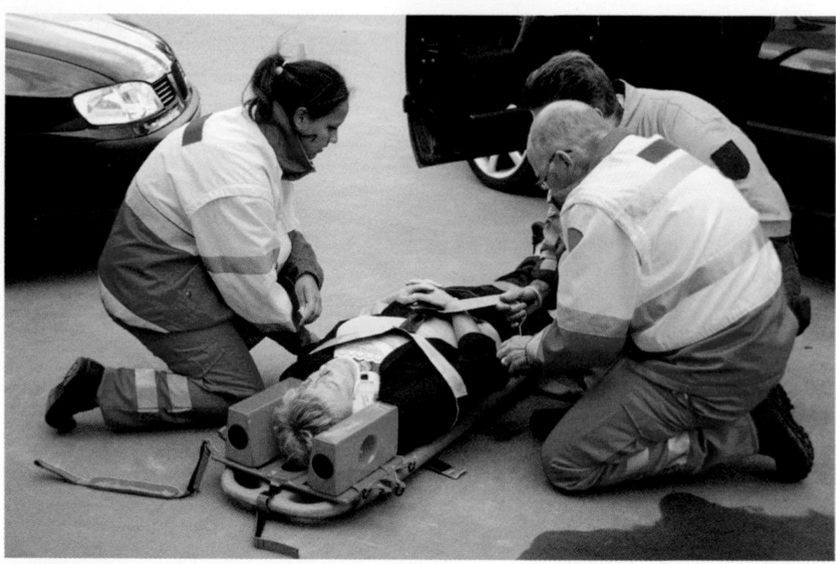

It is important know how to call for emergency help when serious accidents or incidents occur.

Your assessment criteria:

P4 Explain possible priorities and responses when dealing with two particular incidents or emergencies in a health or social care setting

Reflect

What might happen if an untrained and inexperienced person tries to perform first aid in an accident or emergency situation?

P4 Getting help

First aid situations are extremely varied. In care settings, all care practitioners should know who to call for help in different situations and how to contact emergency services. The names and telephone numbers of first aiders are usually displayed on posters or notice boards in public areas of the care setting. If a situation is serious, a 999 call should be made. The emergency operator will ask for the following kinds of information:

- which services are required (police, ambulance and/or fire service)
- the caller's name and the number of the phone they are calling from
- the location of the accident or incident
- the number of casualties involved
- what has happened (including signs, symptoms and state of casualties)
- whether any of the casualties is unconscious.

It is important for the caller to listen carefully to the emergency operator, to provide the information they ask for and to remain as calm as possible, even though this may be difficult in the circumstances. It can be helpful to have someone holding the phone and relaying instructions from the operator, who may provide help and advice on dealing with the casualty.

Accident reporting and incident review

The Health and Safety Executive recommends that employers should provide appointed first aiders, not just to administer first aid treatment, but to record any accidents, incidents or health emergencies in a log book. Useful information that might be recorded in the first aid book includes:

- the date, time and place of an incident
- the name and job of the injured or unwell person
- details of the injuries or illness and any first aid provided
- what happened to the person immediately after being given first aid – went home, went back to work, went to hospital, for example
- the name and signature of the first aider or the person who dealt with the incident.

Effective reports describe what happened clearly and accurately, avoiding emotional statements and without attributing blame. The information provided in accident reports is often used in subsequent investigations, so clear and accurate descriptions are very helpful. Accidents and incidents should always be reported using the appropriate forms or reporting procedures as soon after the event as possible.

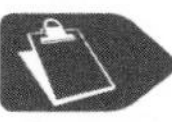

Case study

Sian, aged 17, is standing by the side of the school playing field with a couple of friends watching the Year 11 rugby team playing against another local school. Sian winces every time the players crash into each other when they make tackles. The game looks very aggressive and dangerous to Sian and her friends. Just as they agree that playing rugby must hurt, two players from the opposing team collide as they run for the ball. There is a loud crack as they bang heads and then fall down. One of the boys has blood running down his face and is groaning as he lies on the floor. The other boy is silent and completely still. The referee hasn't noticed what has happened and the game is continuing further up the field. Sian is trying to remember her recent lesson about first aid and the emergency response procedure.

1. What should Sian do now?
2. Which casualty should Sian go to first (explain why)?
3. How could Sian check that the unconscious player is breathing?

Other incidents and emergencies

P4 Suspected or actual abuse

A range of different forms of **abuse** can occur in care settings (see page 104). Care practitioners should know that members of care staff and people receiving care can be affected by abuse. If you suspect that a child, vulnerable adult or a colleague may be experiencing abuse, you should let your supervisor or mentor know about your concerns. They are in a much better position to investigate any suspicions than you are because of their position of authority.

If a child discloses that they have been abused or ill-treated, you should listen carefully and note what they say as accurately as possible. It is important to reassure the child so they understand that they are not to blame for the situation and that members of staff will protect them. However, you must also tell the child that you have to pass on what they've said to your supervisor or manager. It is important not to dig for details, not to question the truth of what they say and to avoid putting pressure on the child to say more.

If an adult tells you they have been abused or ill-treated, it's best to encourage them to report this to the person in charge of their care or to the manager of the care setting. If they are unable to do (or incapable of doing) this, you should let your supervisor or manager know about your concerns.

Infections, chemicals and spillages

Care practitioners need to be aware of the sources of infection (such as **MRSA** and *C. difficile*) that exist in care settings and of the risks associated with hazardous wastes, cleaning fluids, medication and other chemical or body fluid spillages. Chemicals can cause burns and irritate the skin if mishandled or spilt. Misuse of medication can lead to adverse reactions and even overdoses, while spillages lead to the risk of slips and falls.

Your assessment criteria:

P4 Explain possible priorities and responses when dealing with two particular incidents or emergencies in a health or social care setting

M3 Discuss health, safety or security concerns arising from a specific incident or emergency in a health or social care setting.

D2 Justify responses to a particular incident or emergency in a health or social care setting.

Key terms

Abuse: *ill-treatment of another person*

MRSA: *Methicillin-resistant* Staphylococcus aureus, *a bacterium responsible for several difficult-to-treat infections in humans*

Discuss

Why does the relationship between a care practitioner and a person receiving care sometimes lead to abuse or neglect? Share your ideas and thoughts about this with a small group of class colleagues. Try to identify reasons why care can sometimes go wrong.

Care practitioners need to be aware of the policies and procedures relating to infection prevention and control, the COSHH policy and medication management procedures. To minimise the risk of acquiring and passing on an infection, care practitioners should:

- wash their hands between touching one person and the next
- use anti-bacterial hand-gels where available
- use disposable tissues, and cover their mouth and nose when coughing or sneezing
- dispose of tissues safely and promptly
- practise good food hygiene, avoiding cross contamination of cooked and uncooked meat, and disposing of out-of-date food, for example
- use protective gloves and aprons where available
- get help to deal with spillages (e.g. body fluids) from staff who are trained to do this
- cover any cuts with waterproof plasters.

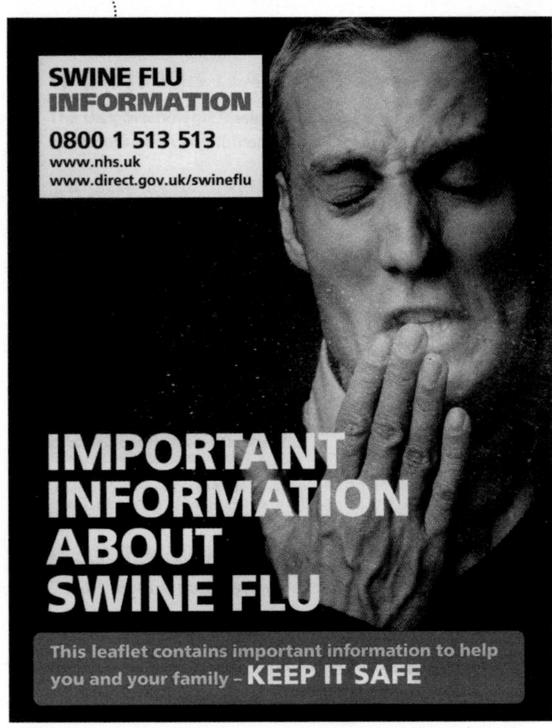

SWINE FLU INFORMATION
0800 1 513 513
www.nhs.uk
www.direct.gov.uk/swineflu
IMPORTANT INFORMATION ABOUT SWINE FLU
This leaflet contains important information to help you and your family – KEEP IT SAFE

Care practitioners should always try to minimise the risk of infection to others.

Intruders

Security is an important issue in any care setting. Care practitioners should understand and follow all security procedures to keep intruders out of care settings. Security policies usually encourage care practitioners to check and challenge the identity of people they don't know, to lock doors and windows and to alert security staff or the police if an intruder is spotted on the premises. Care organisations generally discourage staff from approaching or directly restraining intruders in order to minimise the risk of harm from violence.

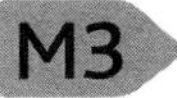

M3 D2 Discussing and justifying responses to incidents and emergencies

Care organisations tend to review what happened during accidents, critical incidents and emergencies to assess emergency procedures, the effectiveness of responses and to learn lessons that may help to prevent similar accidents or emergencies occurring in future. Accident and critical incident reviews may lead to a change in policy or procedure, or may identify the need for better training or improved communication systems, for example.

P4 Aggressive or dangerous encounters

Your assessment criteria:

P4 Explain possible priorities and responses when dealing with two particular incidents or emergencies in a health or social care setting

Aggression and violence does sometimes occur in care settings. This may be the result of an individual's mental health, alcohol or substance misuse problems, but can also result from fear, frustration and anger about services. As a student on placement in a care setting, you would not be expected to help deal with any aggressive or violent incidents. If you do observe any of the following behaviours you should be non-threatening, talk slowly but assertively, and leave the area to alert a member of staff as quickly as you can:

- tense, agitated behaviour (such as pacing around)
- loud, high-pitched voice
- abrupt, hostile speech
- muscle tension in a person's face
- hands closing to make a fist
- lack of eye contact or excessive, fixed eye contact
- invasion of personal space, pushing or deliberately blocking people.

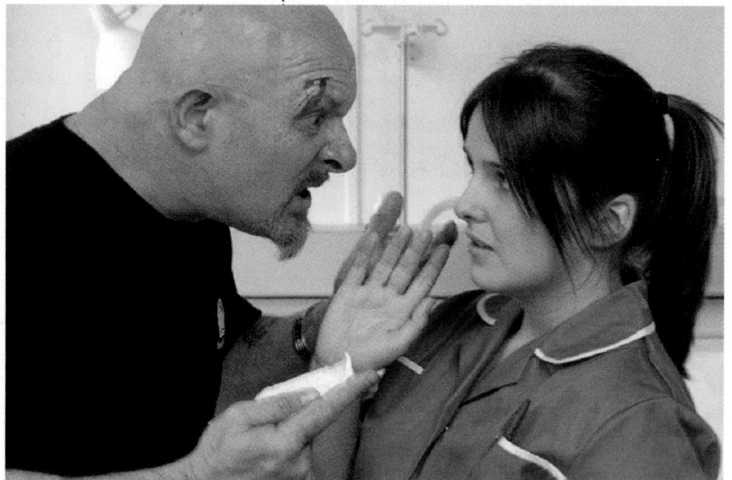

Anger and aggression are sometimes directed at care practitioners when people become frustrated, frightened or are made to wait a long time for treatment.

Fire incidents

Fires are very rare events in care settings. However, staff in every care setting should be prepared for the possibility of fire. Care organisations have a responsibility to produce detailed policies and procedures, and to install fire safety systems. Care practitioners should be aware of the policies and procedures, should take part in regular fire drills and should know how to use all of the fire safety systems. A care practitioner's role during a fire incident is to keep themselves and others safe. Where possible they should help people to escape a fire, but must not put anybody (including themselves) at risk. The person in charge of the care setting usually has responsibility for contacting the emergency services, organising any evacuation and for undertaking a head count when people leave the building.

Major disasters

Major incidents and natural disasters such as floods, loss of water supply and civic emergencies may affect a care setting. In each of these situations, the manager of the care setting has overall decision-making responsibility.

A care setting may flood because of an internal leak (such as a burst pipe) or due to an external deluge of water (such as heavy rainfall or a river bursting its banks). Both would cause major disruption that would be distressing to service users. Staff in a care setting should be aware of a flood policy and a set of evacuation procedures. When a decision is taken to evacuate a care setting, residents are usually moved to a designated evacuation centre run by the local authority.

Loss of water supply is a significant problem for a care setting as many day-to-day activities require a water supply, from flushing toilets, and giving baths and showers, to cooking, as well as maintaining residents' fluid intake. The manager of a care setting would normally deal with the loss of water supply by arranging an emergency supply (such as via a tanker) to ensure that hygiene and basic care needs can be met.

Civil emergencies such as industrial action (strikes), terrorism or public unrest may also lead to the loss of services. The manager of a care setting would have the responsibility of deciding how to respond to such a situation. Protecting the staff and service users, equipment and property would be priorities.

Investigate

Have a look around your work placement setting or the areas of your school or college where you spend most of your time. What fire safety information and equipment are provided there? Would you know what to do in the event of a fire breaking out? If not, find out what the correct fire response procedure is.

What do you know?

1. Identify three different types of incident or emergency that may occur in a care setting.
2. What would you do if you suspected that a child had been abused or ill-treated at your work placement setting?
3. Outline an effective way of responding to an accident or emergency situation in your care setting.
4. Identify the main aims of first aid.
5. What can a care practitioner do to minimise the spread of infection in a care setting?
6. What kinds of behaviours suggest a person is feeling aggressive and may become violent?

Assessment checklist

Your learning and level of understanding of this unit will be assessed through assignments given to you and marked by your teacher or tutor. Before you submit your assignment work for assessment you should make sure that you have produced sufficient evidence to achieve the grade you are aiming for.

To pass this unit you will need to present evidence for assessment which demonstrates that you can meet all of the pass criteria for the unit.

Assessment Criteria	Description	✓
P1	Explain potential hazards and the harm that may arise from each in a health or social care setting.	☐
P2	Outline how legislation, policies and procedures relating to health, safety and security influence health and social care settings.	☐
P3	Carry out a risk assessment in a health or social care setting.	☐
P4	Explain possible priorities and responses when dealing with two particular incidents or emergencies in a health or social care setting.	☐

You can achieve a merit grade for the unit by presenting evidence that also meets all of the following merit criteria for the unit.

Assessment Criteria	Description	✓
M1	Describe how health and safety legislation, policies and procedures promote the safety of individuals in a health or social care setting.	☐
M2	Assess the hazards identified in the health or social care setting.	☐
M3	Discuss health, safety or security concerns arising from a specific incident or emergency in a health or social care setting.	☐

You can achieve a distinction grade for the unit by presenting evidence that also meets all of the following merit criteria for the unit.

Assessment Criteria	Description	✓
D1	Make recommendations in relation to identified hazards to minimise the risks to the service user group.	☐
D2	Justify responses to a particular incident or emergency in a health or social care setting.	☐

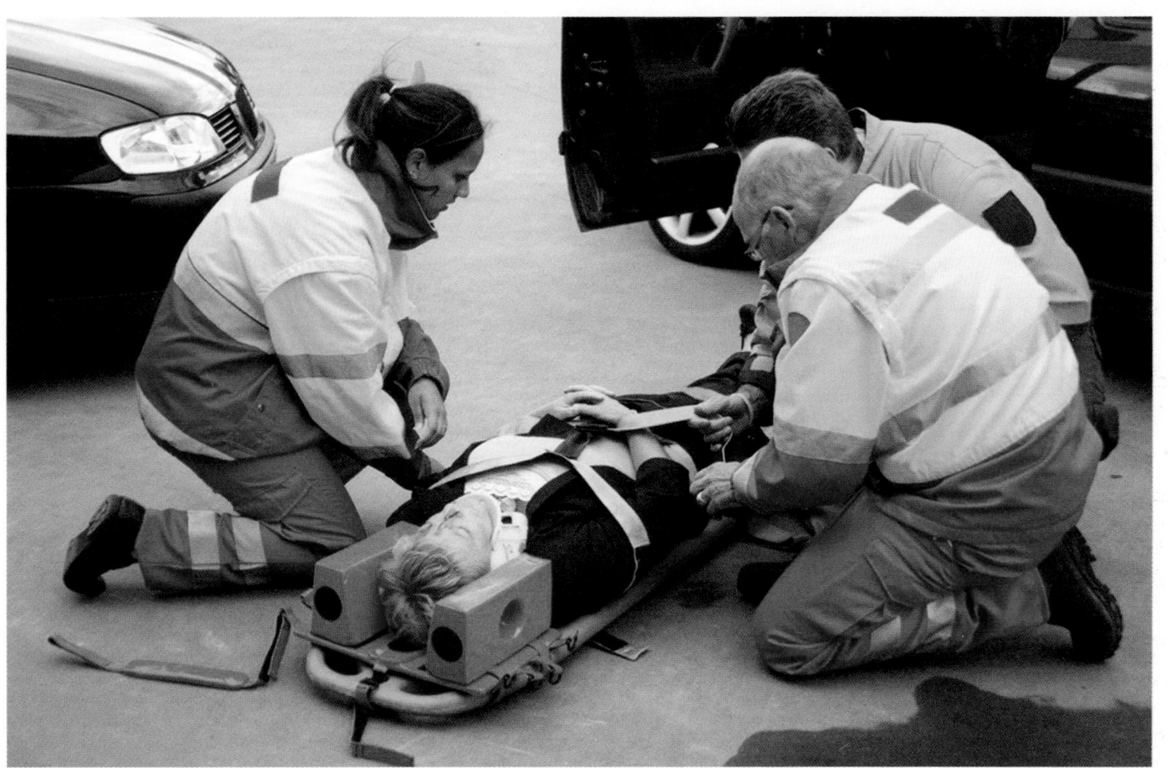

4 | Development through the life stages

LO1 Know stages of growth and development throughout the human lifespan

- life stages from conception to the final stages
- definitions associated with growth and development
- different types of development, and arrested or delayed development

LO2 Understand potential effects of life factors and events on the development of the individual

- the nature–nurture debate
- effects of life factors, such as genetic biological, environmental, socio-economic and lifestyle factors
- major life events

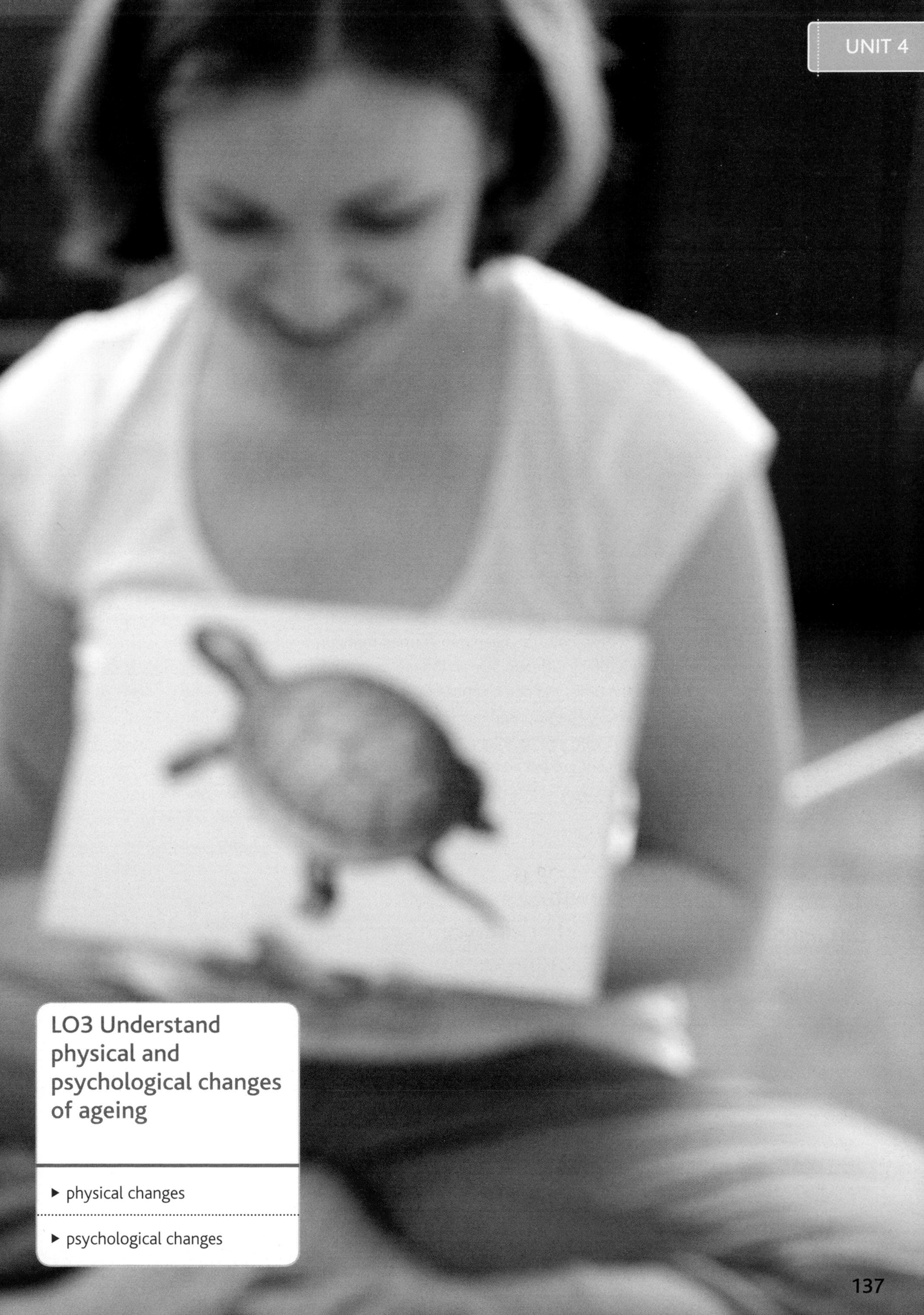

LO3 Understand physical and psychological changes of ageing

- physical changes
- psychological changes

Understanding human growth

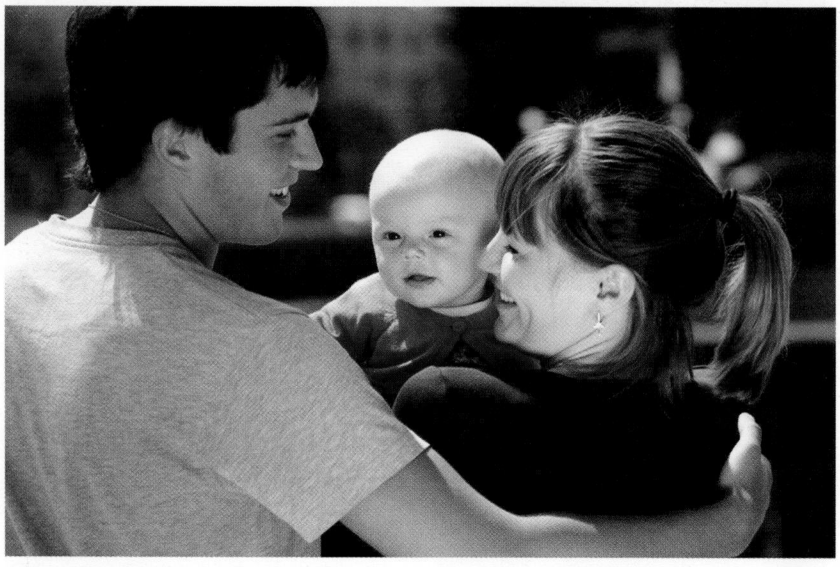

Human growth and development is a lifelong process.

In all sorts of ways, you're not the person you used to be! A lot has happened to you since your birth. Your body, for example, has been transformed through continuous physical growth; you're a totally different size and shape compared to when you were a baby. Most of the time, you don't notice how much you are changing and developing as a person. The surprised reactions of relatives, family friends and people who haven't seen you for a long time provide an indication of the speed and extent of your growth and development during infancy, childhood and adolescence.

Your assessment criteria:

P1 Describe physical, intellectual, emotional and social development for each of the life stages of an individual

P1 What is human growth?

Human beings experience **growth** when they increase in physical size or **mass**. Gain in height is a gradual process that occurs from birth until a point in early adulthood when we reach our maximum height. As you are no doubt aware, some people don't stop getting bigger just because they've stopped getting taller! The physical process of human growth involves both height and weight gain. However, once we reach our maximum height, other aspects of our physique are also usually fully developed and we have reached a point of physical **maturity**. Eating and drinking too much, together with being inactive, can result in further weight increases once our body has reached this point of physical maturity. However, increases in size for these reasons are not part of the normal or expected pattern of human growth.

Key terms

Growth: *an increase in a person's physical size or 'mass'*

Mass: *the quantity of something*

Maturity: *the state or point of being fully developed as a human being*

Reflect

Think about a friend or relative who you have known since childhood (ideally since you were both infants). How have they changed since this point in their life? Complete a table like the one below with your ideas.

	What was the person like when you first knew them?	What are they like now?
Physically		
Intellectually		
Emotionally		
Socially		

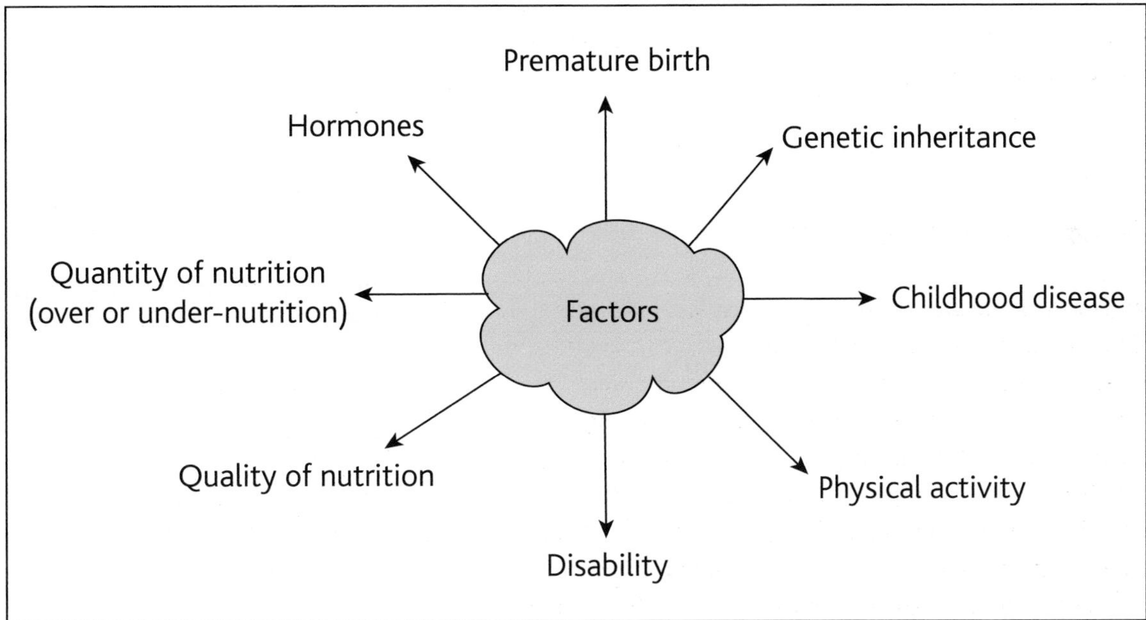

Figure 4.1 Factors affecting human growth.

Understanding human development

P1 What is human development?

Human development refers to changes in the complexity, sophistication and use of a person's capabilities and skills. As a result, human development includes changes that go beyond improvements in our *physical* capabilities and skills. From the moment of birth, human beings experience a continuous process of physical, intellectual, social and emotional development, so that development is never complete.

Developmental norms

In most cases, the processes of human growth and development follow a fairly predictable pattern. For example, observation, experience and research tell us that specific growth and development changes tend to occur within particular time periods (see Figure 4.2). We also know that human growth and development usually follow a predictable sequence. We know, for example, that after babies sit up without support, they will next develop the ability to crawl, followed by the ability to stand up and then the ability to walk. Linking this sequence of expected growth and development events to an expected timeframe enables us to talk about **developmental norms** or **milestones**.

Figure 4.2 Examples of developmental norms.

Milestone	Age
Baby can sit unaided	6–9 months
Baby can crawl	8–10 months
Baby can walk unaided	12–13 months
Infant can say a few words	9–12 months
Puberty begins	10 (girls) 12 (boys)
Menopause occurs in females	45–55 years

Knowledge of developmental norms provides a useful way of assessing a child's growth and development. However, you should also know there is variation in the times when infants and children achieve their developmental norms or milestones. Furthermore, it is incorrect to say a child is 'abnormal' if they reach growth and development norms later than expected. There may be a variety of reasons why a child's general pattern of growth and development is more advanced or delayed than the typical pattern.

Your assessment criteria:

P1 Describe physical, intellectual, emotional and social development for each of the life stages of an individual

Key terms

Developmental norm: *the point at which, on average, an infant or child is expected to achieve a particular skill or developmental change*

Milestone: *a significant event or point in the development of an infant or young child*

Reflect

Find out whether you reached any of these infant milestones at the expected point.

Developmental problems

An infant or child under the age of five may be described by health and social care professionals (health visitors, GPs, social workers) as having **delayed development** if their pattern of physical, intellectual, emotional or social development is significantly and persistently slower than expected for a child of their age. A child with delayed development may receive specialist care or support to promote a particular aspect of their development. **Arrested development** is an old-fashioned term; since it is now considered inappropriate, it is rarely used by health and social care workers. It was used in the past to describe people with complex disabilities, especially learning disabilities and brain damage, whose development seemed to have stopped. It is now recognised that even people with the most complex disabilities and damaged brains are always changing and developing, just at a significantly slower pace.

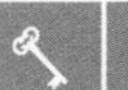

Key terms

Arrested development: *the absence of development, an out-of-date term*

Delayed development: *a pattern of development that is significantly slower than expected*

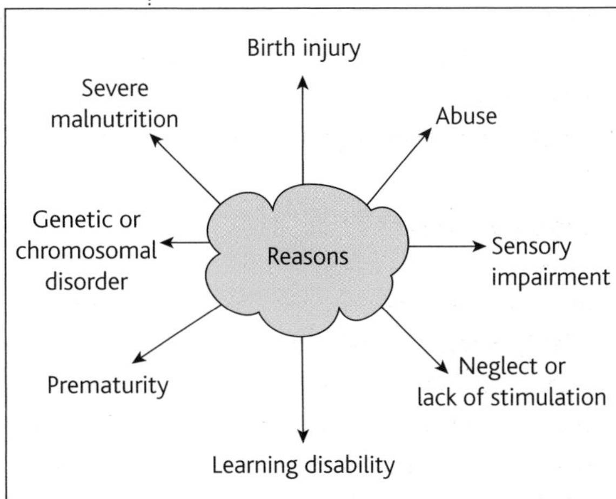

Figure 4.3 Reasons for developmental delay.

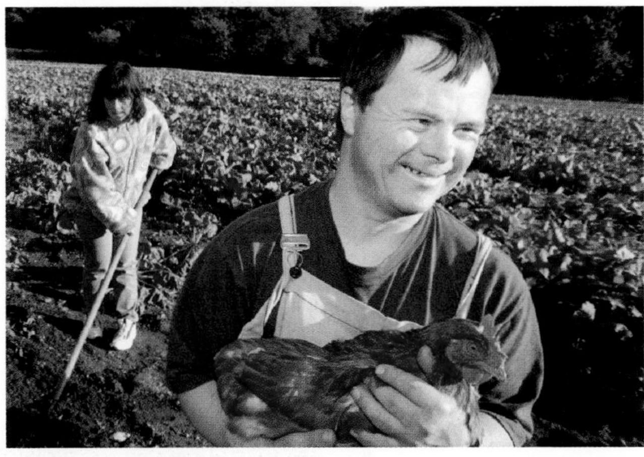

A person with a learning disability usually has some form of arrested development.

Continuity as well as change

When considering human growth and development we tend to think about change. This is understandable as both processes cause a bewildering variety of changes throughout life. However, it is important to appreciate that human growth and development depend on a number of *continuities*. For example, the genes that we inherit from our parents, the values that we learn as children and the patterns of behaviour that we use when we're faced by new situations are all examples of continuing influences on our growth and personal development. In addition, the development of new skills and abilities often depends on the maintenance and continuing use of capabilities and skills that we developed earlier in life.

Understanding life terms

Life is a frequently used word in any book on human growth and development. Typically, it is associated with a variety of other words. Examples of these 'life terms' are life stage, lifestyle (see page 180), life course, life expectancy and life span. The various life terms have different and specific meanings when applied to human growth and development.

Your assessment criteria:

P1 Describe physical, intellectual, emotional and social development of each of the life stages of an individual

P1 Life stages

A life stage is an age-related period of growth and development. Each human life stage is thought to encompass a distinctive pattern of human growth and development. The classic human life stages that are referred to here are:

- infancy (0–3 years)
- childhood (4–9 years)
- adolescence (10–18 years)
- adulthood (19–65)
- older adulthood (65+).

Dividing human growth and development into stages, like those shown in Figure 4.4, is a common way of identifying the main developmental patterns and points of transition that most people experience.

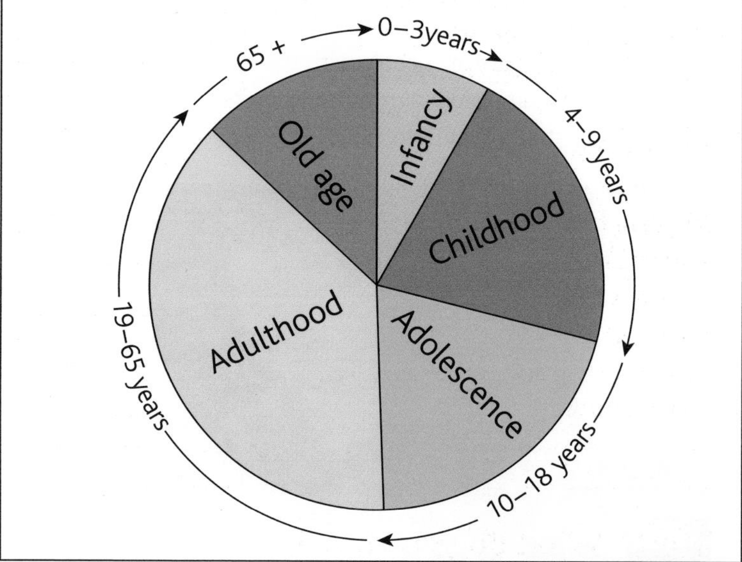

Figure 4.4 Life stages.

The life course

The concept of the human **life course** refers to the ***unique*** pattern of events, experiences and influences that affect an individual during their existence. The idea of a life course encourages us to think about how one person's development is shaped by a unique combination of factors, influences and events. It is the way in which we experience events and influences during our life course that causes us to become the individual we are. This partly explains why brothers, sisters and people from very similar backgrounds may develop in very different ways.

Reflect

Create a life stage table or diagram and identify family members, friends and neighbours who fall into each life stage category. Would it be obvious to people meeting your family, friends and neighbours for the first time which of them belongs in which life stage? Reflect on this and consider why some individuals may be harder to place than others.

Key terms

Life course: *the unique pattern of events and experiences that a person goes through during their existence*

Life span and life expectancy

Life span is the length of time between a person's birth and their death. According to valid and credible records the maximum human life span ever achieved is 122 years. It is very unusual for human beings to survive to such an advanced age. A more typical human life span is, in fact, revealed by another concept – **life expectancy**. This refers to the number of years that a man or woman living in a specified country can expect to live at any given point in time. The life expectancy at birth for men born in the United Kingdom in 2006 was 77. It is slightly longer, at 82 years, for women born in the United Kingdom in 2006.

Life expectancy at birth has increased significantly for both men and women over the last century (see Figure 4.5) and is continuing to increase slowly. Despite the fact that more of us will live to be older, the length of the maximum human life span has not changed much over time; it is still not possible to live forever or to hang on to eternal youth! Human beings inevitably age and eventually die.

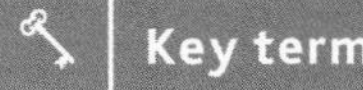

Key terms

Life expectancy: *the number of further years a person can expect to live from a given age point*

Figure 4.5 Life expectancy has increased over the last century.

Year of birth	Males at birth	Females at birth
1911	50.4	53.9
1931	58.0	62.0
1951	66.1	70.9
1971	68.8	75.0
1991	73.2	78.8
1997	74.6	79.6
2011	77.4	81.6
2021	78.6	82.7

What do you know?

1. Can you identify the two things that change as a result of physical growth?
2. If a Health Visitor wanted to check a newborn baby's physical *development*, should she weigh the baby or assess the baby's physical reflexes? Explain why.
3. Can you name five different life stages in which human growth and development occur?
4. Do you know the difference between the human life span and the human life course?
5. In what sense is human growth and development about continuity as much as change?
6. Can you describe what has happened to human life expectancy over the last 300 years?

Conception

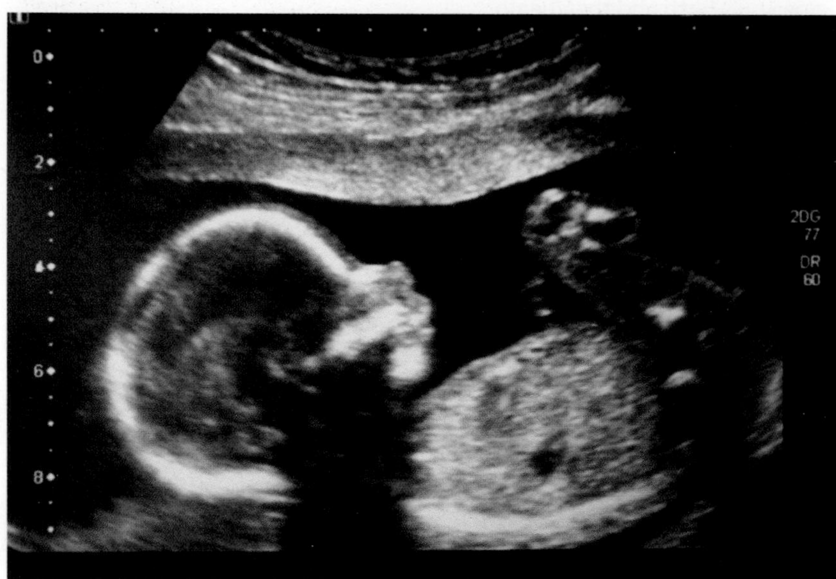

Rapid physical growth and development occurs from the moment of conception.

Your assessment criteria:

P1 Describe physical, intellectual, emotional and social development for each of the life stages of an individual

Key terms

Conception: *fertilisation of the female ovum (egg) by the male sperm*

Ovulation: *the release of an ovum from the ovary*

P1 The start of human life

In biological terms, human life begins with the process of **conception**. Both the male and female reproductive systems need to be functioning effectively for conception to take place naturally.

The female sex hormones oestrogen and progesterone are produced by the ovaries and control the female menstrual cycle. An average menstrual cycle lasts 28 days. During the first part of the cycle, the lining of the uterus (womb) thickens. Around day 14 of the cycle, a female ovum (egg) is released from the ovary into the fallopian tube, a process called **ovulation**. If the ovum is not fertilised by a male sperm, it will be expelled with the lining of the uterus as a menstrual bleed.

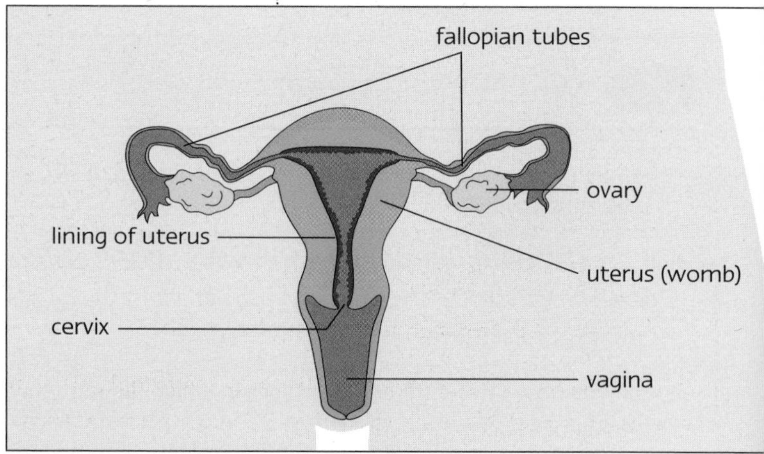

Figure 4.6 The female reproductive system.

The testes produce the male sex hormone testosterone, which stimulates sperm production. Sperm are made in the testes and stored in the epididymis.

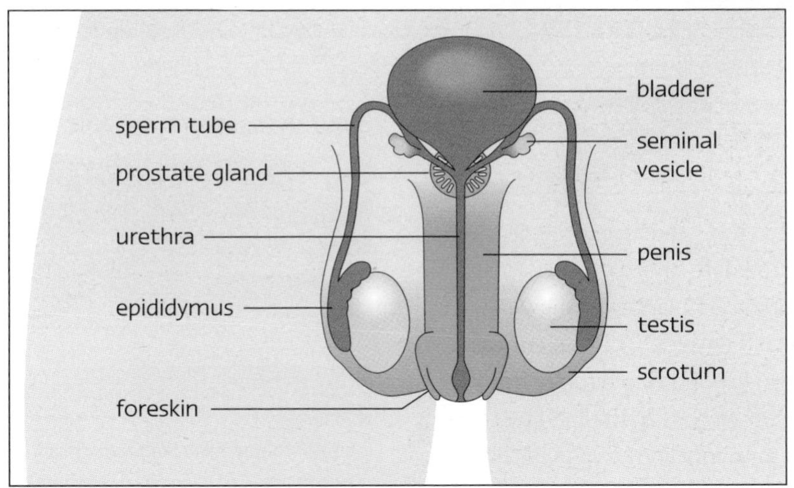

Figure 4.7 The male reproductive system.

When a man becomes sexually aroused, his penis becomes erect and sperm are released from the testes. The sperm mix with semen from the seminal vesicle and are ejected from the penis in an ejaculation. During sexual intercourse, sperm are deposited in the vagina and swim up through the female reproductive system to reach the fallopian tubes.

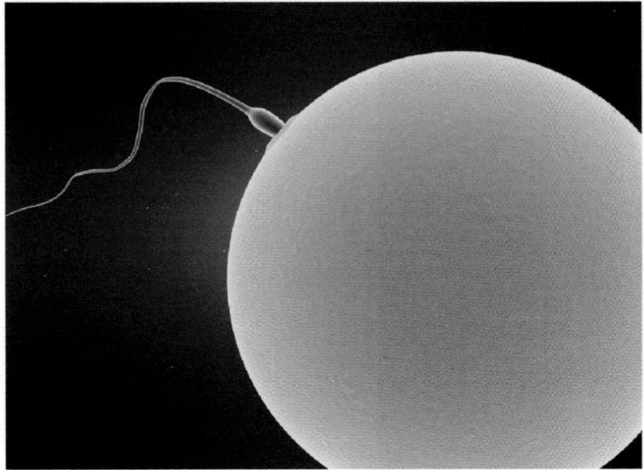

Figure 4.8 Fertilisation and implantation.

After ovulation, the ripe ovum travels along the fallopian tube to the uterus. This journey usually takes 5 to 7 days. If sexual intercourse takes place during this time, the egg may become fertilised by a male sperm in the fallopian tube. The fertilised ovum will then attach itself to the wall of the uterus. This is called implantation. The fertilised egg starts to develop into an **embryo** and begins to grow rapidly. The growth and development of the baby in the uterus is one of the most eventful periods of human growth and development. It usually takes place over 37 to 42 weeks (full-term pregnancy) and can be divided into three different phases known as **trimesters**.

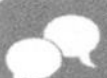

Discuss

Why are some men infertile? In a small group, identify as many reasons for male infertility as you can. Add to your ideas by researching this issue in textbooks and using online sources so that you understand the causes of male infertility.

Key terms

Embryo: *a fertilised ovum from conception to the eighth week of pregnancy*

Trimester: *a period in pregnancy, roughly equivalent to 12 weeks*

Investigate

Using online and library resources, find out how uniovular and binovular twins are conceived. Describe what happens during conception and what the differences are between these two types of twins.

Pregnancy

P1 The first trimester

The first 12 weeks of pregnancy are referred to as the first trimester. The starting point of the first trimester is the date of the mother's last menstrual period. Once the fertilised ovum has implanted in the wall of the uterus, the embryo begins to grow and develop. This is a critical time in the pregnancy. The growing embryo is nourished directly from the mother's blood through the placenta, to which it is attached by the umbilical cord. The embryo receives both nutrients and oxygen in this way, so does not breathe normally or need to digest food. It is protected in the uterus within the amniotic sac, surrounded by amniotic fluid. This protective environment keeps the embryo at a constant temperature and helps to prevent some infections.

From the eighth week of pregnancy, the embryo is referred to as a **foetus**. Most of the major body organs are formed during the first trimester, although they will take more time to reach full maturity. By 12 weeks, an average foetus measures 6 cm and weighs 9–14 g.

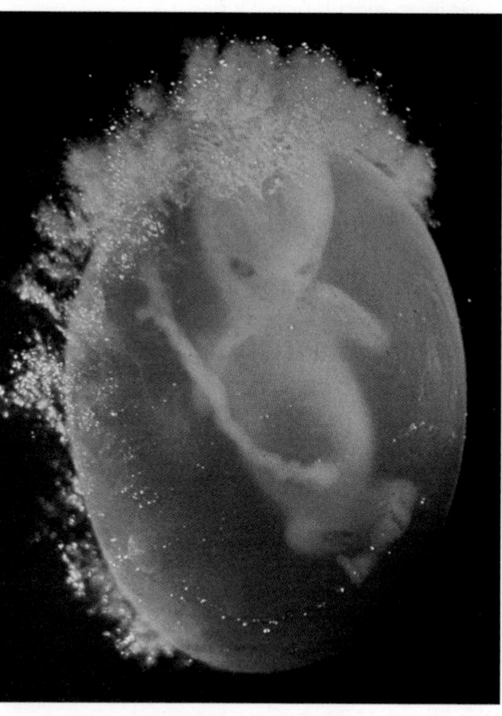

Figure 4.9 A foetus at 12 weeks.

The second trimester

The second trimester of pregnancy occurs between weeks 12 and 25. It is a period of rapid foetal growth and from about week 20 a pregnant woman can usually feel the foetus kicking. By 24 weeks, the foetus is considered to be viable, or able to survive on its own outside of the uterus. At this stage, an average foetus measures 21 cm and weighs 700 g. Most women will appear noticeably pregnant during this trimester as the uterus increases in size and the breasts also enlarge.

Your assessment criteria:

P1 Describe physical, intellectual, emotional and social development for each of the life stages of an individual

Key terms

Foetus: *the developing baby from the eighth week of pregnancy until birth*

Investigate

Use the internet, library or other resources to investigate some of the factors that can adversely affect the growth and development of the embryo and foetus in the first trimester of pregnancy. Make a chart that highlights:

- *the factor*
- *the possible effects on the embryo or foetus*
- *how these effects could be prevented.*

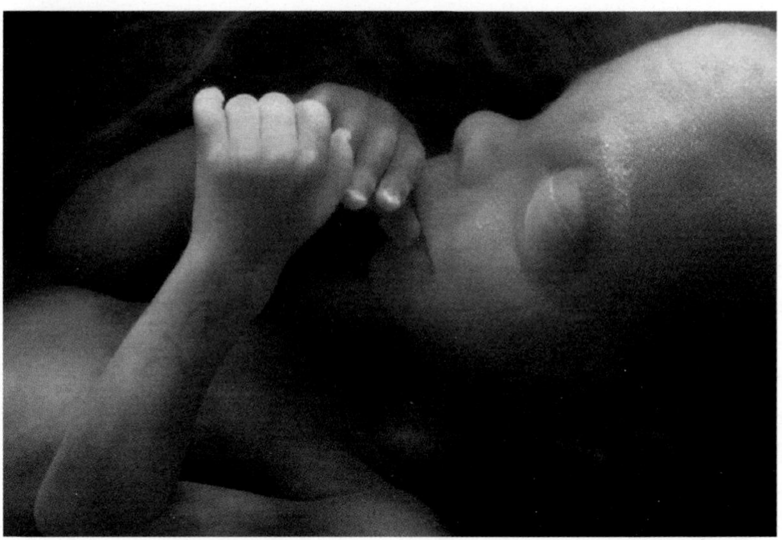

Figure 4.10 A developing foetus.

The third trimester

This is the period from week 25 until full term (between 37 and 42 weeks). The foetus grows very rapidly during this time, in preparation for birth and life outside of the uterus. Towards the end of the third trimester, the baby will settle low in the uterus with the head facing downwards (it is said to be engaged). Occasionally, the baby will settle with its bottom or legs and feet facing downwards (breech position), but in most cases it will turn around before birth. At full-term, an average baby measures 55 cm and weighs 3.5 kg or 7lb 7oz. Many women experience tiredness and backache at this stage in the pregnancy as the foetus is quite heavy.

Investigate

Find out about the major milestones of growth and development in each trimester and create a 'Pregnancy Timeline' from conception to full-term. Present this as a table, poster or diagram.

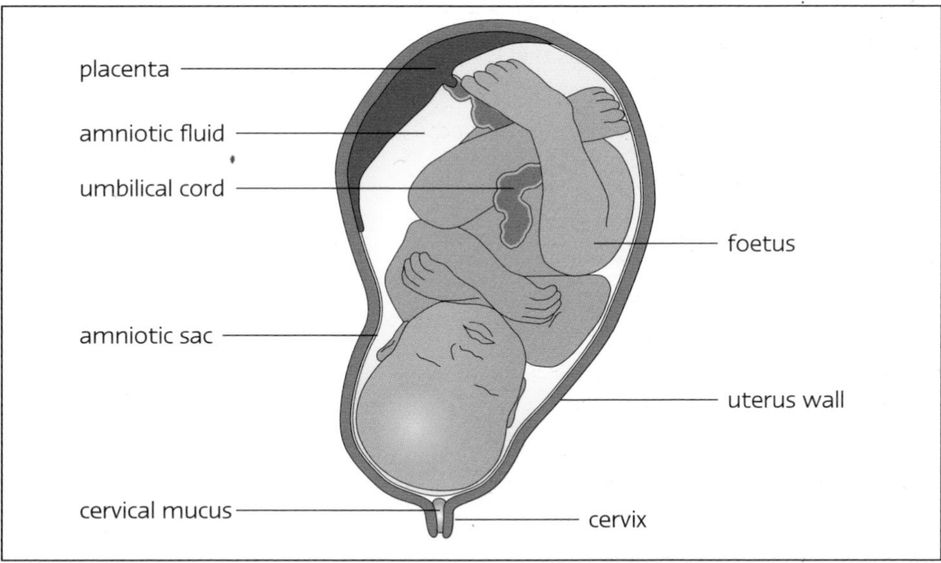

Figure 4.11 Full-term foetus.

Birth

P1 The process of labour

The process of birth is called labour and is well named; the woman's body works hard to push the baby out of the uterus. Birth is the first big event in every human being's life. Approximately 9 months of rapid foetal development culminates in the moment when a new human being enters the world! Labour usually lasts for several hours and can be an anxious time.

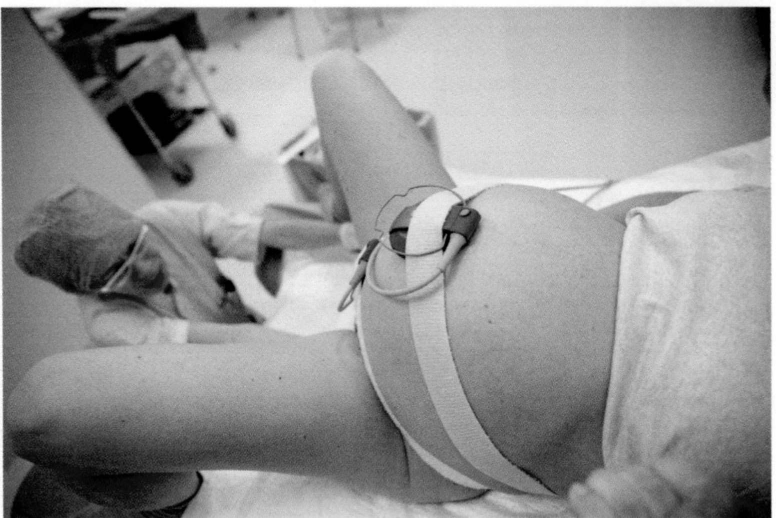

The length of labour varies from woman to woman and can't be predicted.

Labour usually begins with contractions (the muscles of the uterus tighten up and get ready to push the baby out). The amniotic sac may also burst, releasing amniotic fluid. This is often referred to as the 'breaking of the waters' and is a common sign of the onset of labour. The woman may also experience a 'show', which is the release of a blood and mucous discharge from the cervix (neck of the uterus). Labour is generally divided into three stages:

- **Stage one** is characterised by steady contractions of the uterus that open the cervix wide enough for the baby to pass through (usually about 10 cm). This stage can take several hours, with the contractions becoming more intense.
- **Stage two** begins when the cervix has fully opened (fully dilated) and involves the strong and frequent contractions that push the baby out. This is a very active stage of labour as the woman pushes with each contraction. She is usually encouraged to use special breathing techniques. A special moment comes when the baby's head finally

Your assessment criteria:

P1 Describe physical, intellectual, emotional and social development for each of the life stages of an individual

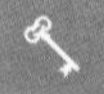

Key terms

Stage one, stage two, stage three: *the three stages of labour*

becomes visible. This is called crowning and is usually a sign that the baby will soon be born.

- **Stage three** consists of expelling the placenta (afterbirth) from the uterus. It is usually a straightforward process guided by the midwife and requires very little effort from the mother. Labour is then complete.

After the birth, mucous is cleared from the baby's nose and mouth to allow him or her to take a first breath. The umbilical cord will then be clamped and cut, permanently separating the baby from the mother. Birth is generally seen as a positive and happy event, even though it may involve some pain, risk and difficulty for both the mother and baby.

Although many births are straightforward and uncomplicated, it can be a difficult and traumatic experience for a baby if:

- labour is very long
- there are complications with the baby's supply of oxygen
- he or she is lying in a position that makes delivery problematic.

All newborn babies are given some immediate physical tests to check that they can breathe and function normally. Birth injuries, inherited disorders and problems due to premature arrival can often be identified shortly after birth. These may affect the baby's subsequent growth and development. However, most babies are born in robust health and will, despite looking quite vulnerable and helpless, experience rapid growth and development over the first few years of life.

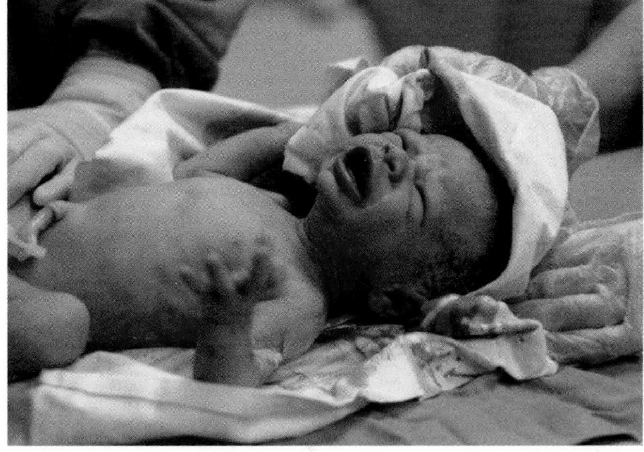

Shortly after birth physical checks are carried out to assess the health of the newborn baby.

What do you know?

1. What is an ovum?
2. Using biological terms, can you describe what happens during conception?
3. Can you explain how an embryo grows into a foetus during the early stages of pregnancy?
4. How does a woman know that she is about to go into labour?
5. What happens when a woman goes into labour?
6. Can you explain why a baby may experience a difficult birth process?

Physical growth and development in the early years

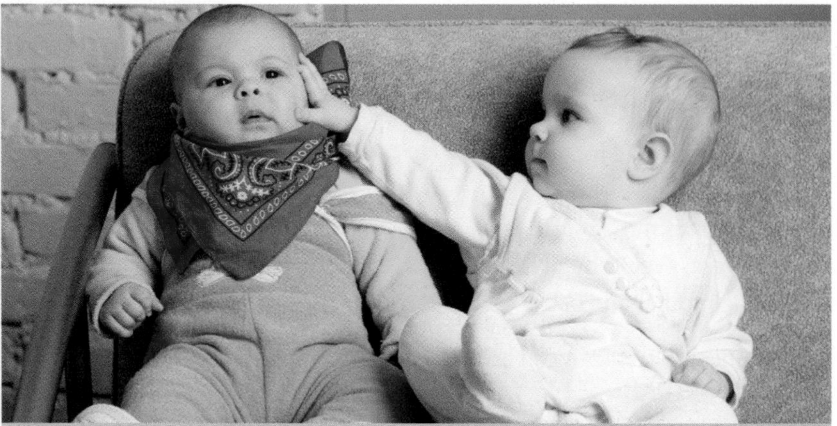

Early infancy is a period of rapid physical growth and change.

Physical growth and development can be observed over relatively short periods of time, particularly in the early years and during adolescence when physical changes are noticeable and occur rapidly. Physical change during adulthood and old age involves less ***growth*** but should not be thought of simply as a period of physical decline.

Your assessment criteria:

P1 Describe physical, intellectual, emotional and social development for each of the life stages of an individual

P1 Infancy (0–3 years)

Infancy is probably the most dynamic phase of growth and development in the human life course. The rapid pace of physical growth and development that began at conception and which continued through 9 months of foetal development shows little sign of slowing when a baby is born. Physical change during the first 3 years of life transforms an infant's appearance. Infants grow taller and generally gain weight very quickly. During the first 18 months of life, an average infant's body weight triples.

An infant's physical growth and development follows a predictable pattern. Physical change occurs from the head downwards (cephalocaudal) and from the middle of the body outwards (proximodistal). An infant first develops gross **motor skills**. These are the basic, unsophisticated movements of limbs, trunk and head that enable children to hold their heads up without support, to hold on to people and large objects, and subsequently to crawl.

In the later stages of infancy, children begin to develop fine motor skills. These are more sophisticated and finely controlled forms of movement. They enable children to eat with cutlery, do up zips and buttons, and tie their shoe laces, for example.

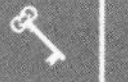

Key terms

Motor skills: *skills related to physical movement*

Figure 4.12 Types of motor development.

Skill Type	Example
Locomotor skills	Pulling, crawling, walking, holding on
Non-locomotor skills	Holding head up, pushing, bending body
Manipulative skills	Reaching, grasping, stacking blocks

Key terms

Centile charts: *graphs showing the normal range of measurements at different ages*

The physical foundations of infant development

The physical growth and changes that occur in early infancy provide an essential foundation for various forms of growth and development that occur later in the human life course. These changes include:

- ossification (hardening) of the baby's soft bones, allowing independent movement and making the infant physically robust
- brain growth, enabling the infant to develop language and thinking skills, later giving the child the ability to build relationships and to use social skills.

Research data on average growth patterns has been used to produce **centile charts** of height and weight for both male and female infants (see Figure 4.13). Health and social care professionals use these to work out whether a child is developing within normal limits for their age.

The red line in Figure 4.13 shows the average trend in weight gain expected in boys in the first 12 months of life. If a 4-month-old boy weights 7 kg, on average 50% of boys of the same age will weigh less than him and 50% will weigh more.

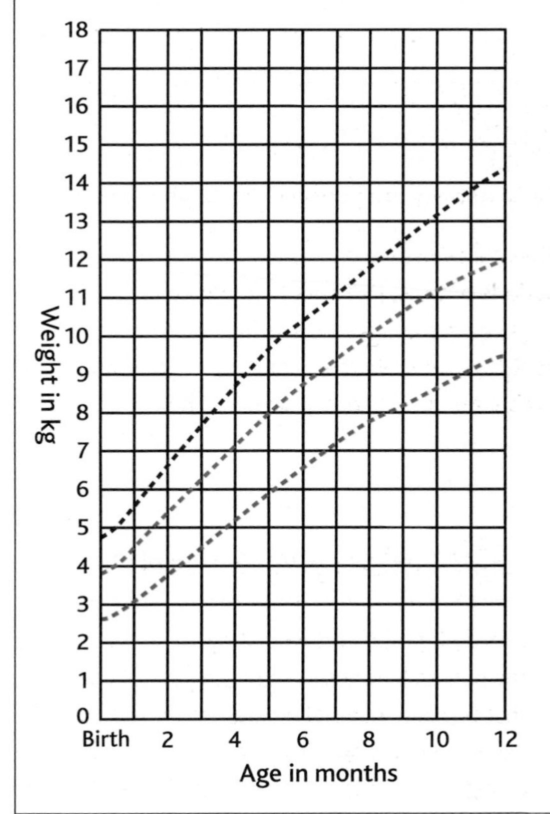

Figure 4.13 Centile chart.

Key:
97 percentile
50 percentile
3 percentile

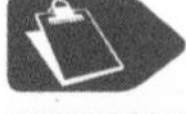

Case study

Jo Michael, Health Visitor, is weighing infants at a baby clinic. Karl, a 9-month-old boy, weighs 12.0 kg. Jo's records tell her that Karl has put on 2.0 kg over the last 3 months..

1. Use the weight centile chart (Figure 4.13) to explain Karl's pattern of growth.
2. Would you be concerned by these figures? Give reasons.
3. What factors might account for Karl's weight at this point in his life?

Physical growth and development in childhood

P1 Childhood (4–9 years)

During childhood, individuals gradually become less physically dependent and immobile, and more physically capable and competent. The pace of physical change experienced by the human body is slower during childhood than in infancy. On average, during each year of childhood a child will:

- grow between 5 and 7.5 cm
- gain about 2.7 kg in weight.

At the same time, motor development is extended and consolidated (see Figure 4.14). Developing children:

- become increasingly physically capable, skilled and robust
- can move easily and skilfully
- develop and use hand–eye coordination.

Improvements in motor skills during later childhood allow children to move with better coordination and complete tasks faster. Girls tend to have more body fat and less muscle tissue than boys at this age, but have very similar abilities in terms of speed and strength. Hormonal changes begin towards the end of this stage, but the effects are not seen until a few years later.

Figure 4.14 Motor development during childhood. Adapted from Bee, Helen *Human Growth and Development* (1994).

Age	Motor skill development
18–24 months old	• able to run at 20 months • walk well at 24 months • push and pull boxes or toys on wheels • stack blocks • pick objects up without overbalancing
2–3 years old	• can now run quite easily • climb onto and get off furniture unaided • move large toys around obstacles • pick up small items • throw a ball forward

Your assessment criteria:

P1 Describe physical, intellectual, emotional and social development for each of the life stages of an individual

Age	Motor skill development
3–4 years old	• can walk up stairs using one foot per step • walk on tip toe • pedal and steer toys with wheels • catch a large ball with both hands • hold a pencil between thumb and forefinger
4–5 years old	• can walk up and down stairs using one foot per step • use a bat and ball • kick a ball • hold a pencil with ease
5–6 years old	• now able to play ball games well • skip using alternate feet • sufficient fine motor control to thread a needle and sew stitches

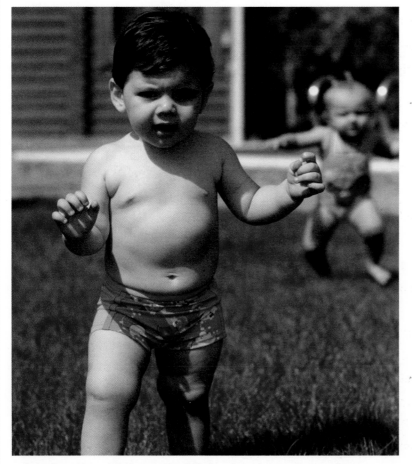

What does this child's motor skill development tell you about his age?

Reflect

How might this kind of knowledge be helpful to health and social care practitioners working with young children?

Physical growth and development in adolescence

P1 Adolescence (10–18 years)

Adolescence is a period of rapid, major physical growth and development. This is in contrast to the slower pace of physical change in late childhood. ***Puberty*** is the term used to describe the period in adolescence when physical changes to the human reproductive system lead to sexual maturity. As a result of puberty, boys can produce sperm and girls can produce eggs that, when fertilised by sperm, can result in a pregnancy and birth of a baby. Girls tend to begin puberty about 2 years earlier than boys.

The influence of hormones

The physical changes that occur during puberty are mainly the result of **hormone** activity. Hormones are the secretions of the endocrine glands. The body produces a number of hormones from several different endocrine glands (see Figure 4.15).

As a result of increased hormone production, primary and secondary sexual characteristics develop in both males and females during adolescence (see Figure 4.16, opposite).

Your assessment criteria:

P1 Describe physical, intellectual, emotional and social development for each of the life stages of an individual

Key terms

Hormones: *chemical substances secreted into the blood by certain glands that stimulate activity in other organs*

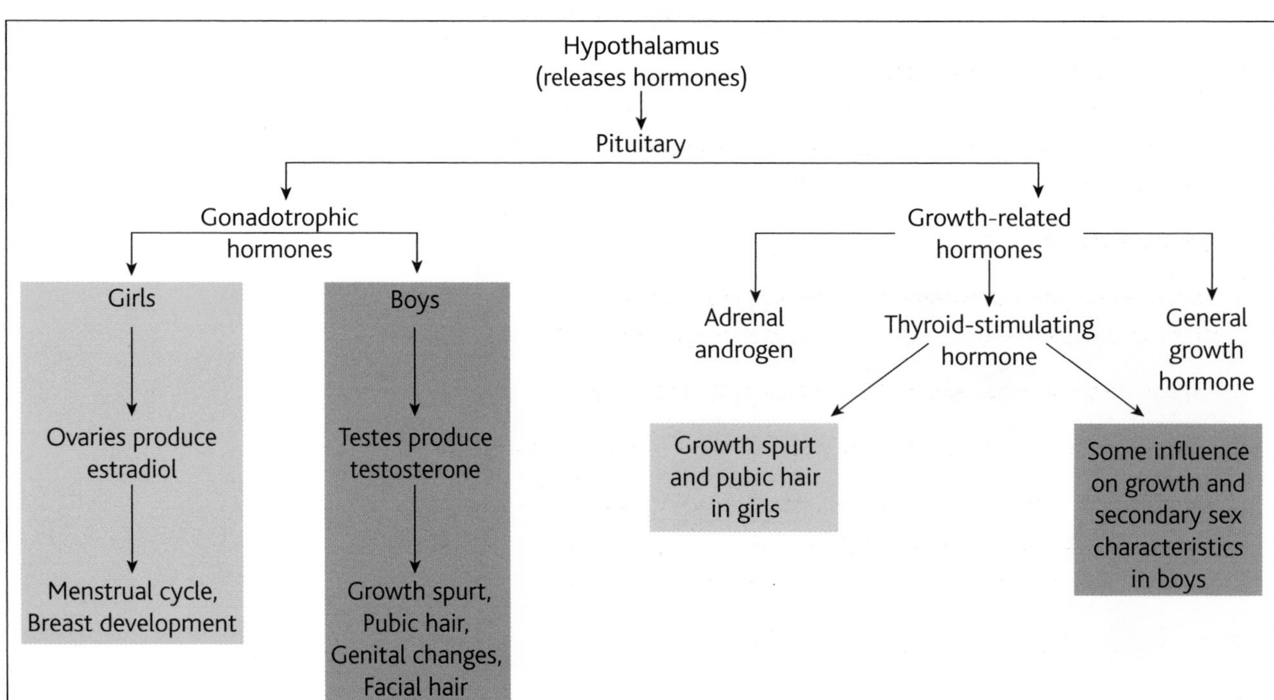

Figure 4.15 Action of the hormones at puberty.

Figure 4.16 Primary and secondary sexual characteristics in males and females.

Sex	Primary	Secondary
Male	Penis Scrotum	Lower voice Facial hair Sperm production Pubic hair Muscle development
Female	Ovaries Uterus Vagina Clitoris Labia	Breasts Wider hips Ovulation and menstruation Pubic hair

Normally, males and females secrete *both* oestrogen and testosterone. However, males generally secrete more testosterone than females and females generally secrete more oestrogen than males. These differences in hormone levels account for differences in physical growth and development during this life stage. At the end of puberty, hormonal activity slows down and the rate of physical change reduces dramatically.

Reflect

A group of primary school children, aged about 10, are to be given simple leaflets to help them understand puberty.

1. *Using a maximum of two sides of A4 and in language that 10-year-olds can understand, create a leaflet giving basic information about puberty for both girls and boys.*
2. *Use charts, drawings and cartoons as appropriate. Try not to be too technical, mind boggling or frightening in the way you explain what happens during this life stage!*

What do you know?

1. Identify three examples of physical development that occur in childhood.
2. What are motor skills?
3. Describe one physical change that only happens to girls and one physical change that only happens to boys during puberty.
4. Explain how hormones effect physical change during puberty.
5. Name two growth-related hormones that stimulate physical change.
6. Describe how a girl's primary and secondary sexual characteristics change and develop during puberty.

Physical growth and development in adulthood

P1 Physical change in adulthood (19–65)

Physical maturity is reached in adulthood. This is the phase of the life course where most people are at their physical peak. As a young adult, a person is likely to have more muscle tissue, stronger bones, better eyesight, hearing and sense of smell, greater oxygen capacity and a more efficient immune system than at any other point in their life.

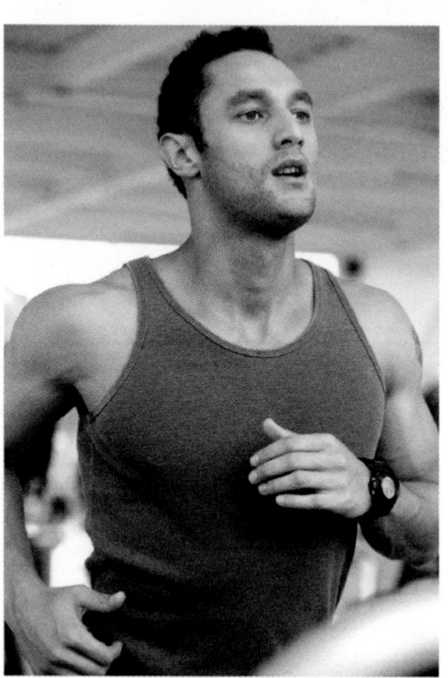

People are usually at their fittest during early adulthood.

In the years leading up to adulthood, physical growth and development has occurred largely as a result of **maturation** (see page 171). From early adulthood onwards, the ageing process takes over from maturation, affecting the way we change physically, as well as our cognitive (intellectual) and psychological functioning.The effects of the human ageing process are much more noticeable in middle adulthood, typically between the ages of 40 and 65. People who are aged 40 are at about the midpoint of their life

Your assessment criteria:

P1 Describe physical, intellectual, emotional and social development for each of the life stages of an individual

Key terms

Maturation: *the gradual process of becoming physically mature or fully developed*

Figure 4.17 Physical changes experienced in adulthood.

Physical function	Age of change	Nature of change
Vision	40–45	Thickening of the lens of the eye leads to poorer vision and more sensitivity to glare.
Hearing	Approximately 50	Loss of the ability to hear very high and very low sounds.
Muscles	Approximately 50	Loss of muscle tissue, especially fibres used for bursts of strength and speed.
Bones	After menopause in women, later in men	Loss of calcium in bones, and wear and tear on the joints.
Heart and lungs	35–40	Decline in most aspects of function when measured during or after exercise, but not at rest.
Reproductive system	Mid-30s for women	Increased risk of reproductive problems and lowered fertility.
Skin elasticity	Approximately 40	Increase in wrinkles due to loss of elasticity.

expectancy and will be aware of some loss of physical ability. For example, they may be aware that they run and walk more slowly and may feel that they have less strength and stamina.

One of the major physical changes experienced by women during adulthood is the onset of the menopause. This occurs when the menstrual cycle ceases because the ovaries no longer produce the hormones that are necessary for ovulation and menstruation. Most women experience the menopause around the age of 50, though there is some variation. From the middle of adulthood onwards, human vision and hearing tend to become less acute, bones become more brittle and less porous, and people become more susceptible to chronic health problems and disability.

Investigate

Do you know anybody who has experienced the menopause? Ask the person what kinds of physical changes they experienced and how this important change affected them emotionally and psychologically.

The final stages of life

The final stages of life are characterised by the gradual loss of function and by physical decline. Biologists and medical researchers have put forward a number of theories to explain why there appears to be a limit to the human life span. These include claims that:

- human body cells can only renew themselves a certain number of times, so that body processes decline and tissue wastage occurs
- the DNA in cells deteriorates over time and, by old age, can no longer be replicated, resulting in cell death
- a gradual decline in hormone production results in the decline of body systems
- body cells become damaged over time, resulting in mutations and the development of degenerative conditions
- toxic substances build up in body cells, gradually damaging them and disrupting the way they work.

What do you know?

1. Identify two ways in which an adult is physically mature.
2. Describe how the human body changes during middle age (40–65).
3. How do menopausal changes affect a woman's body during middle adulthood?
4. Describe and explain how the human body changes during the final stages of life.

Intellectual and language development in infants and children

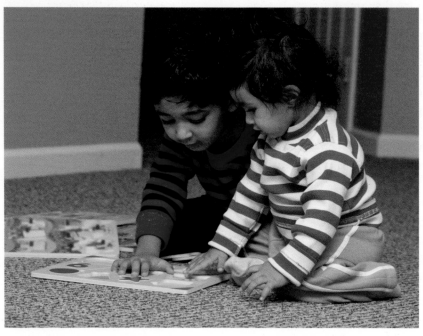

Intellectual development helps people to solve problems and communicate more effectively.

Your assessment criteria:

P1 Describe physical, intellectual, emotional and social development for each of the life stages of an individual

P1 Intellectual potential

Intellectual development affects the ability of the human brain to think, use language and remember; human intellectual development affects both the quantity and the quality of what an individual can do with their brain. People used to believe that a child was born with a mind like an empty book that gradually filled up with knowledge as the child experienced the world. However, scientific research has shown that babies start learning in the womb, having some basic abilities and lots of potential at the moment of their birth. Jean Piaget (1896–1980), a Swiss psychologist, first put forward the theory that we are born with basic intellectual abilities which improve as we experience different stages of intellectual development during infancy, childhood and adolescence.

Infant intellectual development

Thinking is an intellectual, or cognitive, activity. An infant's ability to think is quite limited. During early infancy babies respond mainly to physical stimuli; they cry when they are wet, cold and hungry, for example. This is a relatively primitive level of intellectual response.

Key terms

Cognitive: *relating to mental processes such as thinking, memory and judgement*

Intellectual development: *the emergence and improvement of thinking and language skills*

Jean Piaget, who studied and wrote about cognitive development, called infancy the sensorimotor stage of intellectual development. He claimed that infants learn about the world by using their senses (touch, hearing, sight, smell and taste – hence 'sensori') and through physical activity (hence 'motor'). There is very limited cognitive or intellectual activity involved in this type of learning. Infants don't use their memories and experiences of events in a conscious way to plan their actions.

Thinking skills gradually improve as an infant grows older and intellectual development occurs. For example, by the end of infancy, a child will learn that people and objects continue to exist in the world even when they can't be seen (object permanence). In contrast, a baby who is less than 8 months old won't usually search for a toy that is hidden from view as they watch. This is because they haven't developed the thinking ability to know that the hidden toy still exists. An older infant or young child will look for a hidden toy because their intellectual development enables them to work out that objects still exist even when they're out of sight.

Investigate

Investigate the concept of object permanence using the internet, psychology or child development books. Try to find out how Piaget and other psychologists tested this concept and summarise their evidence.

Figure 4.18 Intellectual development during infancy.

Age	Developmental change
Birth	Explores, using senses to learn.
1 month	Able to recognise parents or main carers by sight and smell.
3 months	Learns by playing with hands, holding and grasping objects.
6 months	Aware of parents' or carers' voices and can take part in simple play activities.
9 months	Recognises familiar toys and pictures, joins in games with familiar people and is able to respond to simple instructions.
12 months	Copies other people's behaviour and is able to use objects appropriately (for example, a brush or spoon).
15 months	Remembers people, recognises and sorts shapes and knows some parts of the body, responding to questions such as 'where's your nose?'
18 months	Recognises self in a picture or reflection, responds to simple instructions and is able to remember and recall simple information.
2 years	Completes simple jigsaws and develops a basic understanding of the consequences of own actions.
2 years 6 months	Usually very inquisitive, asks lots of questions, knows their own name and can find details in pictures.
3 years	Can usually understand time, is able to recognise different colours, can compare the size of different objects (bigger, smaller) and is able to remember the words to their favourite songs and rhymes.

P1 Developing language skills

Learning the basics of a spoken language is an important part of intellectual development during infancy. Babies begin developing communication skills almost straight from birth. Smiles, movements and noises are early ways of communicating with care-givers. However, words don't usually become a feature of communication before an infant is 1 year old and first words are preceded by lots of babbling. Once an older infant begins using words, their vocabulary improves quickly and they can put words into short sentences.

Researchers such as Noam Chomsky (1959) and Steven Pinker (1994) claim that human beings are born with the capacity to develop a verbal language. They argue that human beings, unlike other animals, are biologically programmed or 'hard wired' to acquire and use language. Evidence to support this theory includes the fact that all children, regardless of the language they're learning, progress through the same step-by-step stages: babbling, saying their first word around the age of 1 year, using two-word combinations by 3 years, and generally accomplishing grammatical rules by 4 or 5 years. A child's early language development is promoted by seeing and hearing other people use language and by being encouraged to make sounds and use words.

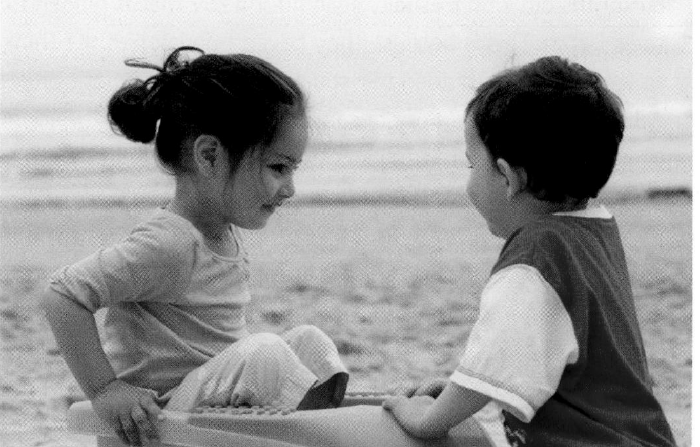

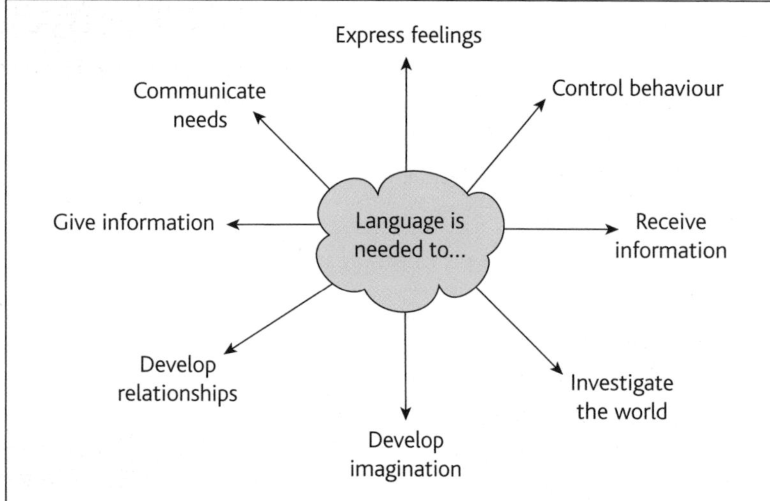

Figure 4.19 The functions of language.

Your assessment criteria:

P1 Describe physical, intellectual, emotional and social development for each of the life stages of an individual

Investigate

How old were you when you first started speaking? Do you know what your first word(s) were? Try to find out from your parents or carers and ask them what they remember about your early language development.

Figure 4.20 Language development during early childhood.

Age	Developmental change
Birth	Communicates through physical movement (moving arms and legs), by crying and through eye contact.
1 month	Makes gurgling sounds, looks at people to get their attention and interacts by making cooing sounds.
3 months	Smiles and makes noises to communicate with familiar people and cries loudly to express discomfort or hunger.
6 months	Makes a number of speech-like sounds ('goo', 'der', 'dhah' and 'ka'), talks by babbling and looks for the source of sounds.
9 months	Uses basic sounds to say simple words, such as 'da da' and 'ma ma'.
12 months	Follows simple instructions and can use simple words such as 'bye bye'.
15 months	Has enough language to join in with nursery rhymes and songs and enjoys having stories read to them.
18 months	Babbles simple sentences, responds to simple questions and more complex requests, and follows instructions.
2 years	Makes two-word sentences ('dog gone'), understands lots of words, can name familiar and everyday objects.
2 years 6 months	Thinks of and asks questions and is able to recall and repeat familiar rhymes and songs.
3 years	Makes longer sentences to describe what they see and to express their feelings, can hold a simple conversation, is able to use about 200 different words and can learn more than one language if they live in a bilingual family.

Childhood intellectual development

Jean Piaget argued that, in early childhood, human beings first develop the ability to use 'symbols' in the form of images and words. As children's intellectual abilities develop, they become better at using these symbols. This pattern of progressive intellectual development can be seen in the way that children's play becomes more sophisticated throughout childhood.

A significant intellectual change occurs during later childhood when children discover that there are some general rules for understanding the world around them. Jean Piaget referred to these rules as 'concrete operations'. An operation is an abstract way of thinking (a scheme), such as reversibility, addition, subtraction and serial ordering, that can be used to understand objects and their relationships. For example, when children develop concrete operational thinking they understand that *adding* to something makes it *bigger* and *subtracting* from something makes it *smaller*.

Key terms

Bilingual: *the ability to speak two languages fluently*

Reflect

If you were a teacher of 7-year-olds in a primary school, how could you test out Piaget's claims about 'concrete operational thinking' with the children in your class?

Intellectual development in adolescence, adulthood and old age

P1 Adolescent intellectual development

During adolescence, a person's ability to think in concrete ways is extended. The level or complexity of an adolescent's thinking, their use of language and their memory ability is significantly greater than it was during their childhood.

Greater intellectual capacity enables people in this life stage to think about objects and situations that they have not directly experienced themselves or which are hypothetical. Abstract thinking, for example, improves an adolescent's ability to:

- contemplate the future
- understand the nature of human relationships
- use foresight to predict possible consequences
- empathise.

Intellectual development in adulthood

Patterns of intellectual development are similar to patterns of physical development during adulthood. For example, intellectual and cognitive processes are at their peak from early to middle adulthood. They begin to decline in various ways, such as in loss of memory capacity, as the individual enters old age.

Nancy Denny (1982) developed a model of change that shows how human cognitive performance rises then falls over the life course (see Figure 4.21).

Your assessment criteria:

P1 Describe physical, intellectual, emotional and social development for each of the life stages of an individual

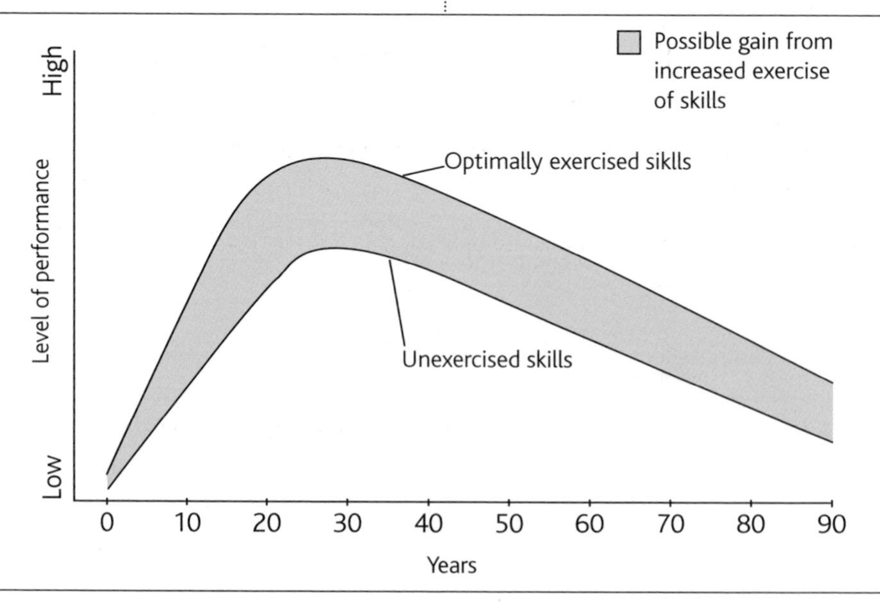

Figure 4.21 Nancy Denny's model of change in human cognitive performance.

Denny's research also showed that, in the middle years of adulthood, a person's cognitive ability can continue to develop if intellectual tasks are based on highly practised skills or specific learning. When people don't use (or under-use) their cognitive skill, the decline in their intellectual abilities is likely to be more noticeable from the middle of adulthood onwards. However, many middle-aged and older adults retain their ability to do high level, productive work and engage in intellectual problem-solving.

Intellectual change in old age

Up to the age of 75, changes in intellectual function are relatively small and hard to detect. From 75 years of age onwards, reduced intellectual functioning tends to be quite noticeable. However, in the majority of older people, this is ***not*** the result of **dementia**-related disease; it is simply a general feature of human ageing. Although there is little change in the quality of an older person's short-term memory, the general pattern is for older people to experience some slowness when recalling information from their long-term memory and for them to be less effective at problem-solving.

Key terms

Dementia: *a degenerative brain disease that causes confusion, gradual memory loss and loss of physical functions*

Reflect

How might an older person benefit from life experience and the wisdom they've acquired when their memory and thinking ability starts to decline?

What do you know?

1. How do infants learn during the sensorimotor stage of intellectual development?
2. Can you describe three examples of intellectual development during the first 3 years of a child's life?
3. What evidence suggests that human language abilities have a genetic basis?
4. Can you explain what 'concrete operational thinking' involves during childhood?
5. What type of thinking ability is usually developed during adolescence?
6. How is cognitive performance and intellectual ability affected by the ageing process?

Social and emotional development in infancy

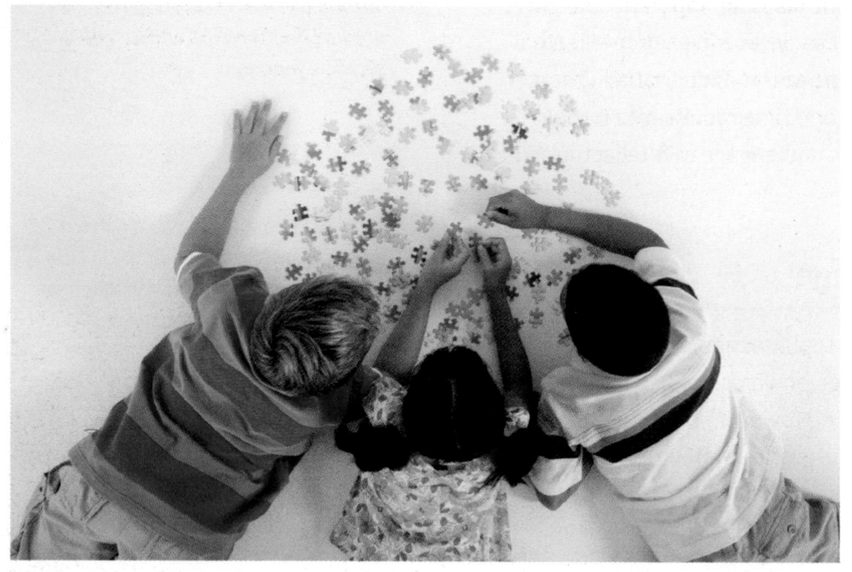

Your assessment criteria:

P1 Describe physical, intellectual, emotional and social development for each of the life stages of an individual

P1 Society, culture and social relationships

Social development is concerned with the ability to form relationships using communication skills. The ways in which individuals develop socially are strongly influenced by the society and culture in which they grow up. **Emotional development** is concerned with a person's feelings and their sense of self or identity. Emotional development and social development are closely linked. A person's social relationships and their ability to communicate effectively with others have a significant impact on how they feel about themselves and on how they are able to express and deal with their feelings.

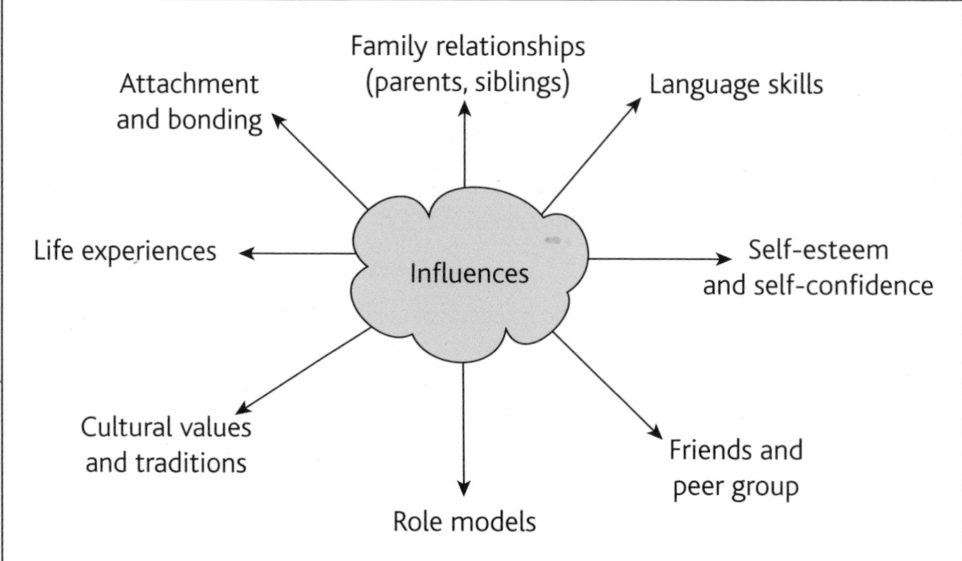

Figure 4.22 Influences on social and emotional development.

Key terms

Emotional development: *the emergence of feelings about self and others*

Social development: *the emergence and improvement of communication skills and relationships with other people*

Early emotional development

An infant's early emotional development plays an important part in their future relationships with others. Ideally, an infant should have opportunities to develop feelings of trust and security during the early years of life. The process of developing a strong emotional link with parents or main care-givers is known as **attachment**. The parent or carer response to this emotional linking is known as **bonding**. It is through attachment and bonding that an infant's first emotional relationship is formed.

Key terms

Attachment and bonding: *processes through which an emotional link is established between a baby and a parent or carer*

An infant's response to other people changes as they develop socially and emotionally:

- Up to 6 months, the baby is content to be held by anyone. He or she may protest when put down. This is known as ***indiscriminate*** attachment.
- Between 7 and 12 months, the baby is usually bonded to her parents and shows fear of strangers. This can be intense for 3 or 4 months. This is known as ***specific*** attachment.
- From 12 months onwards, the baby's attachments broaden to include other close relatives and familiar people. This is known as ***multiple*** attachment.

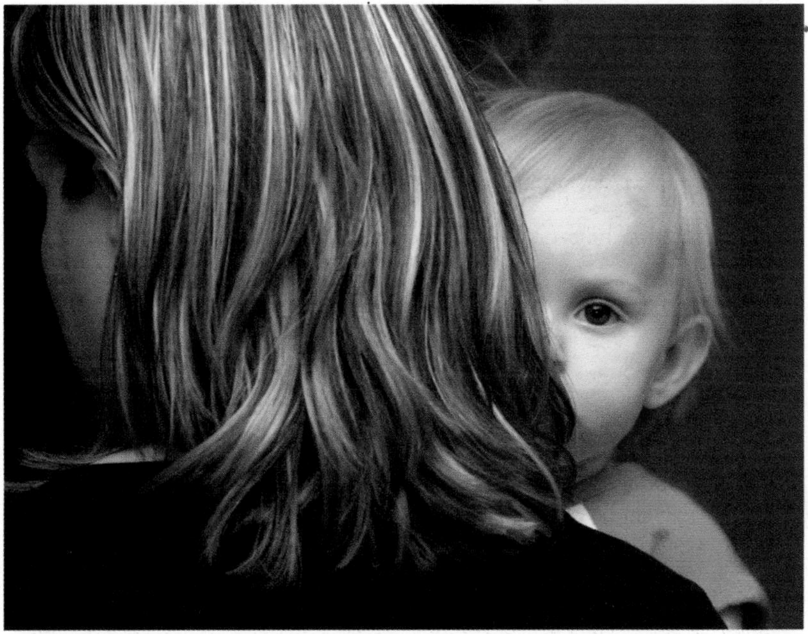

Between 7 and 12 months, the baby is usually bonded to her parents and shows fear of strangers.

It is thought that our first experience of attachment and bonding provides a blueprint for subsequent relationships. Poor or faulty attachment, or problems with parental bonding, may lead to feelings of insecurity and difficulties in forming and maintaining relationships later in life.

As their social and intellectual abilities develop and their life experience increases, infants are increasingly able to communicate and interact with other people. However, making friends and playing co-operatively also require some practice. Opportunities to mix and play with other children have a positive effect on the development of an infant's relationship-building skills.

Discuss

In a small group, share ideas about ways in which the parents of a newborn baby can promote attachment and bonding with their child. Do you have any experience of friends or relatives who have done this? Discuss strategies that you think are effective in promoting a baby's emotional development.

Social and emotional development in childhood and adolescence

P1 Childhood

Emotional and social development during childhood builds on the foundations established during infancy. During childhood, children form new relationships with new people in new situations – such as with teachers at school and with their friends.

Significant features of social development that occur during childhood include:

- the development of further communication and relationship-building skills
- an increase in the number and variety of relationships with people outside the family
- a greater degree of independence from parents
- an improvement in the ability to use social and language skills to manage personal relationships.

Children gradually develop greater awareness of who they are and how they are similar to and different from others. A child can usually identify their own sex (boy or girl) by 2 years of age. However, it is not until they reach 5 or 6 years that most children realise this feature of their identity is fixed! This concept, known as **gender constancy**, forms an important part of a child's developing sense of self.

Your assessment criteria:

P1 Describe physical, intellectual, emotional and social development for each of the life stages of an individual

Key terms

Gender constancy: *the notion that a person's sex (male or female) is fixed and will not change*

Self-concept: *the combination of self-image and self-esteem that produces a sense of personal identity*

Children's ideas about self

A child's sense of self – who they are – is relatively simple. In early childhood, children don't tend to reflect on their self-worth. Instead, they tend to think about who they are in terms of their visible characteristics and can say how good they think they are at familiar physical, intellectual and social tasks. For example, a child might say, 'I'm no good at counting, but I am good at running.' Children develop a clearer **self-concept** as they progress through childhood. By the end of this life stage, children usually have an awareness of their own internal qualities, beliefs and personality traits. They will now be able to make judgements about their self-worth and self-esteem.

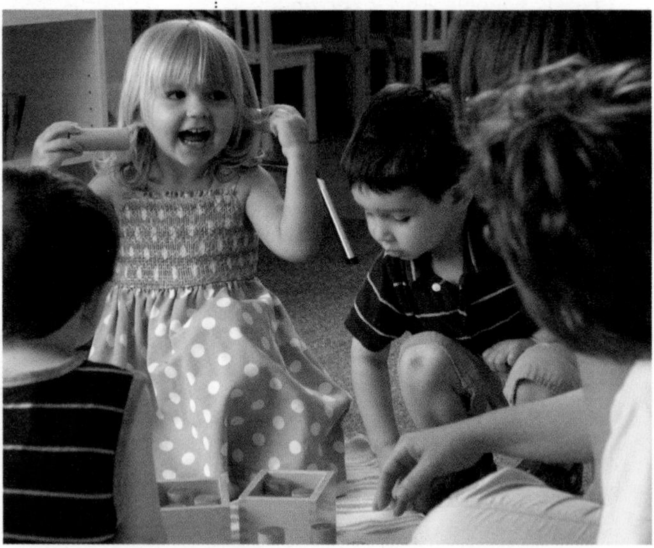

Ideas about self-concept gradually become more sophisticated during childhood.

Relationships with friends become increasingly important during childhood. In fact, by the middle of childhood many children prefer to spend time with their peers rather than with their parents and can become quite embarrassed by parental attention when their friends are around! Childhood friendships tend to be sex-segregated with boys preferring to make friends with other boys and girls establishing friendships with other girls.

Reflect

Can you remember who your first or best friend was during childhood? How did you meet this person? Think about how and why they were important to you.

Adolescence

Adolescence is often seen as an emotionally difficult and stormy life stage. Teenagers' turbulent hormones are often blamed for their moodiness and emotional sensitivity.

Two of the key emotional concerns of adolescence are:

- coping with the physical effects of puberty
- forging a sense of personal identity.

Issues
Who am I?
What do I think?
What do others think about me?
What is happening to my body?
How do I look?
Am I normal?
Why do I feel like this?
How can I be more independent?

Figure 4.23 Issues for adolescents.

The significant physical changes that adolescents experience often trigger concerns about what is normal development and about self-image. Adolescents tend to need reassurance about their growth patterns. They may seek this from friends, parents, teachers, magazines and other media. Social and emotional development and physical maturation during adolescence are intertwined. For example, early maturation can result in increased attention and extra responsibility, especially for boys. For girls, it can result in unwanted sexual attention, pressure and awkwardness. Alternatively, late maturation can damage self-confidence and self-esteem in some adolescents who may be teased or bullied.

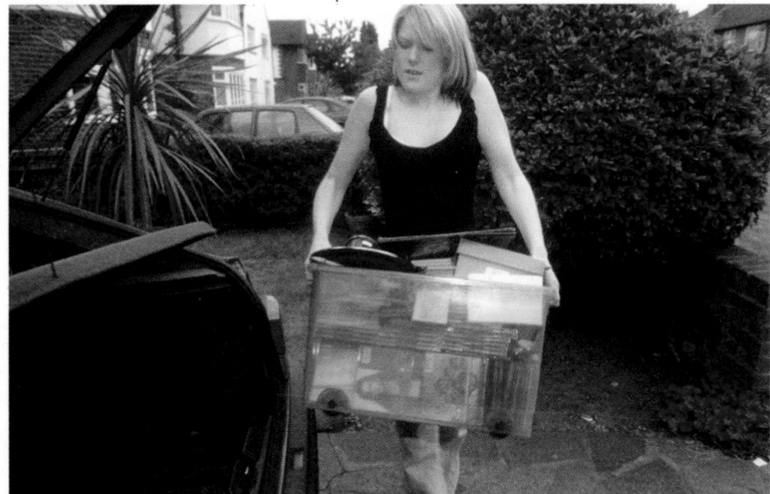

Leaving home is a pivotal moment in the life of many young people.

Friendships in adolescence

Relationships with friends play a very important role in social and emotional development during adolescence. Friendships are more stable and adolescents generally spend more time with their peers than they did during childhood. An adolescent's friendship group becomes a means of transition from family to independent, adult life. It is by using increasing social opportunities and the ability to choose and make new relationships with peers that adolescents gradually separate from their parents.

Social and emotional development in adulthood and old age

P1 Adulthood

People typically leave home to live independently of their family in early adulthood. Greater independence from the family requires new relationships. Often young adults make new friendships through work and social life, focusing on finding a partner and sustaining an intimate relationship. New responsibilities and an extension of the person's social circle may also result from marriage or cohabitation. Much of adulthood is concerned with trying to find a balance between the competing demands of work, family and friends. Each of these types of relationship contributes to social development by giving the person a sense of connection and belonging to others.

New parenthood is also a common feature of early adulthood. For most people it appears to be an experience that brings profound satisfaction, a greater sense of purpose and increased self-worth. It also introduces a number of role changes. Sex roles and spouse relationships tend to change when children arrive. The birth of a child appears to result in a drop in partners' relationship satisfaction and an increase in 'role strain' because the roles of parent and spouse are partly incompatible.

The multiple roles of adulthood (partner, parent and worker) change as an individual progresses through this life stage. When children leave home, the role of parent is affected. Work tends to be less demanding and there are usually fewer potential promotion opportunities by middle age. Relationships, especially partnerships, are likely to be given more time and assume a new significance. Partnership satisfaction tends to rise in mid-life, possibly due to the reduction in role strain. Effectively, partners have more time to spend together in mid-adulthood. Also, poor marriages tend to have ended by this point.

Older adulthood

Older adulthood is a time when considerable changes in roles and relationships are experienced. Many long-standing roles are shed. The role of worker is largely lost as people retire. The role of spouse is lost when a partner dies. The role of son or daughter is lost when parents die. The roles that remain are less complex and usually involve fewer duties. There can be less structure to life as a result.

Partner relationships in later life tend to be based on loyalty, familiarity and mutual investment in the relationship. Partners tend to spend more

Your assessment criteria:

P1 Describe physical, intellectual, emotional and social development for each of the life stages of an individual

time with each other, but may live alone when a partner dies. Many older people see their adult children regularly for purposes of practical help and emotional support. Continuity and adaptation are the themes of later adulthood relationships. Bee (1995) refers to the creation of a 'convoy' of stable relationships throughout life: 'a protective layer of family and friends who surround us and help us to deal with life's challenges'. People tend to choose friends who have similar social and psychological characteristics and who are at the same life stage.

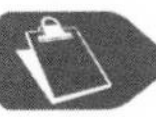

Case study

June and Bert have been married for 38 years. June is 62 and Bert 64 years old. They have three grown-up children. Bert is in his last year of working for a printing company. He has worked there for the last 29 years. June works for 7 hours a week as a dinner lady.

1. Make a list of the issues and changes that June and Bert may experience in retirement.
2. Using your list, write down some suggestions to help them deal successfully with these issues and changes.
3. Think of someone you know well who has retired. Without revealing personal details about them, describe the ways in which their retirement has been a positive or negative experience.

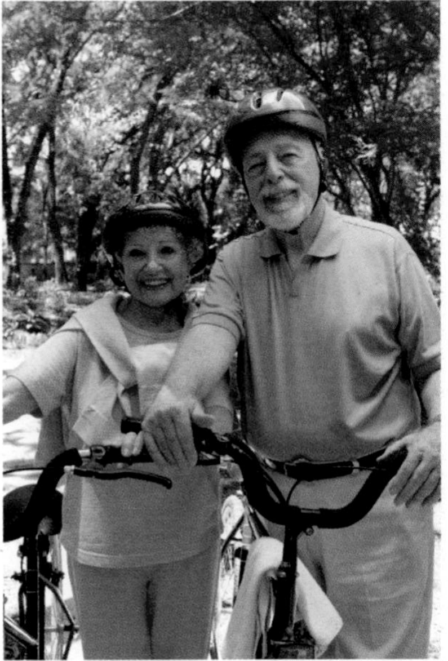

What do you know?

1. Identify the key psychological process that affects early relationships in infancy.
2. Describe the pattern of social and emotional development that occurs during childhood.
3. How does an individual's sense of self or identity tend to change during childhood?
4. What part do friends play in social and emotional development during adolescence?
5. Identify two factors that influence emotional and social development during adulthood.
6. Explain how a change in life roles can affect emotional and social development during older adulthood.

Explaining human development – nature or nurture?

As well as *describing* patterns of human growth and development, professionals try to explain *why* they happen. These explanations can have important implications for how we provide care for people.

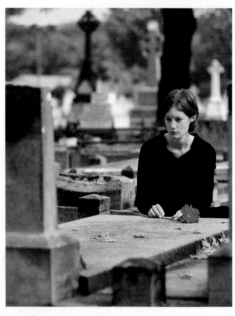

Death is one of the few universal experiences that all human beings encounter.

Your assessment criteria:

P2 Explain the potential effects of five different life factors on the development of an individual

M1 Discuss the nature–nurture debate in relation to the development of an individual

D1 Evaluate how nature and nurture may affect the physical, intellectual, emotional and social development of two stages of the development of an individual

M1 Nature–nurture explanations

The nature–nurture debate contrasts two important ways of explaining human growth and development:

- The *nature* approach suggests that people are born with qualities, abilities and characteristics that determine the kind of person they will become.
- The *nurture* approach argues it is the way a person is brought up and their circumstances that are more important influences on the kind of person they become.

Nature influences on human growth and development include genetic factors and biological processes that affect the person from within. People who take an extreme nature viewpoint argue that we are pre-programmed by our genes and biological processes to develop and behave in certain ways. By contrast, **nurture influences** are non-biological, environmental factors that affect the person from outside. People who take an extreme nurture viewpoint argue that human beings are not programmed to develop in a specific way because we have free will, can make lifestyle choices and are influenced by a complex range of psychological, social, geographic and economic factors.

 Key terms

Nature influences: *biological factors and processes that influence growth and development*

Nurture influences: *external environmental influences on growth and development*

The nature–nurture debate is often presented as an argument between two extreme viewpoints. However, researchers and health and social care practitioners are now more likely to adopt a third approach that takes account of both types of influence:

- Biological influences (nature) are important for ***universal*** forms of development, for example learning to walk.
- Environmental influences (nurture) are prominent in ***particular*** forms of development, for example, learning to speak with a Liverpool accent.

If you agree with this third approach, you would accept that genes enable most of us to learn to walk, but only a Liverpool upbringing leads to a person developing a genuine Liverpudlian accent.

Reflect

Which aspects of your own growth or development are best explained by nurture influences?

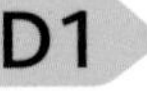

D1 Evaluating the impact of nature and nurture influences

Nature and nurture influences on human growth and development can also be thought of as internal and external influences. Internal (nature) factors, such as genes, determine how a person grows and develops because they have a direct biological influence on the person. These internal nature-type influences tend to have their strongest impact on growth and development during infancy, adolescence and old age. Basic, biological processes cause irreversible physical changes to the human body during these life stages.

External environmental (nurture) influences, on the other hand, have a less direct effect on human growth and development. They tend to shape rather than determine a person's emotional, social and intellectual development and life course. External environmental influences are important, for example, in promoting social development during childhood and adolescence, and emotional development during infancy and adolescence.

Discuss

What role does effective parenting play in the way a child behaves towards others? Can parents inhibit a child's aggressive disposition through nurturing, or are some children just naturally more aggressive than others? Reflect on the nature–nurture debate and discuss this issue with class colleagues.

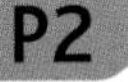

P2 The process of maturation

Maturation theory is an example of a nature approach to human growth and development. This claims that maturation is a predictable sequence of changes in human growth and development that is controlled by genes. For example, during adolescence a girl's genetic programming ensures that she grows breasts, experiences changes in her body shape and begins menstruation. Similarly, maturation in adolescent boys results in the growth of facial hair, a range of changes to their physique and a deepening of the voice. In later life, maturation ensures that we all develop wrinkles in our skin. These physical changes that unfold in a relatively predictable way lead some people to refer to human beings as having a 'biological clock'.

Key terms

Maturation: *the gradual process of becoming physically mature or fully developed*

Explaining human development – biological factors

P2 Genetic inheritance

When you see a baby, you are looking at the unique product of two different, but now combined, sets of genes. In purely biological terms, a baby consists of cells. With the exception of egg and sperm cells, each cell of the human body contains 46 chromosomes arranged in 23 pairs.

In turn, chromosomes contain **genes**, units of heredity information. That is, they pass on information which affects biological characteristics like eye colour and predispositions to particular conditions (see Figure 4.24). We know this from scientific research that has identified and isolated specific genes.

Because you have 23 pairs of chromosomes, you have matching pairs of genes for nearly every biological trait. Twenty-two of the pairs are known as **autosomes**. For these 22 chromosomes, the instructions of the **dominant genes** are followed. The instructions of a **recessive gene** are only followed if neither in the pair is dominant. So, the majority of features and characteristics that a person inherits are genetically dominant.

The **sex chromosomes** make up the twenty-third pair. A woman's egg cells only carry X chromosomes. The sperm cells from the father can carry an X or a Y chromosome. It is, therefore, the fertilising sperm cell that determines whether a child will be male or female. If the sperm cell that fertilises the egg cell carries an X chromosome, the XX combination will make the child female. If the sperm cell carries a Y chromosome, the child will have an XY combination and will be male.

Figure 4.24 describes a number of conditions that some people are predisposed to because of the genes they've inherited from their parents.

Advances in genetic research are continually revealing how genes work in combination with one another and with environmental factors. It is fair to say that genes do exert a powerful influence on the physical growth

Your assessment criteria:

P2 Explain the potential effects of five different life factors on the development of an individual

Key terms

Autosomes: *chromosomes that are not sex chromosomes – there are 22 pairs of them in humans*

Dominant gene: *a gene with characteristics that are always expressed*

Gene: *the basic unit of heredity in a living organism*

Recessive gene: *a gene with characteristics that are only expressed in the absence of a dominant gene*

Sex chromosomes: *the X and Y chromosomes responsible for determining the sex of a human being*

Figure 4.24 Examples of conditions with a genetic component.

Condition	Symptoms	Causes
Cystic fibrosis	Thick, sticky mucus affects the lungs and digestive system; an increased risk of fertility problems	Inheritance of faulty disease-carrying gene
Coeliac disease	Indigestion, bloating, abdominal pain and weight loss	Intolerance to gluten resulting from inherited gene
Brittle bone disease	Bone pain, twisted or mis-shapen limbs and risk of fractures	Inherited mutated gene

and development of human beings. However, lots of other factors also interact with our genetic predispositions to influence the way we develop. For example, while an individual might inherit a genetic predisposition to a particular form of cancer or to heart disease, the person's lifestyle can make it more or less likely that the disease will actually occur. So, while genes play an important part in determining how we grow and develop, the environment is also very influential.

Biological influences before birth

Researchers now recognise that the environment in a pregnant woman's womb has a significant influence on the development of her growing baby. For example, if a woman smokes or drinks alcohol during her pregnancy, she will introduce nicotine and alcohol into her womb. These substances are absorbed into the blood supply to the baby and may slow or alter foetal development (see Figure 4.25).

Figure 4.25 Biological influences affecting development before birth.

Condition	Causes	Effects
Foetal alcohol syndrome	Low birth weight, heart defects, behavioural and learning disorders, problems with emotional development, facial deformities	Excess alcohol consumption by mother during pregnancy
Infections during pregnancy	Hearing and visual impairment	Rubella
	Baby may acquire infection	Hepatitis B, herpes and HIV

What do you know?

1. Identify an example of one nature influence and one nurture influence on human growth and development.
2. What is the nature–nurture debate?
3. Explain how nature influences on development differ from nurture influences.
4. Give an example of a physical change that occurs because of maturation.
5. Using an example, explain how diseases and health conditions can be inherited.
6. Describe two biological influences and the effects they can have on an individual's pre-natal development.

Explaining human development – environmental factors

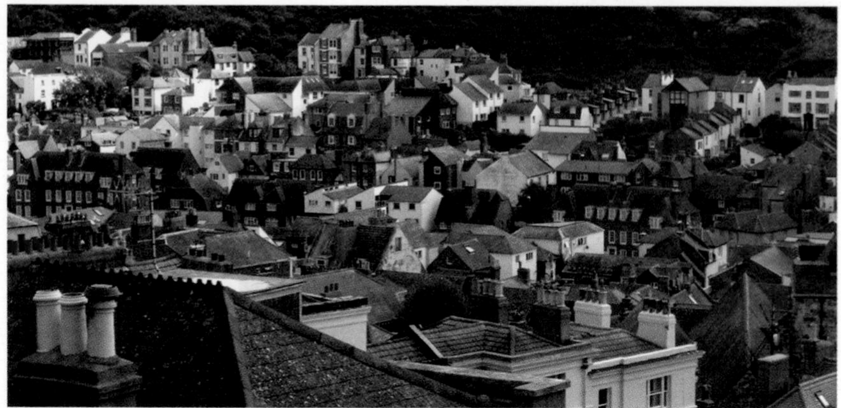

The physical or built environment can influence a person's development in various ways.

Your assessment criteria:

P2 Explain the potential effects of five different life factors on the development of an individual

Environmental factors have an indirect and variable impact on human development, compared to genetic influences. However, it is possible to predict in general terms the likely effects that, for example, pollution and poor housing conditions can have on human growth and development.

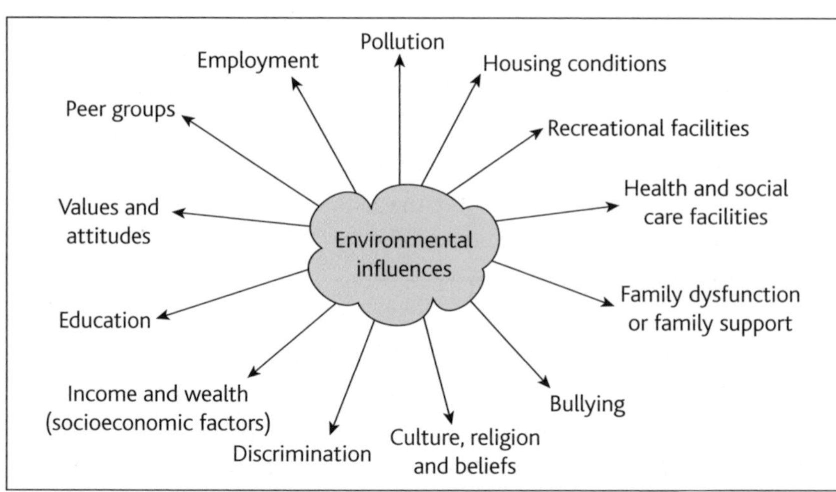

Figure 4.26 Environmental influences on human development.

P2 Pollution

Physical growth and development can be directly affected by the presence of pollution in the atmosphere. The level of air pollution in the United Kingdom has changed very little since the early 1980s. As a result, air pollution continues to contribute to the higher levels of respiratory problems (including asthmatic symptoms and bronchitis) that are prevalent in urban areas. Carbon monoxide and other harmful gas emissions from vehicles, aircraft, ships and factories can be particularly damaging to a person's respiratory system. Babies and children can experience restricted growth potential, though people at all stages of life can have their physical health damaged by poor air quality.

Noise pollution from vehicles, aircraft and crowded environments can damage a person's hearing and affect their psychological wellbeing. Unwanted noise is associated with high stress levels, sleep disturbances and high blood pressure. Noise pollution is usually worst in built-up, urban environments.

Housing conditions

Housing provides shelter and protection and is important for physical health and development. A person who lives in poor conditions – where there is inadequate heating, dampness and overcrowding for example – is at risk of developing respiratory disorders, allergies, inflammatory diseases, stress and mental health problems. Children who live in overcrowded homes are more likely to be victims of accidents.

Older people with low incomes sometimes have to choose between buying food and heating their homes. Hypothermia can result from insufficient heating; normal body temperature is 37°C and hypothermia is defined as a fall in body temperature to below 35°C. It is important to note that a person's home provides them with a sense of emotional wellbeing and psychological security, so housing conditions influence an individual's emotional development too.

Reflect

What features of housing do you feel are important in making a person's home 'healthy'?

Access to recreational facilities

If you want to live a healthy life, it is important to have a balance between work and non-work activity. Leisure time, including having hobbies, enjoying a social life and simply relaxing, is part of a healthy life. The recreational activities that people take part in contribute to their growth, development, health and wellbeing by:

- helping them to form social relationships
- providing opportunities to communicate with and feel valued by others
- enabling them to develop social skills
- providing opportunities to develop and use physical and intellectual abilities and skills, depending on the recreational activity
- providing them with an important sense of belonging to a group or team.

Having access to a range of recreational facilities promotes development because it provides people with opportunities to establish a healthy work–life balance, to explore their interests and develop a range of physical, intellectual and social skills.

Discuss

What kind of recreational activities do you take part in? What impact does your choice of recreational activity have on your health and wellbeing?

P2 Access to health and social care services

We are all likely to use health care services at some point. Effective health care services are obviously necessary when people experience life threatening health emergencies. In the UK, the National Health Service offers a variety of free emergency care services.

Access to ongoing health care services is also important for people who experience chronic health problems or disabilities that require regular treatment and support. Specialist health and social care services may be required by people who need additional help or specialist intervention to promote, support or sustain their physical, social or intellectual development. This can occur during any life stage and, for some people, is a requirement throughout their whole life course.

Your assessment criteria:

P2 Explain the potential effects of five different life factors on the development of an individual

Bullying

Bullies are people who abuse others. A bully behaves in an abusive way in order to gain power over another person. **Bullying** behaviours can include:

- repeated mocking, taunting or teasing
- physical intimidation or assault
- offensive, degrading or humiliating comments
- less favourable treatment (discrimination) at work or in social situations
- manipulating, isolating or excluding a person.

Key terms

Bullying: *exposure, repeatedly and over time, of an individual or group to negative actions by others that are designed to inflict injury or discomfort*

Bullies usually see themselves as having greater social or physical power than the people they target. Their behaviour is designed to bring about a submissive response from their victim. Bullying can occur in families, at school, in the workplace and in social situations. Victims of bullying have a higher risk of developing stress-related illnesses, suffering damage to their self-esteem and sense of self-worth, experiencing loneliness, depression and anxiety, and may even consider committing suicide. Efforts should always be made to tackle incidents of bullying before the victim suffers serious developmental harm.

Family dysfunction

In dysfunctional families the needs of family members are not met and relationships are inappropriately aggressive, manipulative or unsupportive. Adults and children living in dysfunctional families may experience high levels of stress, have poor communication skills, feel neglected and emotionally unsupported, have low self-esteem and a negative sense of self-worth.

Effects of culture, religion and beliefs

The United Kingdom is a multicultural society, being ethnically and religiously diverse. **Culture** can affect physical growth and development when cultural beliefs or practices influence food choices, patterns of exercise and use of health care services, for example. Social development may also be affected when cultural beliefs or practices influence attitudes, values and opportunities to develop and experience friendships and other non-family relationships. Emotional development may be influenced by extended family structures, by the closeness or expected pattern of relationships within the family and by a person's identification with their cultural heritage. In these different ways, culture can play a very important, though often unseen, role in shaping our personal growth and development.

Key terms

Culture: *common values, beliefs and customs or way of life*

Discrimination

Unfair discrimination involves treating an individual or group less favourably. Discrimination can affect an individual's development by:

- damaging a person's self-image and self-esteem
- undermining a person's self-confidence and inhibiting them from achieving their potential
- causing emotional distress and fear
- resulting in physical assault and injury
- preventing a person from having equal opportunities in education, work or areas of their social life
- acting as a barrier to an individual getting the care services, social support or treatment they need.

Socioeconomic factors

Personal development can be affected by a number of money-related or **economic factors** which influence quality of life and access to opportunities. Income refers to the money that a household or individual receives; expenditure is how much of that money is spent. People receive money from working, from pension and welfare benefits, and from other sources such as investments. People with a high income are likely to have better educational and leisure opportunities and to live in better circumstances. Having better opportunities and reduced money-related stress allows these individuals and families to make the most of their abilities and potential. The reverse is usually the case for people experiencing poverty.

Key terms

Economic factors: *money-related factors (e.g. income, wealth, employment)*

P2 Education

Nurseries, schools, colleges and universities are places where people experience a great deal of social and emotional development, making and experimenting with a variety of different social relationships. These may be formal relationships with authority figures such as teachers and tutors, as well as informal relationships with fellow students.

Relationships in school, college or university with same-sex and opposite-sex friends and colleagues may be positive, supportive and rewarding. Many people make strong, life-long friendships at school or college and meet people who become their role models. However, educational experiences can also be negative for those who find themselves bullied, excluded from friendship groups or who find education a stressful and unrewarding experience. We should recognise that many people have a mixed experience of education, finding that it has influenced their personal development in both positive and negative ways at different points in their life.

Values and attitudes

We acquire our **values** and **attitudes** through **socialisation** in the family and in other important settings such as at school and in the workplace. People's values and attitudes are an important influence on their development because they affect lifestyle choices, health behaviours and the way in which they form and maintain their personal and social relationships.

Peer groups

Friends of approximately your age and other people with whom you share similarities, important links or with whom you identify are members of your **peer group**. Gender, ethnicity and leisure interests could, therefore, form the basis of non-age related peer groups.

Peer groups are an important influence on human development during childhood and adolescence. Emotional and social development during adolescence is closely linked to relationships with same-sex and opposite-sex friends, for example. An adolescent's attitudes and values, ways of behaving and sense of self-worth are significantly affected by their friendships and peer group expectations. This is largely because adolescence involves a search for a sense of personal identity. Taking cues from and being like friends are strategies that many teenagers use as they try to achieve this important sense of self. This doesn't mean to say that friendships in childhood, adulthood or old age don't influence personal development. They do, but not usually in such a powerful and formative

Your assessment criteria:

P2 Explain the potential effects of five different life factors on the development of an individual

Key terms

Attitudes: *assumptions that affect an individual's ways of thinking and behaving*

Peer group: *a group of people who share common characteristics*

Socialisation: *the process of learning the attitudes, values and culture (way of life) of a society*

Values: *moral principles*

way. Friendships are very important in children's social and emotional development and play a vital role in supporting and sustaining an adult's sense of identity, belonging and sense of self-esteem.

Employment status

A person's employment status has a bearing on their **social class**. Usually, people in higher status employment belong to higher social class groups, and vice versa. As well as providing income, a person's job status influences their self-concept and their intellectual, social and emotional development. Having higher status employment and stimulating work is likely to have a positive effect on personal development. Working in very difficult or stressful conditions, in a lower status job or in an environment where employers and colleagues are not supportive or friendly may have a negative effect on self-esteem and personal development.

Key terms

Social class: *a group of people who are similar in terms of their income, wealth and job status*

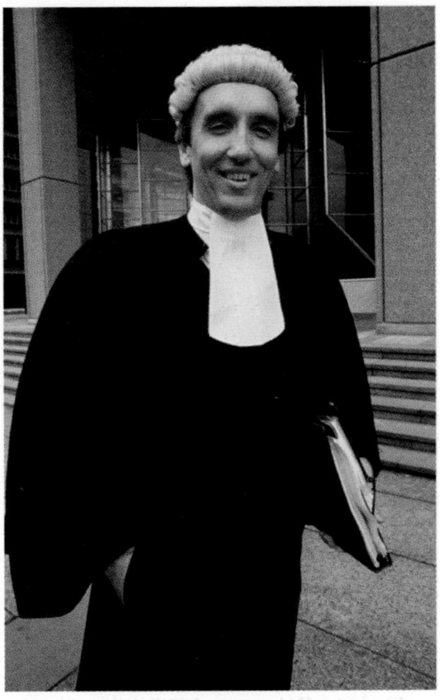

With which social class do you associate lawyers?

What do you know?

1. Identify four environmental factors that can affect an individual's development.
2. Describe how a person's housing conditions may affect their development.
3. What is bullying and how can it impact on an individual's development?
4. Identify three socioeconomic factors that can affect an individual's development.
5. Describe the links between income and expenditure and human development.
6. Explain how an individual's peer group can influence their growth and development.

The effects of lifestyle factors on development

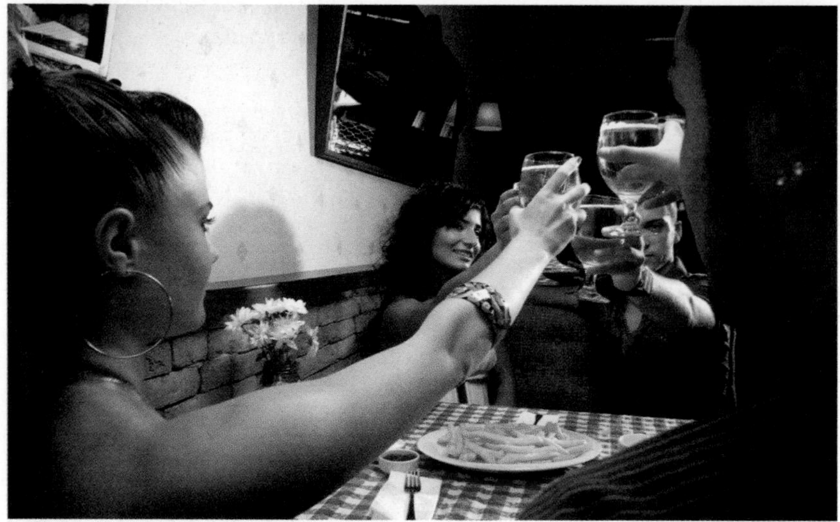

A person's lifestyle can have both positive and negative effects on their health and development.

Your assessment criteria:

P2 Explain the potential effects of five different life factors on the development of an individual

The term **lifestyle** is sometimes used to refer to the particular attitudes and habits that a person has or which are typical of a defined group of people. In this sense, the lifestyles of 'healthy' people are seen as distinctive and different from the lifestyles of 'unhealthy' people. The term *lifestyle* is also associated with the consumption or use of a whole variety of things that affect human health and development, ranging from the foods we consume, to the use of alcohol, drugs and cigarettes. So, lifestyle factors refer to both our ***attitudes*** and to our ***behaviours***.

Key terms

Lifestyle: *the way a person lives*

P2 Nutrition and dietary choices

Our dietary requirements change as we progress through life, though we always need ***adequate nutrition*** to meet our specific health and growth needs depending on our life stage. ***Adequate nutrition*** is the key issue in debates about nutrition and lifestyle. Food that contains a high level of fat, sugar or salt is likely to be of poor overall nutritional quality. Regardless of life stage, a diet based on these types of food doesn't contain the balance of nutrients that a person needs to sustain their health and development.

A person's dietary intake is an aspect of their lifestyle because they choose what to eat on the basis of what they like and enjoy. However, other factors also play a part in dietary choices. For example, the cost and availability of different foods, cultural traditions, knowledge of nutrition

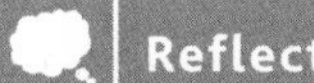

Reflect

What nutritional or dietary choices do you make (or are you considering) as a way of promoting your health and wellbeing?

and the power of advertising all influence our food choices. It is overly simplistic to blame people for 'bad' lifestyle choices when they may not be able to make more positive decisions about their diet.

Alcohol intake

Alcohol is used widely within the adult population in the UK. It is an important part of leisure activities and, for many, plays a significant role in cultural events, such as birthday, Christmas and wedding celebrations. *Alcohol misuse* occurs when a person becomes dependent on regular alcohol consumption or consumes excessive amounts through 'binge drinking'. There is a variety of physical and mental health risks associated with these problematic patterns of drinking. For example, regular consumption of excessive amounts of alcohol increases the risk of developing high blood pressure, coronary heart disease, cancers of the mouth and throat, and liver damage. Depression and obesity are also associated with high levels of alcohol consumption.

Investigate

How does consumption of excessive amounts of alcohol affect an individual's physical and mental health and wellbeing? Using online and library sources obtain information on the consequences of both binge drinking and chronic (long-term) alcohol misuse. Produce a poster or leaflet outlining your findings.

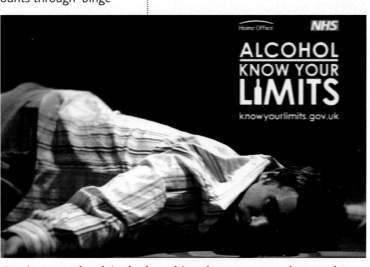

Getting very drunk is the last thing that some people ever do.

Use and misuse of substances

While drug misuse is not as prevalent as alcohol misuse in the UK, the NHS Information Centre's annual survey of drug misuse in England revealed that in 2009–10 8.6 per cent (2.8 million people) used illicit substances. This is part of a downward trend from an all-time high of 12.3 per cent in 2003–04. Cannabis is the most commonly used drug among adults with 6.6 per cent of 16 to 59-year-olds admitting to using it in 2009–10. The use of Class A drugs such as heroin has dropped from 3.7 per cent in 2008–09 to 3.1 per cent. in 2009–10.

Drug misuse can become part of a person's lifestyle for a variety of reasons. For example, people use drugs because of peer pressure, as an 'experiment', as a way of coping with difficulties and pressures in life, and as part of leisure activities. Drugs may offer short-term 'highs' but are highly likely to damage health and development in the medium and long term. Even in the short term, depending on the drug being used, there is the danger of overdosing or causing lasting health damage. Ultimately, substance misuse doesn't promote health or personal development and carries with it significant risks, whatever life stage a person is in.

The effect of life events on development

The events that a person experiences in their life influence how they develop and change in each life stage. A **life event** can change the direction of a person's life, affecting their personal development. **Predictable life events**, such as starting school, going through puberty and retiring from work, often mark a transition from one stage of life to another, acting as milestones in our personal development. **Unpredictable life events**, such as sudden illness or injury, redundancy or the death of a friend or relative, occur unexpectedly and are often associated with loss, but may also lead to positive change in a person's life.

Your assessment criteria:

P3 Explain the influences of two predictable and two unpredictable major life events on the development of an individual

Key terms

Life event: *an event that causes a change in a person's development or has special significance for them*

Predictable life event: *an expected life event*

Sibling: *a brother or sister*

Unpredictable life event: *a life event that occurs unexpectedly*

P3 Birth and parenthood

The birth of a child is a life event for both the parents and any siblings of the baby. New relationships are formed and existing relationships, parent–parent and parent–child, change as a result of the addition to the family. For many children, the birth of a **sibling** is an exciting and happy event. However, sometimes siblings become jealous and may compete for their parent's affection.

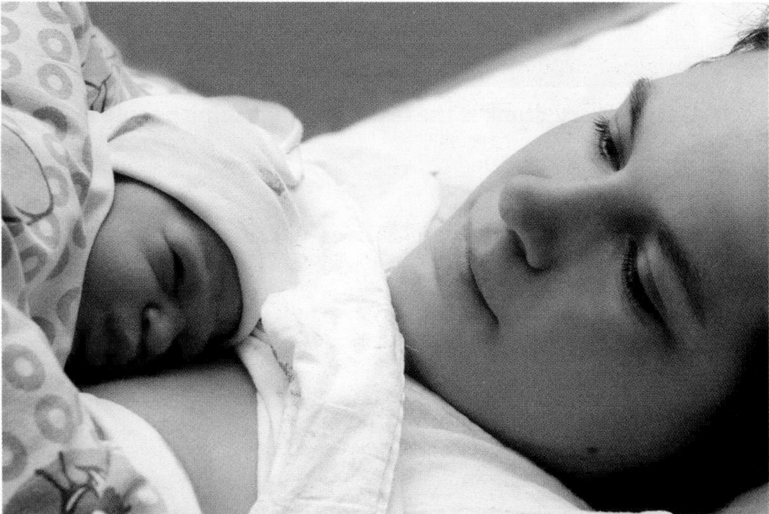

The moments following birth are thought to be very important for mother-baby attachment and bonding.

Becoming a parent is a very positive, emotionally fulfilling moment for many people. However, parenthood can be a cause of stress, mental health difficulties and relationship problems for some couples. New parents have to adapt their roles and relationship to cope with the needs of a dependant child. Some couples are adaptable, with partners offering each other practical and emotional support. Others are unable or unwilling to do this and relationship difficulties or breakdown may result. Parenthood also results in a major change to a person's identity, as they take on their new 'mum' or dad' role.

Leaving home and leaving care

Leaving home or care can be a stressful life event for many people. Home is usually a place that offers safety, security and stability. Leaving can mean a break with the past, with family or well-known carers and with friends. The practical demands of organising the removal of possessions, arranging finance to cover the cost of moving, finding money for rent or perhaps buying somewhere to live and possibly moving to an unfamiliar area all add to the emotional strain of this life event. However, leaving home and leaving care also mark a transition to independence and can have a very positive effect on an individual's sense of identity and self-esteem.

Discuss

What do you think are the benefits and drawbacks of leaving home to live independently at the end of adolescence? Share your ideas with a couple of class colleagues and try to identify ways in which this could have a positive impact on your development.

Illness or serious injury

Illness or serious injury may have a temporary or a permanent impact. For example, accidents and some types of illness can result in a disability, such as loss of sight or hearing, or the loss of a limb. A person who acquires a disability in this way will have to adapt their skills and lifestyle to cope with their new situation.

Serious illness may be unexpected and can result in massive lifestyle changes as the person tries to cope with the effects of the illness. A person's everyday routine, their relationships with others and their need for practical and emotional support may all change because of their illness.

Starting school or nursery

Going to school or nursery for the first time is a big event for most children. Families and schools often go to great lengths to prepare children for this life transition. Talking about what happens at school, meeting staff, going for short visits and then for extended sessions can all help a child prepare for nursery and school. However, even the most well prepared child may be reluctant to be left by their parents on their first day. Teachers and other staff can usually provide enough support and reassurance to help young children settle.

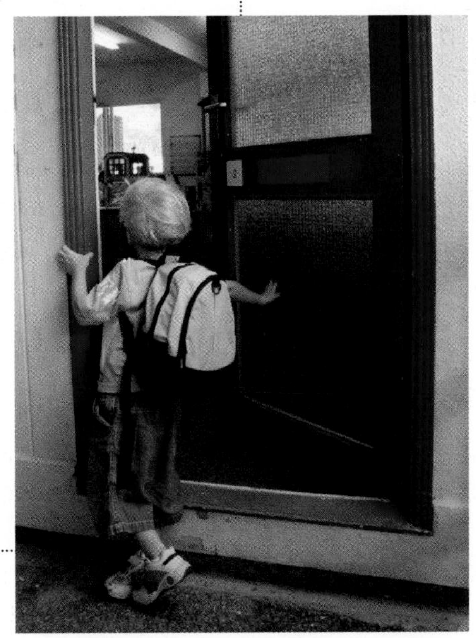

Starting nursery and starting school are key life events during childhood.

P3 Employment

Your assessment criteria:

P3 Explain the influences of two predictable and two unpredictable major life events on the development of an individual

Beginning work or changing jobs may affect development by:

- promoting individual responsibility and personal independence
- promoting intellectual development through training and the development of work-related skills
- leading to new social relationships and the development of social skills
- boosting self-confidence and changing an individual's identity as they gain experience, are promoted and improve their employment status (see page 179).

Work can also affect personal development when a person loses their job because they are made **redundant**. Redundancy can lead to:

Key terms

Redundant: *job roles that are no longer required*

- loss of self-confidence and self-respect
- loss of status and identity
- increased stress levels
- problems with sleeping, eating and mood
- loss of social relationships with work colleagues
- increased strain in personal and family relationships.

However, redundancy can lead to positive outcomes for some people; they may be motivated to learn new skills, start a small business or change their lifestyle in a way that causes them to feel happier and more satisfied in the long term.

Bereavement

Bereavement can cause a major change in a person's life, affecting their social and emotional development, as well as impacting on their self-concept. If a person has lived to a great age or has a terminal illness, we may anticipate and prepare ourselves for their death. In other cases, however, a person's death may be sudden and unexpected. In either case, the sense of loss that follows a death can be profound; powerful emotions of disbelief, sadness, anger and guilt may be very difficult to deal with. Bereavement can be especially traumatic when a person dies suddenly or dramatically because of an accident, serious injury or suicide, for example. A sense of bereavement can cause both short-term and long-term developmental problems.

Key terms

Bereavement: *deep feeling of loss experienced when a partner, relative or friend dies*

Marriage and divorce

Marriage is usually a positive life event, celebrated by hundreds of thousands of people each year. It can involve major adaptations for both partners and their close relatives and friends. Ideally, the couple will establish a deeper emotional commitment to each other. Marriages alter family relationships; the roles of family members change and new members are introduced into family groups. For example, in-laws become part of a wider family network and relationships between original family members may weaken when a son or daughter moves away to live with their new partner. This can cause a sense of loss for the parents of the new couple and for the partners themselves as they move away from their birth family.

People do not marry intending to get divorced, but divorce is now relatively common in the United Kingdom. One in three marriages ends in divorce. Despite being relatively common, divorce is an unexpected life event. It often has a major emotional impact on the couple and on other family members, particularly on any children. Marriage breakdown and the process of divorce usually have major financial and practical consequences too, such as having to find different accommodation and independent sources of income. Children may be affected by their parents' divorce as they adapt to new living arrangements, changing relationships and sometimes step-parents. Though divorce can have a negative impact on the lives of those affected, it may still be preferable to being in a stressful and unsatisfactory relationship.

Investigate

Use the website of the Office for National Statistics (www.statistics.gov.uk) to find the latest data on patterns of marriage and divorce in the UK. Are fewer people getting married or more people getting divorced than in the past?

What do you know?

1. Identify three lifestyle factors that can affect an individual's health and development.
2. Describe how an individual's use of alcohol could have a negative impact on their health and development.
3. Identify two predictable and two unpredictable life events.
4. Explain how the birth of a child can be a positive life event for some people, but a negative life event for others.
5. What is bereavement and how can this affect an individual's development?
6. Explain why marriage is seen as an important life event that influences personal development.

Theories of ageing

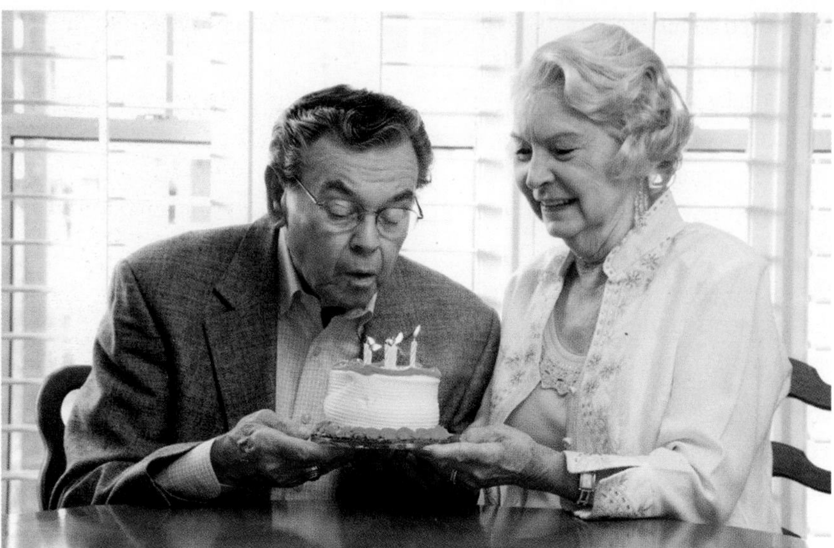

An increasing proportion of the UK population now live well into 'old age'.

Your assessment criteria:

P4 Explain two theories of ageing

Reflect

What physical and mental characteristics do you associate with the following age groups?

- *65+*
- *18–64*
- *12–17*
- *0–11*

Key terms

***Disengage:** to become disconnected from something*

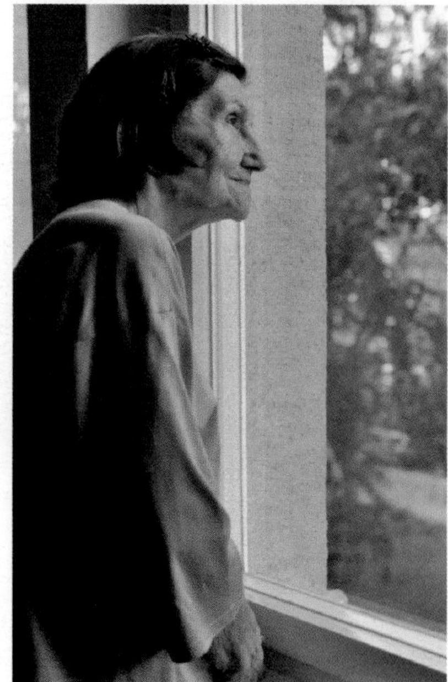

Is old age still associated with loneliness and isolation?

P4 Understanding ageing

The ageing process is an inevitable part of human growth and development. Various attempts have been made to explain the process of ageing and to identify the key influencing factors. Health and social care practitioners often work with older people and need to understand how individuals adapt to life during old age.

What is disengagement theory?

Cumming and Henry (1961) proposed disengagement theory as a way of explaining behaviour and development in old age. They suggested that when people reach their sixties they began to **disengage** from active roles in society for a variety of reasons, for example:

- ill-health
- retirement from work
- loss of friendships and social support, through illness and death of partners, friends and relatives
- lack of access to travel facilities
- inability to use communication technology (email, internet, ICT systems).

Cumming and Henry argued that disengagement in old age occurs voluntarily and with the approval of the younger generation because it frees up employment opportunities. This, they suggest, is a normal and appropriate response that has benefits for society and for older people.

Disengagement theory has been criticised for promoting acceptance of the **social exclusion** of older people. For example, it could be argued that ageism, ageist policies and ageist practices restrict the ability of some older people to remain active citizens and that withdrawal from active social roles is imposed, not a choice. Cumming and Henry's (1961) original research has also been criticised as it was based on a small sample of American adults who were taken to be typical of all older people everywhere! Other evidence also suggests that many older people remain engaged with their family and friends and are often more socially active in these groups once they have retired from work.

What is activity theory?

This theory proposes that, in contrast to disengagement theory, the more active an older person is, the more satisfied they will feel. Activity theorists such as Fennell, Phillipson and Evers (1989) argue that older people often resist disengagement from important aspects of their life by maintaining a 'middle-age' lifestyle. Many older people take part in social and educational activities as a way of staying mentally and physically healthy, for example. Enjoying the company, support and friendship of others and having hobbies and interests are ways of avoiding stagnation and preventing the loss of mental and physical skills.

Activity theory has been criticised on the grounds that it may be a way of explaining the response to ageing of some people, but that it fails to take the diversity of the older population into account. Being socially active and engaged may be possible for those with certain personality characteristics living in certain circumstances. However, other people may not have the financial resources, good health or drive to maintain an active lifestyle in old age. Activity theory has been criticised on the grounds that it may be a way of explaining the response to ageing of some people, but that it fails to take the diversity of the older population into account. Being socially active and engaged may be possible for those with certain personality characteristics living in certain circumstances. However, other people may not have the financial resources, good health or drive to maintain an active lifestyle in old age.

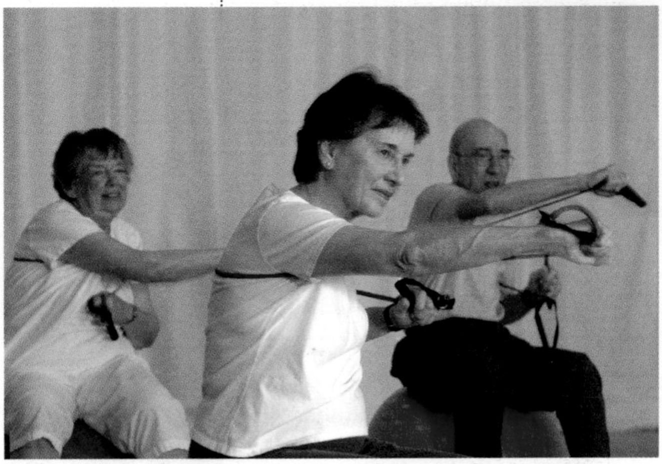

Many older people live active, healthy lives long into their 'old age'.

Key terms

Social exclusion: *being on the edge of or outside mainstream society*

Reflect

1. *Can you think of any older relatives, neighbours or family friends who have disengaged as they have aged? Bearing confidentiality in mind, describe how the person's behaviour, relationships or activity levels have changed as they have disengaged.*
2. *Can you also think of older relatives, neighbours or friends who haven't disengaged from society during old age? Again, bearing confidentiality in mind, describe how these people have maintained their social connections and activity levels.*
3. *What do you think about disengagement theory as a way of explaining responses to ageing? Is it helpful and realistic or an unhelpful, inadequate way of explaining responses to ageing?*

P4 Continuity theory

This approach argues that it is important for ageing individuals to maintain a continuous sense of self, as well as the same habits, interests, contacts and lifestyle as in earlier years. Continuity theorists, like Atchley (1989) argue that older people make adaptations to achieve this sense of continuity, promoting and maintaining their self-esteem, self-concept and wellbeing in later life. Continuity theory accepts that people have different approaches to their old age. Some wish to withdraw and disengage from a previous lifestyle and can do this without losing their sense of self. Others are energised and motivated by active involvement with family, friends and need to stay engaged.

Contemporary theories

Contemporary theories are critical of both disengagement and activity theory. Both are seen as rigid and uncritical of society's role in structuring ageing.

A political economy perspective draws attention to the impact of social and economic structures on the financial status, isolation and opportunities open to people in later life. It is argued that the cumulative effect of earlier advantages and disadvantages in life impact on people in old age. For example, women with small incomes due to earlier part-time work and disrupted career patterns often have to live on low incomes later in life. The result is a polarisation of older people into poor, socially excluded and 'young-at-heart', fit and wealthy groups.

Social **gerontologists** also argue that subjective experience of ageing is important. In this sense the historical background to a person's life, as well as their position in society, is important. Ageing is an integrated process where the life a person has lived gives meaning to their experience of old age.

M2 Explaining development in older adulthood

The various theories of ageing provide a number of ways of explaining development in older adulthood. The main claims of each theory can be evaluated by applying them to the development of a particular individual. Asking older people about their experiences of ageing in the context of each theory will produce material that will allow you to compare and contrast the accuracy of the claims being made and the usefulness of each theory.

Your assessment criteria:

P4 Explain two theories of ageing

M2 Discuss two major theories of ageing in relation to the development of the individual

D2 Evaluate the influence of two major theories of ageing on health and social care provision

Key terms

Gerontologist: *a person specialising in the health and social care of people in old age*

Figure 4.27 Using theories of ageing in practice.

Disengagement theory questions	Activity theory questions	Continuity theory questions
• How has your life changed in older adulthood? • Have you given up any roles or responsibilities during this time? • Do you feel any less active or involved in society than you did in middle age? • Overall, has there been much change in the quality of your life since early adulthood?	• Do you feel that you are more or less busy since you retired? • What do you do with your time now? • How have your activities and goals in life changed in older adulthood?	• In what ways, if any, have your sense of identity and self-esteem changed in older adulthood? • Can you think of any ways in which you have adapted your lifestyle to cope with the changes of older adulthood? • Why did you make these adaptations to your lifestyle?

D2 The influence of ageing theories on care provision

Ideas about age and the ageing process affect the way health and social care services are provided for older people. Most older people live at home and are active, with or without support. Others choose supported forms of accommodation or are in need of 24-hour care.

Services seek to promote choice and are respectful of older people's preferences and wishes. Health and social care practitioners generally recognise that older people should be able to choose their preferred level of activity and might need to be supported to achieve this. Care practitioners shouldn't force people to be active or engaged in ways they don't wish to be. An individual should be able to maintain continuity over their own life and choose their own level of activity.

What do you know?

1. Can you identify three different theories of ageing?
2. Using your own words, briefly describe the main claims disengagement theory makes about ageing.
3. Discuss the weaknesses of disengagement theory as a way of explaining social responses to ageing.
4. How does activity theory explain older people's responses to ageing?
5. Why should care practitioners see ageing as a life-long process, rather than something that happens in the person's final life stage?
6. Explain how theories of ageing can influence the provision of health and social care services for older people.

The process of ageing

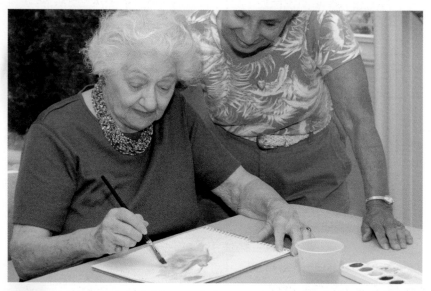

Creative and leisure activities can help to maintain physical, intellectual and social skills during later life.

Your assessment criteria:

P5 Explain the physical and psychological changes which may be associated with ageing

P5 Physical change in old age

Improvements in our standard of living over the last 200 years have resulted in an extension to average life expectancy (see page 143). One consequence of this is that UK health and social care practitioners now work with a growing number of people who are experiencing the physical and psychological effects of the ageing process.

During later adulthood people experience gradual physical decline in both the structure and functioning of their body.

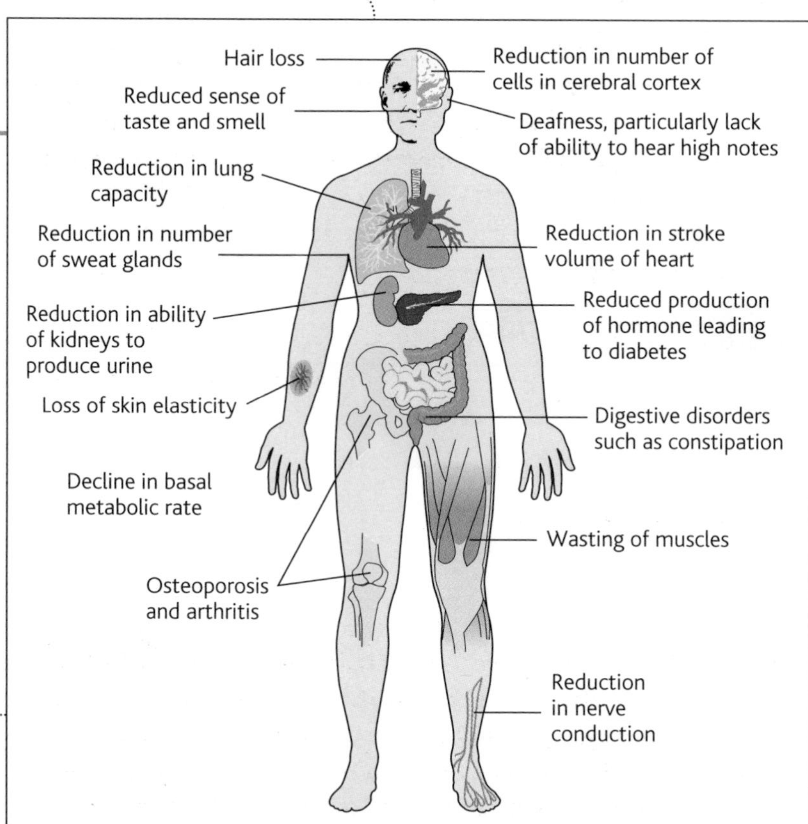

Figure 4.28 Various changes affect the human body in old age.

These changes in structure and function are part of the normal ageing process. For most people, the pace of physical change and the age-related decline in their physical abilities quickens between the ages of 60 and 70 years, and accelerates rapidly between 75 and 80 years of age. Changes occur in the physical structure of the brain, as well as in the body.

Hormonal changes

Menopause in middle age leads to a reduction in oestrogen production in women, causing osteoporosis (thinning of the bones). Some women are **genetically predisposed** to develop this condition, but regular exercise can reduce the risk of bone fracture.

Key terms

Genetically predisposed: *more likely to experience a condition because of genetic inheritance*

Cardiovascular system changes

Older people tend to develop narrower arteries due to higher cholesterol levels and the build up of fatty deposits. This can lead to raised blood pressure, and increased risk of stroke and heart attack; fatty deposits can break away and partially block important arteries. The result can be coronary heart disease with symptoms of breathlessness and chest pain. A heart attack will occur if blood flow is stopped by a blockage in an artery.

Respiratory system changes

An individual's respiratory muscles tend to decline in strength with age. A person's lungs may also become less efficient. Older people are more likely to have chronic respiratory diseases such as chronic obstructive pulmonary disease (COPD), emphysema and bronchitis which damage the respiratory system.

Investigate

Using the internet and other reference sources, find out about the causes and symptoms of emphysema and chronic obstructive pulmonary disease. Create an information leaflet that describes the background to each condition and explains why older people are at risk of these conditions.

Nervous system changes

Loss of the nerve cells that activate muscles and a decline in the effectiveness of **neurotransmitters** during older adulthood increase an individual's risk of:

- developing motor neurone disease
- experiencing sensory loss
- changes to cognitive functioning.

Changes to the nervous system may impair an older person's sense of taste and smell, for example, and can mean they are less sensitive to the cold. This increases the risk of hypothermia. Hearing also tends to deteriorate slowly as people age. Quiet and high-pitched sounds (such as voices) become more difficult to hear. Sight is affected because the lens in the eye loses its elasticity. The result is that older people find it harder to focus on close objects.

Key terms

Neurotransmitters: *chemicals that transmit nerve impulses from one nerve cell to the next*

Your assessment criteria:

P5 Explain the physical and psychological changes which may be associated with ageing

M3 Discuss the effects on self-esteem and self-confidence of the physical changes associated with ageing

P5 Muscular–skeletal changes

Physical changes to the body can result in muscle wastage, a decline in strength, stamina and mobility, and the development of arthritis. Because calcium and protein are lost from the bones, older people can become physically frail and experience fractures. The thinning and compacting of the discs in the spine can also lead to some older people becoming shorter or developing a curved spine in later adulthood.

Changes to the skin

Ageing results in a loss of elasticity in the skin and the development of wrinkles. Older people may also show the signs of damage from ultraviolet light on their skin in the form of age spots, wrinkles and a 'leathery' appearance.

Effects of smoking

Smoking can lead to lung and other cancers that develop in later adulthood. Smoking is also associated with:

- cardiovascular disease, as it causes the arteries to harden and narrow
- damage to the respiratory system in the form of COPD and emphysema
- damage to the skin, leading to a lined and leathery appearance.

M3 Psychological changes associated with ageing

It is difficult to generalise about the psychological changes associated with ageing as each person's experience is unique. However, psychologists have observed some common patterns. For example, psychologists who use disengagement theory suggest that older people gradually disengage or separate from society as a result of ageing. Erik Erikson (1968) saw old age as the final stage of psychosocial development in which people develop a sense of 'ego integrity' to avoid despair about the futility of their lives. Those who achieve ego integrity have a clear sense of identify and a stronger sense of self-esteem than those who don't.

Ego integrity and a stronger sense of self-esteem can be achieved through reminiscence about past experiences and achievements. Older people who are able to do this with family, friends or in social groups have their identities and lives **validated**. Older people who have little support may become lonely and isolated, being unable to retain their sense of self. They may lose confidence and have a lower sense of self-worth as a result.

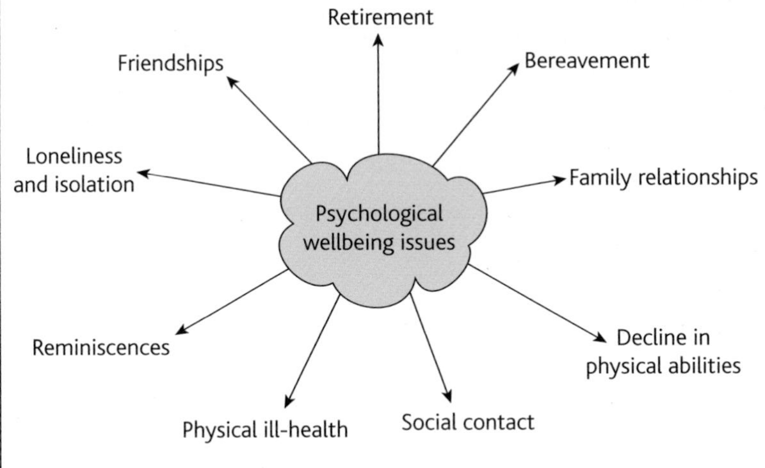

Figure 4.29 Issues affecting psychological wellbeing in older adulthood.

Key terms

Validated: *supported by a positive response from others*

What do you know?

1. Identify three physical changes that occur as a result of the ageing process.
2. What is the menopause and why does this occur in middle or older adulthood?
3. Explain why older people are more at risk of coronary heart disease than younger people.
4. How might smoking earlier in life have an impact on an older person's physical health?
5. Describe how an older person may experience psychological change in later life.
6. Explain how an older person can maintain their confidence and self-esteem in later life.

Assessment checklist

Your learning and level of understanding of this unit will be assessed through assignments given to you and marked by your teacher or tutor. Before you submit your assignment work for assessment you should make sure that you have produced sufficient evidence to achieve the grade you are aiming for.

To pass this unit you will need to present evidence for assessment which demonstrates that you can meet all of the pass criteria for the unit.

Assessment Criteria	Description	✓
P1	Describe physical, intellectual, emotional and social development for each of the life stages of an individual.	☐
P2	Explain the potential effects of five different life factors on the development of an individual.	☐
P3	Explain the influences of two predictable and two unpredictable major life events on the development of an individual.	☐
P4	Explain two theories of ageing.	☐
P5	Explain the physical and psychological changes which may be associated with ageing.	☐

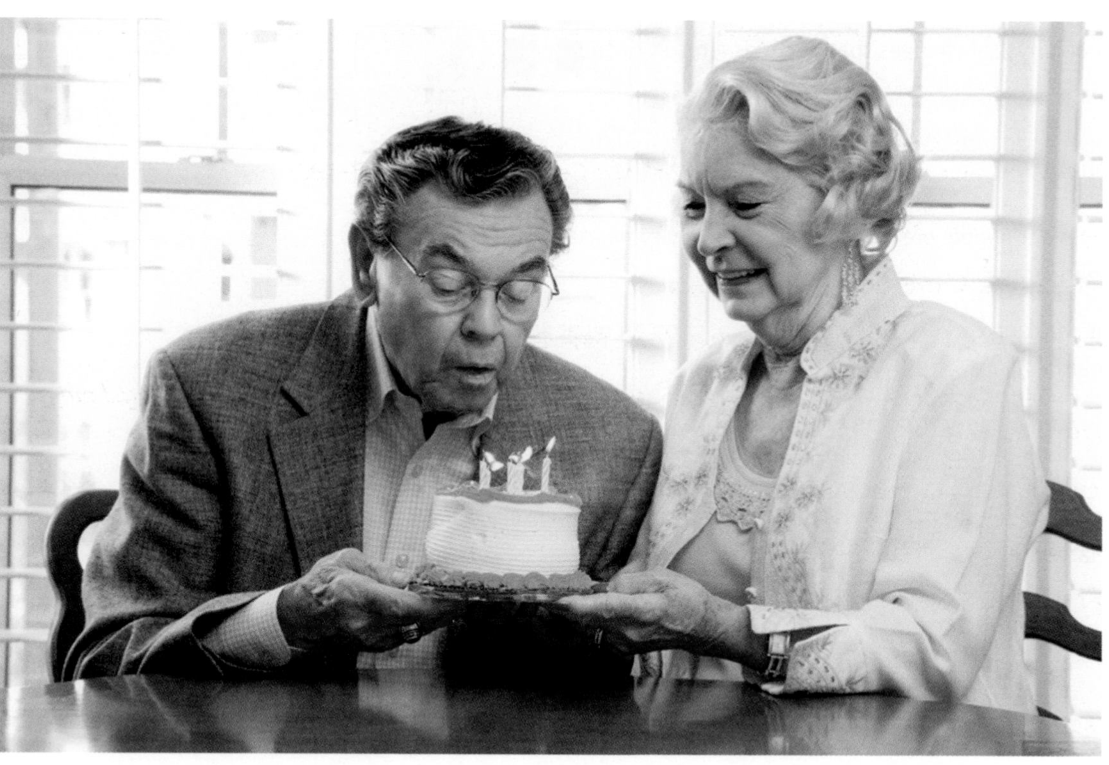

You can achieve a merit grade for the unit by presenting evidence that also meets all of the following merit criteria for the unit.

Assessment Criteria	Description	✓
M1	Discuss the nature–nurture debate in relation to the development of an individual.	☐
M2	Discuss two major theories of ageing in relation to the development of the individual.	☐
M3	Discuss the effects on self-esteem and self-confidence of the physical changes associated with ageing.	☐

You can achieve a distinction grade for the unit by presenting evidence that also meets all of the following distinction criteria for the unit.

Assessment Criteria	Description	✓
D1	Evaluate how nature and nurture may affect the physical, intellectual, emotional and social development of two stages of the development of an individual.	☐
D2	Evaluate the influence of two major theories of ageing on health and social care provision.	☐

References

Atchley, R.C. (1989) 'A continuity theory of normal ageing', *The Gerontologist*, 29, 183–190

Bee, H. (1995) *The Developing Child*, Harlow, Longman

Chomsky, N. (1959) *Syntactic Structures*, London, Mouton

Cumming, E. and Henry, W.E. (1961) *Growing Old*, New York, Basic Books

Denny, N. (1982) 'Ageing and cognitive changes' in Wolman, B. (ed) (1982) *Handbook of Developmental Psychology*, New Jersey, Prentice Hall

Erikson, E. (1968) *Identity: Youth and Crisis*, New York, Norton

Fennell, Phillipson and Evers (1989) *The Sociology of Old Age*, Milton Keynes, Open University Press

Pinker, S. (1994) *The Language Instinct*, London, Penguin

5 Anatomy and physiology in health and social care

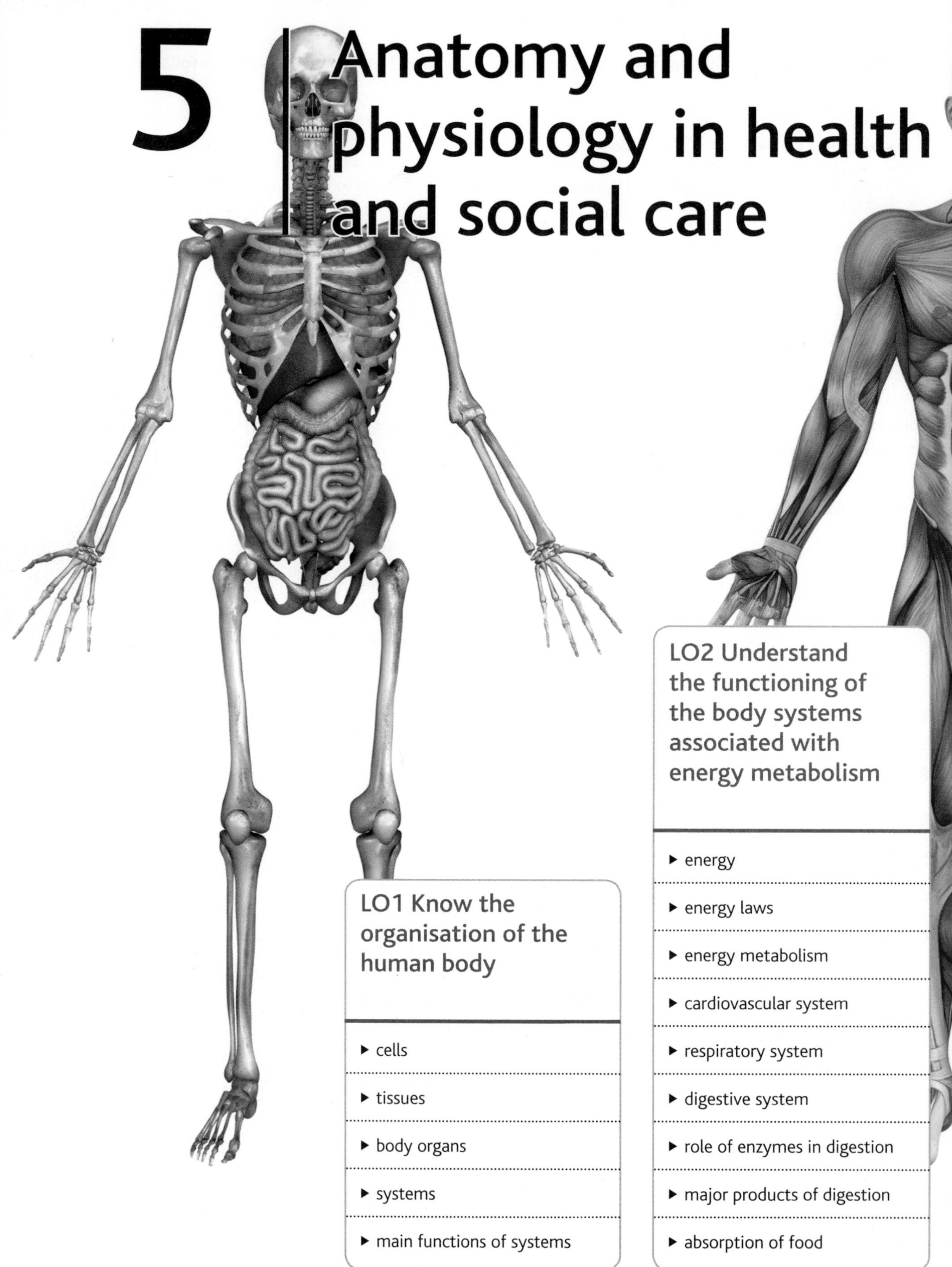

LO1 Know the organisation of the human body

- cells
- tissues
- body organs
- systems
- main functions of systems

LO2 Understand the functioning of the body systems associated with energy metabolism

- energy
- energy laws
- energy metabolism
- cardiovascular system
- respiratory system
- digestive system
- role of enzymes in digestion
- major products of digestion
- absorption of food

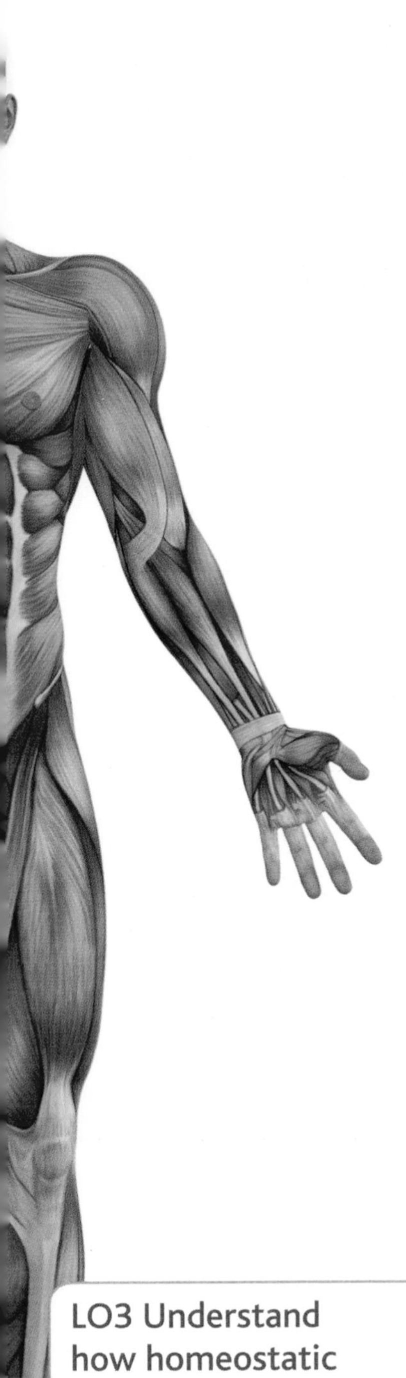

LO3 Understand how homeostatic mechanisms operate in the maintenance of an internal environment

- homeostasis
- homeostatic regulation

LO4 Be able to interpret data obtained from monitoring routine activities with reference to the functioning of healthy body systems

- measurement
- normal variations
- data presentation and interpretation

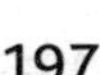

Organisation of cells in the human body

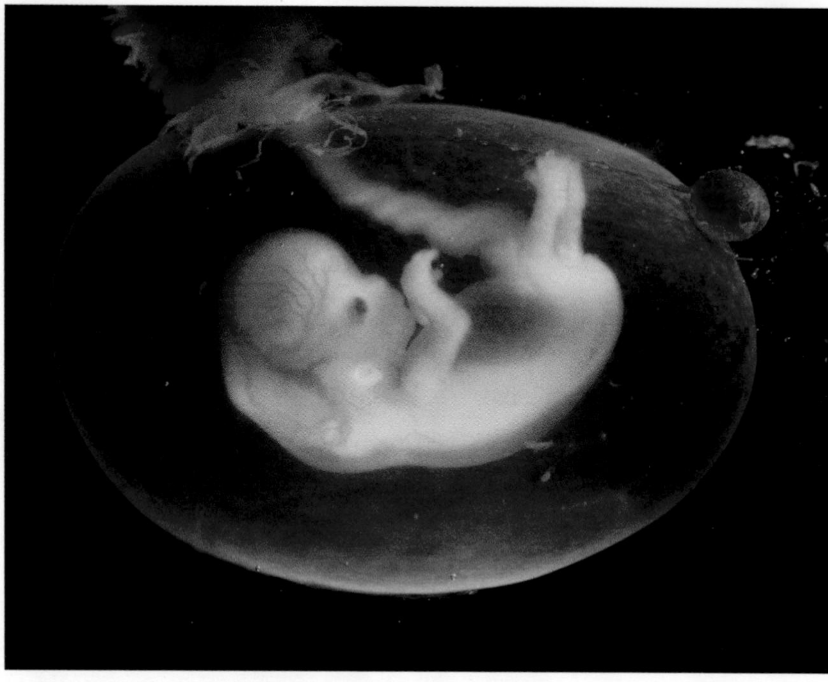

Human life begins at the cellular level.

Your assessment criteria:

P1 Outline the functions of the main cell components

Looking at the human body as if it were a machine, an engineer might ask two questions:

1. What is it made of?
2. What do the different parts do?

The first question requires an answer about *structure*. The second question requires an answer about *function*. Health and social care practitioners need to understand the organisation of the human body as a whole – in terms of both structure and function and how these features of human anatomy and physiology combine.

Discuss

In groups, discuss why health and social care practitioners need to know how the human body is organised.

P1 What is a cell?

There are about 50 trillion (50 million million) cells in your body. You began life as a clump of just eight very special **stem cells**. These eight cells made up the human embryo from which you developed. Each of these stem cells had the potential to develop into any of the different cells that make up your body. Over time, they divided and differentiated into specialist cells types – nerve, bone and muscle cells, for example – each with a specific function.

Key terms

Stem cells: *cells that are capable of renewing themselves and becoming many different cell types*

Cells are the smallest elements of the body, visible only with a microscope (see below). Each cell has three main parts:

1. a nucleus that controls the way the cells works – as a nerve cell, a muscle cell or a white blood cell, for example
2. cytoplasm, a jelly-like substance containing the internal structures that enable the cell to function (see page 200)
3. a **membrane** surrounding and protecting the cell.

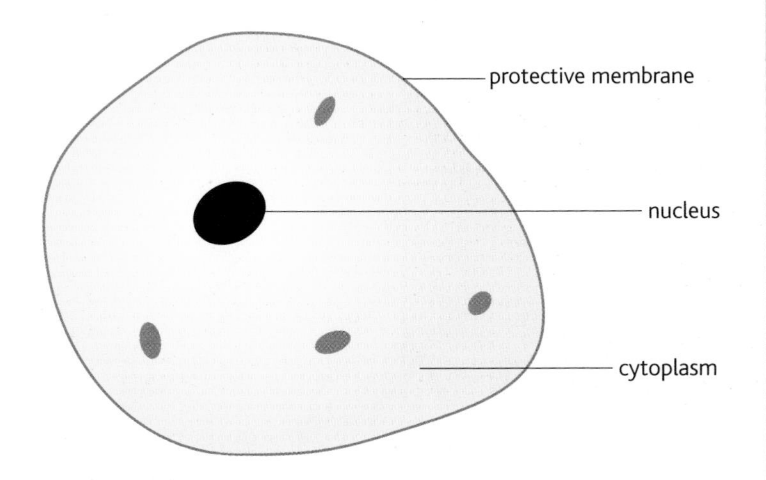

A human cell.

Key terms

Membrane: *the outer boundary of a cell*

The nucleus

The nucleus is the largest structure in a cell. Usually, there is only one nucleus in each cell, though there are some types of cell that have more than one nucleus (for example, muscle cells), and some red blood cells and bacterial cells have no nucleus at all. In general, the nucleus, found in the centre of the cell, is spherical in shape and contains the cell's **DNA**. The nucleus is surrounded by a **selectively permeable** plasma membrane that allows proteins and nucleic acids to pass through. The nucleus is the control centre of the cell, coordinating all of its functions.

Key terms

DNA: *the abbreviation of* Deoxyribonucleic acid, *a nucleic acid that contains the genetic instructions for the development and function of all known living organisms and some viruses*

Selectively permeable: *allowing some molecules to pass through gradually*

Your assessment criteria:

P1 Outline the functions of the main cell components

P1 Cytoplasm

Cytoplasm is the gel-like substance found between the outer cell boundary and the membrane surrounding the nucleus. It is where the various chemical reactions that make up the cell's metabolism occur. Cytoplasm contains a complex mix of chemicals and nutrients that are the basic living materials needed by the cell. Embedded in the gel, cytoplasm also contains a variety of cell organelles (see below).

Cell organelles

Cell organelles are various structures within a cell, each having their own distinct function. In some ways they are like mini-versions of the organs of the human body – hence the term 'organelles'. Key organelles include:

- mitochondria
- the endoplasmic reticulum
- the Golgi apparatus
- lysosomes.

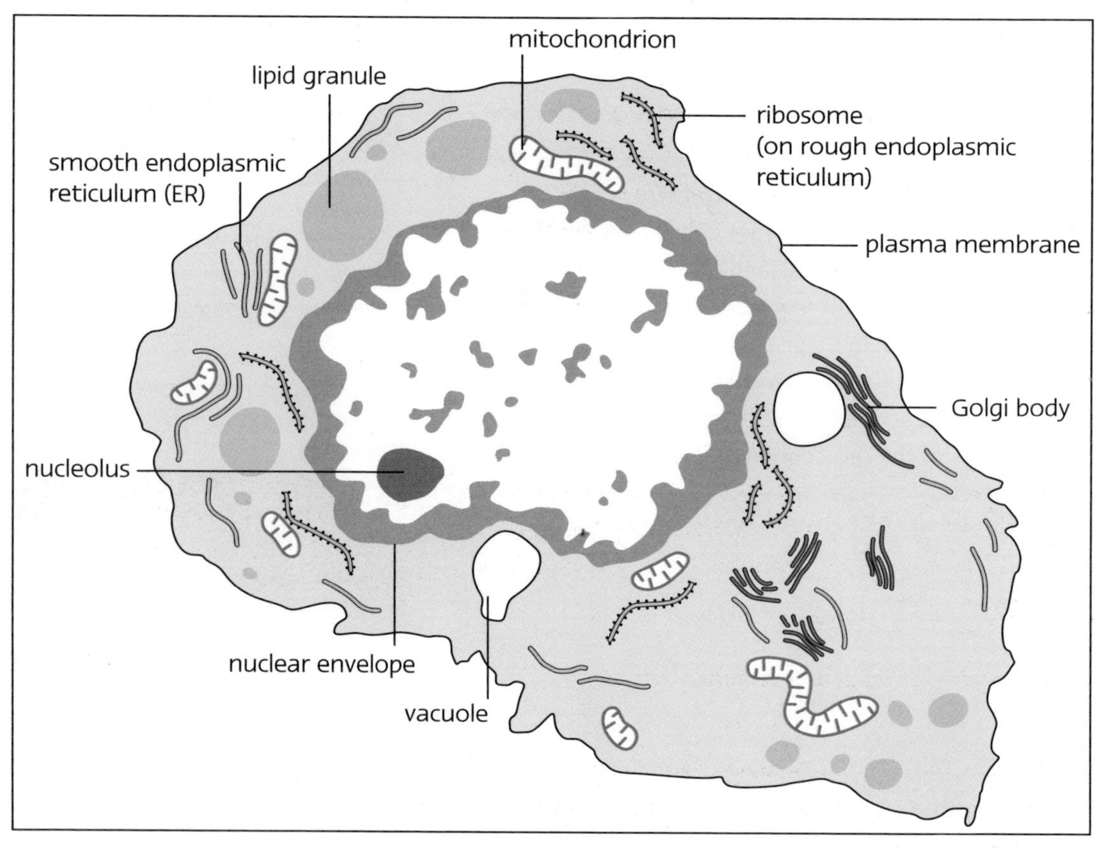

Figure 5.1 A typical human cell with organelles.

Mitochondria

These are bigger organelles that appear in large numbers in most body cells. They are usually sausage-like or spherical in shape. Their function is to make **ATP** through aerobic respiration. ATP is a molecule that provides chemical energy to cell processes. Mitochondria have an unusual double membrane structure: a smooth outer layer and a folded inner layer. The large internal surface of the inner layer enables the complex processes of aerobic respiration to take place.

The endoplasmic reticulum

Endoplasmic reticulum (ER) is a system of complex tunnels or channels spreading throughout the cytoplasm. The outside surface of the ER is known as 'rough ER'. This is because it has **ribosomes** attached to it, giving it a studded, bumpy or grainy appearance under a microscope. The function of the rough ER is to collect together and transport proteins made on the ribosomes. The second type of ER is known as 'smooth ER'. This doesn't have any ribosomes attached to it and is responsible for steroid (lipid hormone) production. It is also a storage site for calcium in skeletal muscle cells and contains enzymes that detoxify a variety of molecules.

The Golgi apparatus

This is a tightly packed group of flattened, fluid-filled cavities or vesicles that shift and change as vesicles are added and lost. The Golgi apparatus is thought to play an important role in synthesising and modifying proteins, lipids and carbohydrates. Proteins that are made on ribosomes attached to the ER are packaged into vesicles . These then join with the Golgi apparatus for protein modification. Once modified, proteins are secreted into lysomes or out of the cell.

Lysomes

These are best described as bags of digestive enzymes. They are found in cell cytoplasm and in small vesicles produced by the Golgi apparatus. They contain powerful **lytic enzymes** that can:

- destroy old or surplus organelles in a cell
- digest material taken into a cell, such as a bacterium or carbon particles
- destroy whole cells and tissues that are no longer required (for example, the muscle cells of the uterus after giving birth and milk-producing tissue after breast feeding finishes).

Key terms

ATP: *the abbreviation of* Adenosine triphosphate, *the major source of energy for cellular reactions*

Ribosomes: *small organelles that make proteins from amino acids*

Investigate

Use library and other resources to investigate the structure and function of a specialised cell. Draw a labelled diagram of the cell and explain its function in the body. How does the specialised cell differ from the typical or generalised cell shown in Figure 5.1?

Key terms

Lytic enzymes: *enzymes that break down materials*

Organisation of tissues in the human body

P2 What is a tissue?

A tissue is a group of cells of the same type, with the same structure and function. For example, the cells lining the inner surface of the gut form a tissue; muscle cells in a muscle form a tissue. There are four main types of human tissue:

1. **Epithelial tissue** consists of thin sheets of cells that line and cover a variety of body structures, such as the intestines for example.
2. **Connective tissue** is tough and fibrous, and holds parts of the body together. Ligaments and tendons are largely connective tissue.
3. **Muscular tissue** is present in all muscles, including the heart, and has the ability to contract, producing movement.
4. **Nervous tissue** consists of **neurons** that conduct electrical impulses, enabling communication between the brain and different parts of the body.

Your assessment criteria:

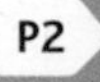

P2 Outline the structure of the main tissues of the body

Key terms

Epithelial, connective, muscular and nervous tissue: *the four types of tissue found in the human body*

Neuron: *a cell that specialises in conducting nerve impulses*

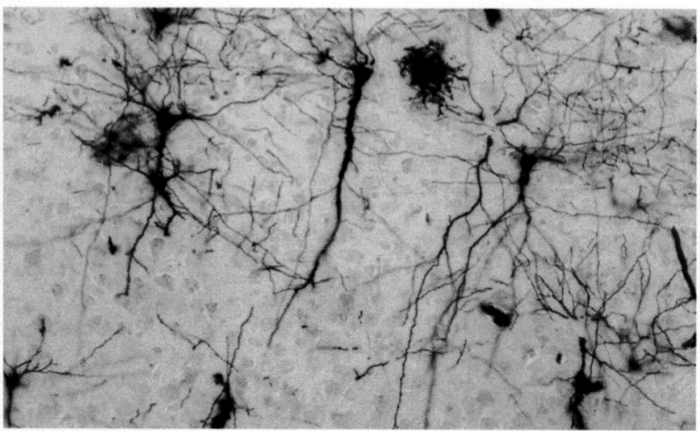

Epithelial tissue

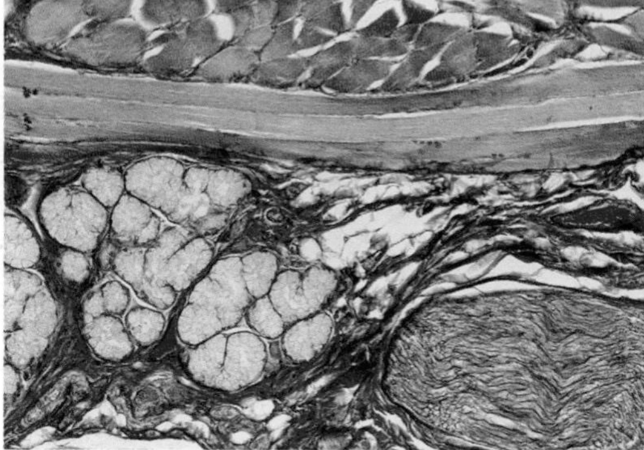

Connective tissue

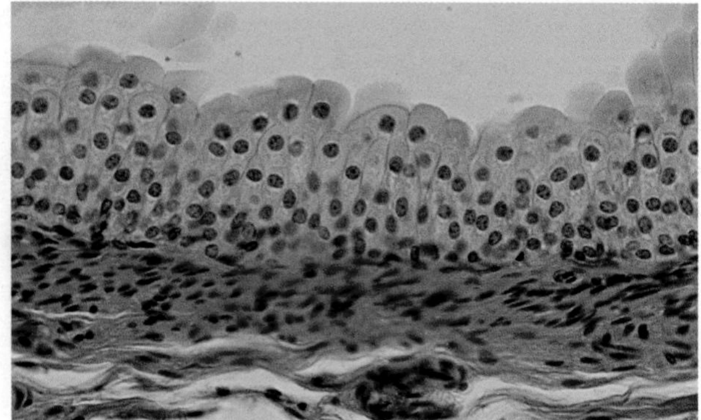

Muscular tissue

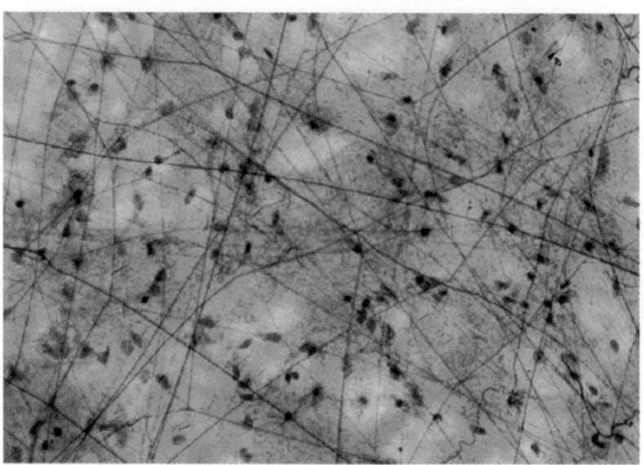

Nervous tissue

Epithelial tissue

Epithelial tissues are continuous sheets of cells that line the structures and cavities of the body. They act as barriers keeping different body systems separate. Different forms of epithelial tissue exist:

- **Simple squamous epithelium** consists of one layer of cells. This tissue can be found on the surface of lung alveoli where gases (oxygen and carbon dioxide) pass through.
- **Stratified squamous epithelium** consists of layers of cells that are replaced continuously. This tissue is found in the skin and in places like the mouth, tongue, oesophagus and vagina.

Ciliated epithelial tissue, a specialised form of simple squamous epithelium, in the nose forms a hair-like carpet that cleans the air going into the respiratory tract. The hairs trap dust and other particles, and remove them in mucous.

Connective tissues

These tissues connect body structures together and can be found throughout the human body (see Figure 5.2). All connective tissues, except blood, have a structural role in the body.

Key terms

Simple and stratified squamous epithelium: *two types of epithelial tissue*

Reflect

Suggest why it is important that squamous epithelial cells are replaced very quickly. (Hint: think about where this type of tissue is found in the body.)

Figure 5.2 The main types of connective tissue in the human body.

Tissue type	Function
Bone	Forms the skeleton, protects and supports body organs and anchors muscles.
Cartilage	Smoothes surfaces at joints, prevents collapse of trachea and bronchi.
Adipose	Stores fat and insulates the body.
Blood	Transports substances around the body.
Areolar	Protects organs, blood vessels and nerves, and strengthens epithelial tissue.

Unlike epithelial cells, connective tissue cells are not packed closely together. Instead, they are separated by a non-cellular matrix (a mesh) with a composition that gives each type of connective tissue its particular characteristics.

Bone

Bone is a specialised connective tissue. It consists of cells and a matrix embedded with fibres. The extracellular matrix becomes calcified, giving bone its characteristic hardness. The function of bone tissue is to:

- provide internal support for the body and sites for tendon and muscle attachment
- protect vital body organs
- store calcium and phosphate.

Bone tissue is formed continuously throughout life.

Cartilage

This is a tough, smooth and flexible connective tissue. Its function is to protect the surfaces of bones at the joints and to maintain the structure of the trachea and bronchus. Most of your nose and ear lobes are also made of cartilage!

Adipose tissue

Another connective tissue, this is body fat. Adipose tissue makes up 15–20% of an average person's weight. There are two types of adipose tissue:

- white adipose tissue provides insulation, stores energy and forms protective pads between organs
- brown adipose tissue generates heat and consumes energy; the percentage of brown adipose tissue reduces with age in human beings.

Adipose tissue is found beneath the skin, around the internal organs, in bone marrow and in breast tissue.

Your assessment criteria:

P2 Outline the structure of the main tissues of the body

Reflect

Can you think of two vital body organs that are protected by bone tissue?

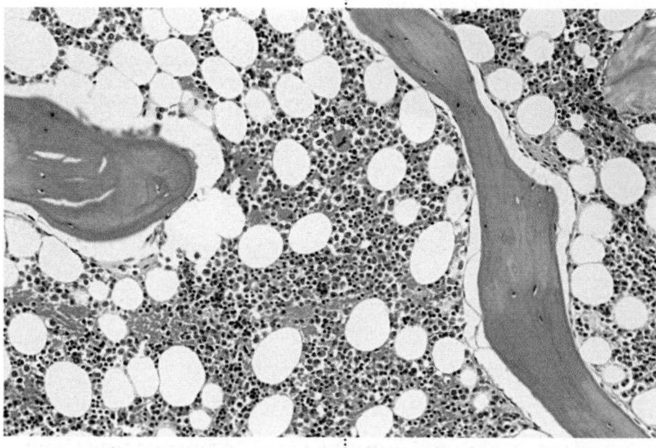

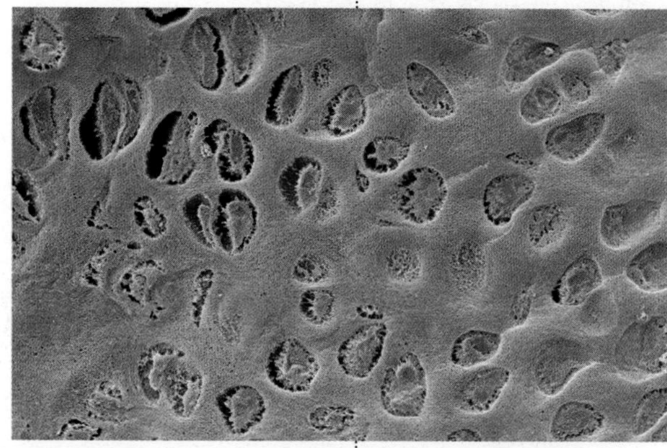

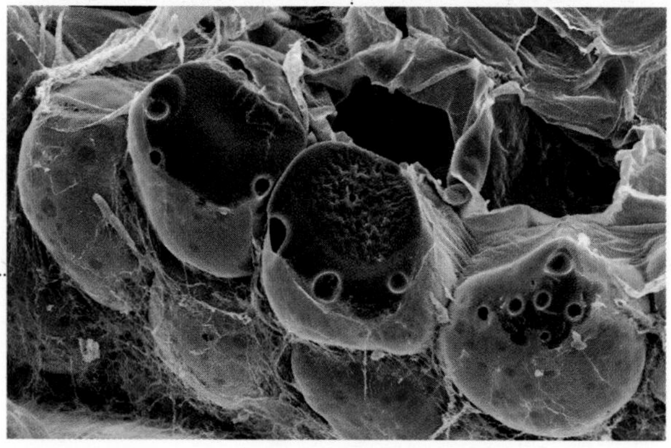

Blood

Blood is a fluid connective tissue in which plasma (a fluid) separates the cells.

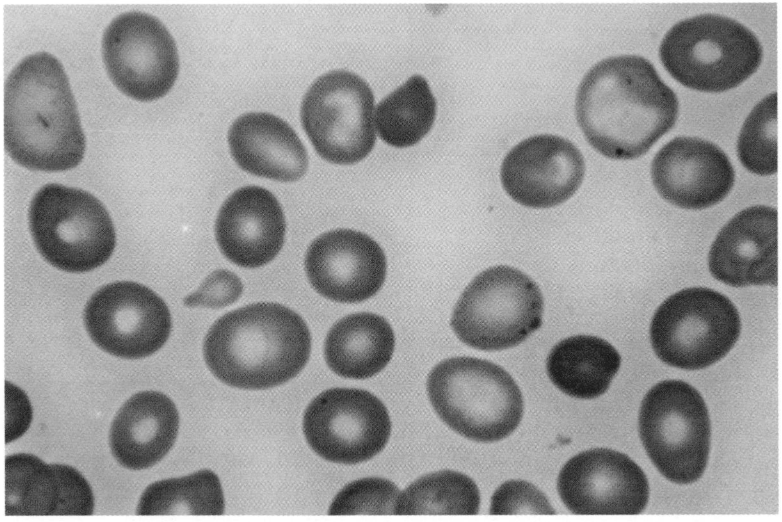

Areolar tissue

This is a loose connective tissue found in many different locations around the body. For example, it is found in the dermis and subcutaneous layers of the skin. Its function here is to bind the outer layers of skin to the muscles beneath. It can also be found around mucous membranes, blood vessels, nerves and the organs of the body.

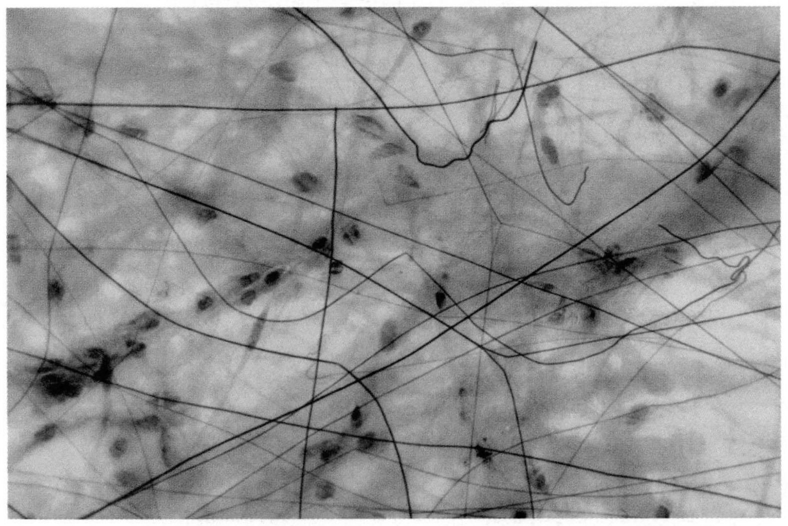

P2 Muscle tissue

Muscle tissues are unusual because they can contract and relax. They contain the protein fibres, actin and myosin. These cause movement when they slide over each other. There are three main types of muscular tissue (see Figure 5.3).

Figure 5.3 The main types of muscular tissue.

Tissue type	Function
Skeletal (striated)	Attached to the skeleton, produces movement and maintains posture. Can contract and relax rapidly and is under voluntary control.
Smooth (non-striated)	Found in tubular organs, glands, bronchioles, the reproductive system and the gut. This muscle tissue controls the movement of substances along tubes. It is not under voluntary control and movement is slow (see peristalsis on page 236).
Cardiac	Found in the heart, this has self-generating (myogenic) contractions that occur rapidly.

Nervous tissue

This contains elongated cells that transmit electrical impulses. The function of nervous tissue is to control and coordinate the activities of the body. Receptor cells (for example in the sense organs: eyes, ears, nose, mouth, skin) detect changes in the external and internal environment and send impulses along sensory neurones to the central nervous system (brain and spinal cord). The brain then processes this information and responds. Impulses that mediate the response are sent along motor neurones to the muscles and glands of the body.

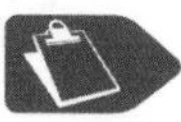

Case study

In the early hours of New Year's day, Andrew Reid, age 19, climbed up scaffolding erected around a building near to his local pub. He fell 7 m from the top of the scaffolding onto a grassy area. When paramedics arrived, they found him lying on his back, unable to move his arms or legs and complaining of neck pain. Andrew was awake, alert and aware of where he was, what day it was and what had happened; he was frightened because he could not feel his arms or legs. Other than scrapes to his arms, he had no other obvious injuries.

Your assessment criteria:

P2 Outline the structure of the main tissues of the body

Investigate

Using online and library resources investigate the following conditions:

- *hypertrophic cardiomyopathy*
- *Duchenne muscular dystrophy.*

Identify the type of muscle tissue that is affected by each of these conditions, the main changes that occur in the muscle tissue and the consequences of this for health.

Andrew was X-rayed on arrival at hospital. The X-ray showed that Andrew had fractured vertebrae in his spine. A few days later, a physical examination revealed that Andrew's vital signs were normal but that there was no change in his ability to move or feel sensations in his arms or legs. Andrew also had urinary incontinence and needed a catheter connected to a urine collection bag.

1. Why do you think Andrew was unable to move his arms or legs?
2. How have Andrew's injuries affected his nervous system's ability to function?

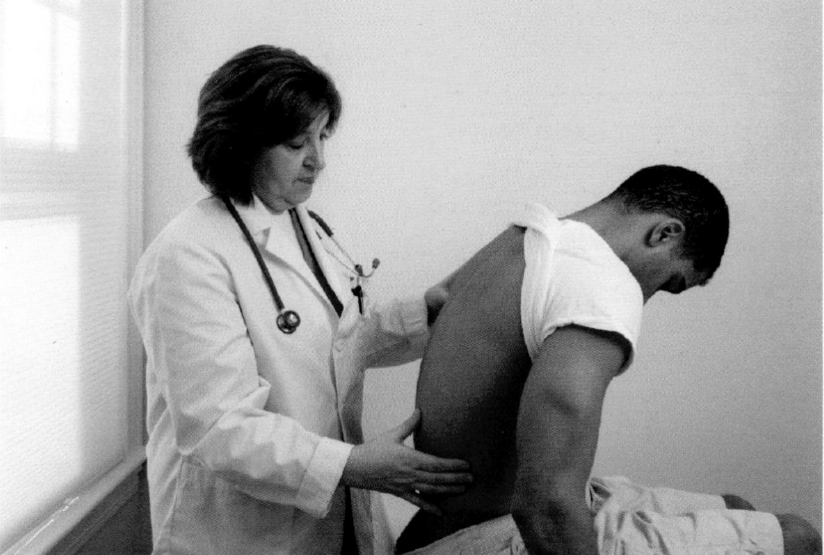

Back injuries can cause damage to both nervous and muscle tissues.

What do you know?

1. Can you identify three different types of body tissue?
2. Describe the purpose of epithelial tissue and identify one place in the body where it can be found.
3. Explain what connective tissue does in general.
4. What is the specific function of bone tissue in the human body?
5. What is adipose tissue and why do human beings need it?
6. Identify the type of muscular tissue that is only capable of slow movement and explain its function in the body.

Human organs

P3 How does the human body work?

One answer to this question is to point to the various **body organs** that carry out the vital functions necessary to sustain life. Each of the organs in the body has a specific function such as absorbing food, pumping blood or producing a hormone. You need to know where the organs are located in the body and also how they work together as **body systems** (see page 212).

Organs in the human body

An organ is a separate, recognisable body part, such as the liver or heart for example. Organs are made up of more than one type of tissue. The different types of tissues within an organ are grouped together in order to perform one or more specific function. Figure 5.4 shows where the major organs are located in the human body.

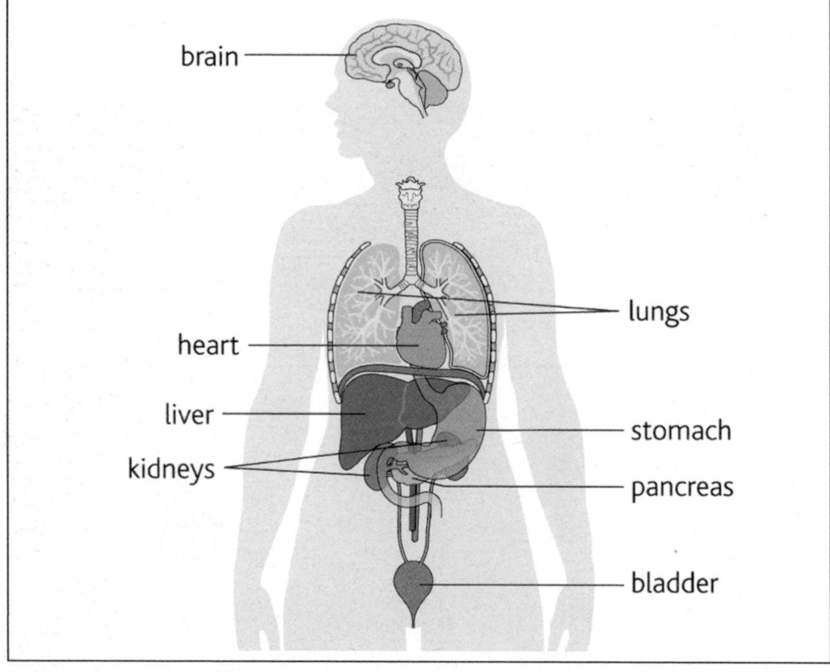

Figure 5.4 The locations of the major organs of the human body.

Your assessment criteria:

P3 Outline the gross structure of all the main body systems

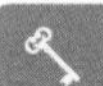

Key terms

Body organ: *a body part that has a particular function, such as the heart or the liver*

Body system: *a network or assembly of body organs that work together to achieve a particular goal, such as the respiratory system or cardiovascular system*

Reflect

How many different organs in the human body can you identify now? Make a list before you read through the rest of this topic!

The heart

The heart's vital function is to pump blood to the lungs and around the body. Blood delivers oxygen, nutrients, hormones and antibodies to all areas of the body, and takes away waste products. A normal size adult human heart is about the size of a clenched fist and is located in the **thoracic cavity** between the lungs. The heart and lungs are protected by the rib cage.

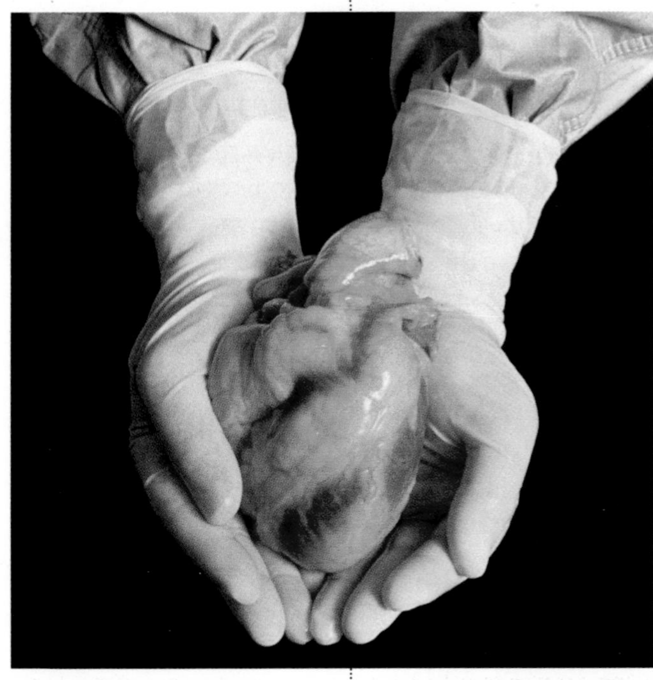

An adult human heart.

The lungs

The two main functions of the lungs are:

1. to transport oxygen from the atmosphere into the bloodstream
2. to remove carbon dioxide from the bloodstream and release it into the atmosphere.

The lungs are located in the chest or thorax, on either side of the heart (see Figure 5.5).

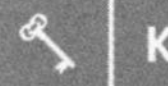

Key terms

Thoracic cavity: *the space between the neck and the abdomen*

The brain

The three main functions of the brain are:

1. to receive and respond to information about a person's environment
2. to coordinate and control physical functions, such as breathing, heart rate, balance and movement
3. to make the individual self-aware and able to think about others.

The brain, located in the skull, is a complex organ which acts as the control centre for nervous system and the body as a whole.

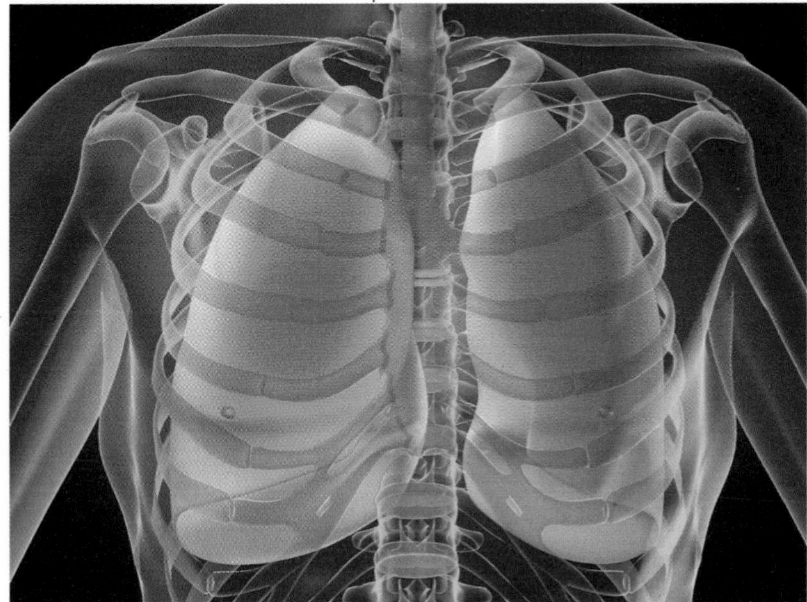

Figure 5.5 The lungs.

P3 The stomach

The main role of the stomach is to store food while some of the processes of digestion take place. In the stomach chewed solids are further broken down and mixed with digestive juices to form a liquid. Digestive **enzymes** in the juices **catalyse** the breakdown of food. Partly digested food moves from the stomach into the small intestine where further enzymes are released to complete the digestion process.

The liver

The liver is the largest internal organ in the human body. It is on the right side of the **abdominal cavity** just below the diaphragm. The liver performs a number of functions including:

- storage of iron and some vitamins
- removal of drugs, alcohol and other toxins from the blood
- in conjunction with other organs, control of glucose in the blood
- production of the heat that keeps the body warm
- production of the bile salts that break down fat in the small intestines.

The intestines

The intestines are part of the alimentary canal, extending from the stomach to the anus. As shown in Figure 5.6, the human intestine consists of two segments, the small intestine (duodenum and ileum)
and large intestine (colon):

- The small intestine is a greyish purple colour, 35 mm in diameter and about 6 to 7 m long in an average adult. The main function of the small intestine is to break down and digest food.
- The large intestine is dark red in colour and about 1.5 m long. It stores undigested food as faeces until it is passed out of the body through the anus.

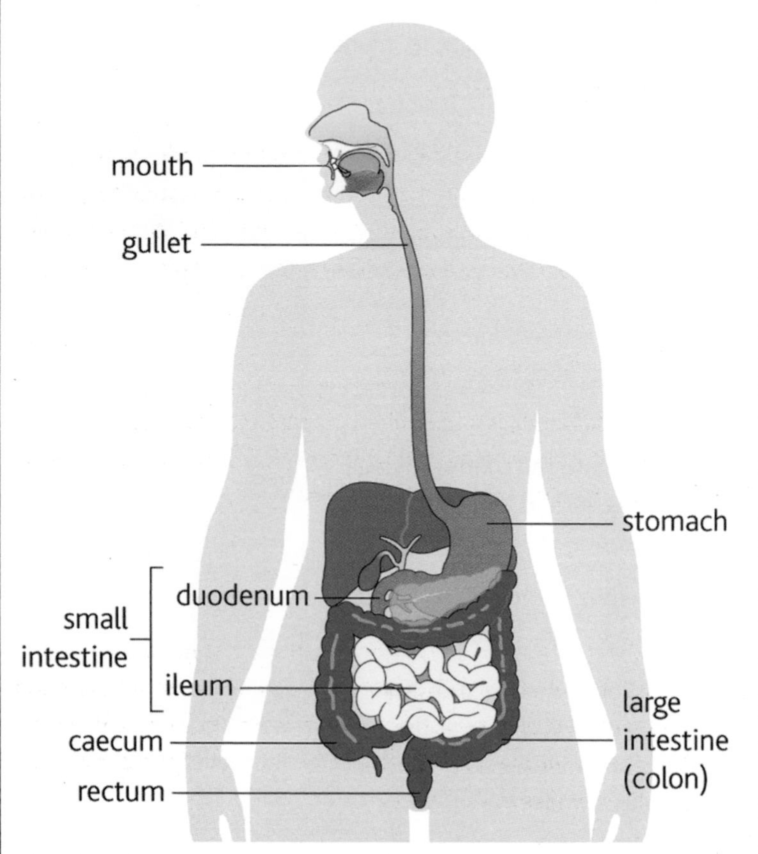

Figure 5.6 The human intestines.

Your assessment criteria:

P3 Outline the gross structure of all the main body systems

Key terms

Abdominal cavity: *the part of the body containing the stomach and the intestines*

Catalyse: *to speed up a chemical reaction using a catalyst*

Enzyme: *a complex protein that acts as a catalyst in specific biochemical reaction, without being changed by the reaction*

The pancreas

The function of the pancreas is to produce some of the hormones that control glucose levels in the blood and to secrete enzymes into the small intestine that help the body to break down and digest food.

The kidneys

The kidneys are located at the back of the abdominal cavity, one on each side of the spine, just below the level of the diaphragm. They are bean-shaped and weigh between 115 g and 170g in adults, with the left kidney slightly larger than the right. The kidneys filter out and remove excess salt, water and waste products from the blood, producing urine; they keep the composition of the blood balanced, maintaining correct levels of minerals, salts and fluids.

The bladder

The bladder's function is to store urine until it is excreted (removed) from the body. The bladder stretches when it fills and contracts when it is emptied.

Ovaries and testes

The testes are the male reproductive organs that produce and store sperm cells, and that manufacture the hormone testosterone. The ovaries are the female reproductive organs that produce and store eggs cells, and that manufacture the hormones oestrogen and progesterone.

The uterus

The uterus, or womb, is a muscular structure that protects and nourishes the baby as it is developing. During labour, it contracts and pushes the baby down the birth canal (see page 148).

The skin

The function of the skin is to protect the body, maintain body temperature, receive and communicate information from the person's environment (through touch, pain and pressure, for example) and to produce the sweat that carries waste products out of the body, as well as being part of temperature control.

Investigate

Using the internet and textbook sources, find out what an ileostomy and a colonoscopy involve, why these procedures are sometimes carried out and how they can affect a person. Produce a diagram or poster to explain how one of these surgical procedures affects the normal functioning of the intestines.

Human body systems

P3 What is a body system?

Particular structures in the body carry out particular functions. Biologists tend to link together into a system the structures that are involved in a particular major function (see Figure 5.7).

Your assessment criteria:

P3 Outline the gross structure of all the main body systems

Figure 5.7 Body systems, organs and functions.

System	Main organs (gross structure)	Main functions
Respiratory	Lungs, trachea, nose and mouth	Breathing and maintenance of oxygen supply
Circulatory	Heart and blood vessels	Transport and supply of materials to cells around the body
Digestive	Gut, liver and pancreas	Digesting and absorbing food materials
Endocrine	Pituitary gland, adrenal glands, thyroid gland, pancreas, testes and ovaries	Coordinating conditions *within* the body, particularly chemical changes
Nervous	Brain, spinal cord and nerves	Controlling and coordinating the body, often reacting to events *outside* the body
Renal	Kidney, bladder and ureters	Eliminating waste products from the body
Sensory system	Eyes, ears, nose, taste buds, skin	Detecting conditions outside the body
Immune	Lymph nodes, spleen, white blood cells	Protecting the body against illness
Reproductive	Penis and testes in males; vagina, uterus and ovaries in females	Producing offspring (reproduction)
Musculoskeletal	Muscles, bones and joints	Muscles and bones move the body; bones also help to protect delicate body parts and produce blood

Thinking about body systems

Thinking about organs arranged into body systems may help us to understand the way the body functions. However, it is not a completely accurate reflection of the way we are:

- The body is ***not* simply** a collection of separate systems. The overlap in function between systems means that changes in one system can produce signs in other systems too. For example, damage to the liver makes the skin look yellow due to an accumulation of a pigment that is normally broken down by a healthy liver. Damage to the nervous system may show itself as a lack of movement – an apparent failure of the musculoskeletal system.

- The body is ***not*** a machine; both structure and function change over time as part of the ageing process. The structures within the body of a human baby will have changed dramatically by the time he or she reaches 70 years of age (see page 190). For example, damaged parts will have been repaired, structures will have grown and overall height will have increased, and the reproductive system will have switched on at the beginning of puberty. In contrast, a washing machine does not age into a tumble drier – and it certainly cannot repair itself!

Organs can function in more than one system

Sorting the structures of the body into systems is not always easy, because some organs have a part to play in more than one system. For example:

- The penis is involved in both the reproductive and the excretory systems.
- The pancreas is an essential part of the digestive system but also produces a hormone, insulin, to control blood sugar levels. This means it is also part of the endocrine system.
- The skin is part of the immune system (it protects against foreign bodies), the sensory system (it is full of sensitive nerve endings) and the excretory system (it produces small amounts of urea in sweat).

What do you know?

1. Write a sentence to explain the scientific meaning of each of the following terms: *body organ* and *body system*.
2. Which is nearer to your head – the abdominal cavity or the thoracic cavity?
3. Identify two body organs found in the abdominal cavity and describe the function of one of them.
4. Describe the location and function of a woman's uterus.
5. Identify the body organs that make up the musculoskeletal system and the purpose of this body system.
6. Which body system is responsible for the maintenance of an oxygen supply?

Energy metabolism and the human body

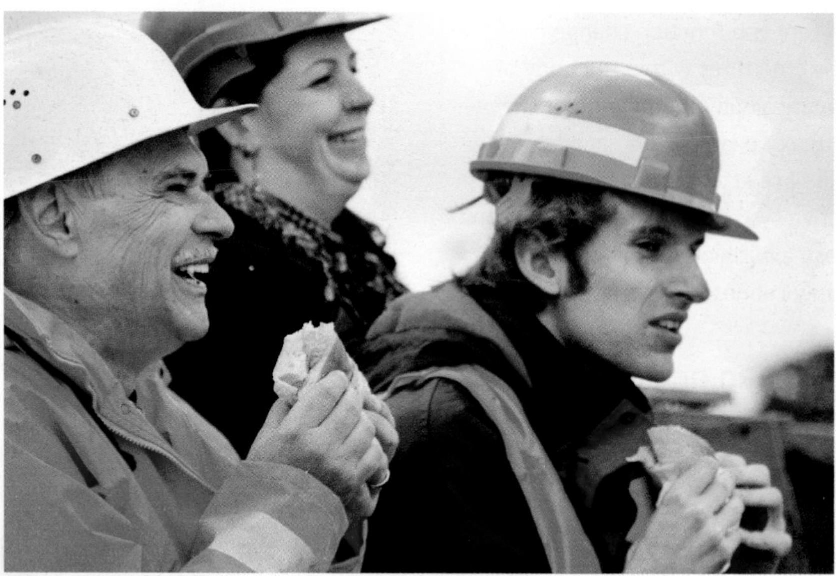

Food is the human body's main source of energy.

Your assessment criteria:

M1 Discuss the role of energy in the body

M1 Energy and the human body

One way of understanding the link between energy and the human body is to think of your body as a machine that won't work without an energy-rich fuel supply. Food is the source of this energy-rich fuel, but it cannot give you energy directly. Firstly, the food you eat must contain the kinds of materials (nutrients) that can be converted into energy. Then a number of processes have to occur to extract the energy from these materials. This process of converting food into energy is called **metabolism**.

The process of metabolism follows the first law of thermodynamics which says that:

Energy can be transformed from one form to another, but cannot be created or destroyed.

Energy exists in several different forms, including chemical, heat, light, sound and nuclear energy. Chemical energy is the main form of energy used by the human body. Chemical energy is found in the bonds between atoms in food molecules. When these bonds are broken, the energy in the bonds is released and the atoms are separated.

Key terms

Metabolism: *the chemical processes of a living body*

What do we need energy for?

The human body needs a constant supply of energy to stay healthy. The body uses energy to:

- grow – building new tissue uses up energy when raw materials are converted into the chemicals found in new cells
- repair – cells need energy to repair any damage
- move – muscles need a supply of energy for movement; the movements you can see and those you can't, such as the movements of heart and gut muscle
- build new chemicals – including the many chemicals made inside the body that you cannot see
- send nerve impulses – nerve tissue requires a constant supply of energy and dies very quickly if energy is not available
- stay warm – production of heat is an essential by-product of metabolism.

Energy is constantly leaving the body as heat. So, what stops the body from running out of energy like a battery in a torch? In biochemical terms the answer is **cellular respiration** (see Figure 5.8). In other words, if you eat and metabolise food you will acquire, convert and release the energy needed by your body! Providing your food supply is sufficient, your body's energy levels will stay topped up and will keep you alive. To summarise: ***nothing*** happens in your body without a supply of energy and that energy ***always*** comes from your food.

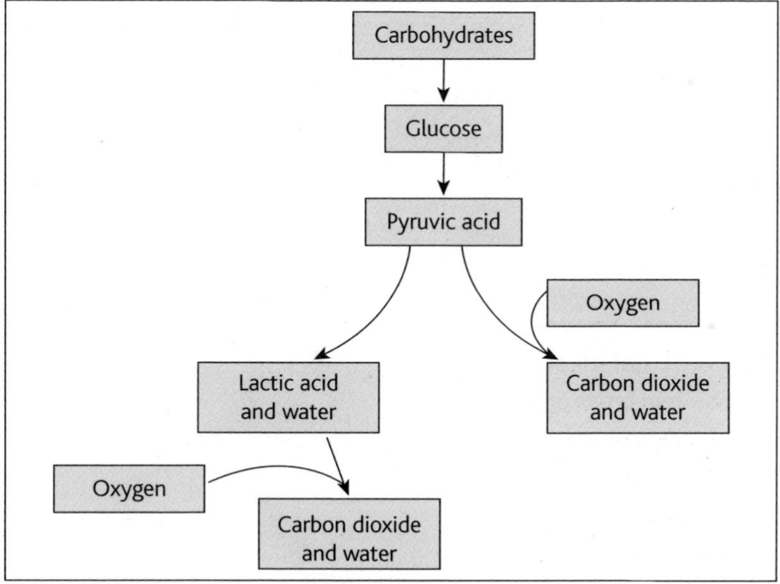

Figure 5.8 Aerobic and anaerobic respiration.

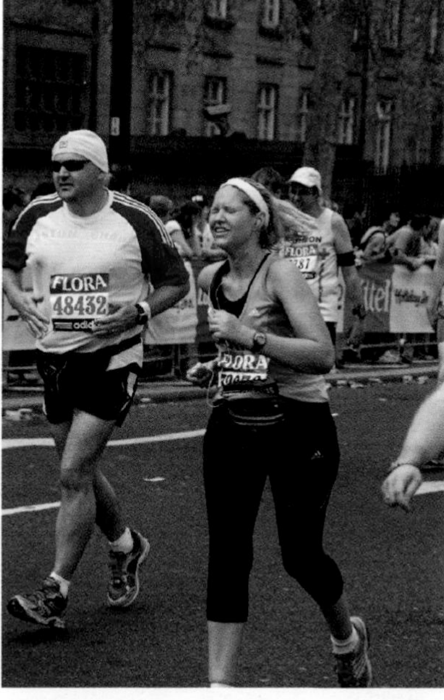

Muscles need an energy supply to function.

Key terms

Cellular respiration: *the breakdown of glucose (a sugar) to release energy in a form the body can use*

Reflect

Why do you think that people who compete in long distance races are usually given a small packet of biscuits or a chocolate bar as they cross the finishing line? How is this connected to their body's energy needs?

M1 Metabolic processes

Metabolism is best described as the set of chemical reactions that happen in the body's cells. Metabolism is happening constantly, with thousands of metabolic reactions all occurring simultaneously to keep cells healthy. There are two types of metabolic process:

- **Anabolism** supports the growth of new cells, the maintenance of body tissues and storage of energy for the future. Anabolism converts small molecules into larger more complex molecules of carbohydrate, protein and fat.
- **Catabolism** breaks down organic matter to harvest energy in cellular respiration and is sometimes referred to as 'destructive metabolism'. Cells break down large molecules (usually fats and carbohydrates) to release energy. This release of energy provides fuel for anabolism, heats the body and enables the muscles to contract and the body to move.

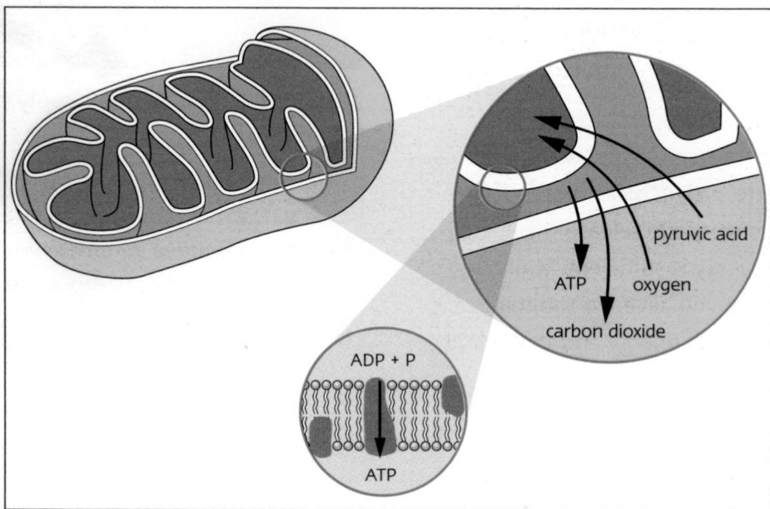

Figure 5.9 Where respiration happens in the cell.

Your assessment criteria:

M1 Discuss the role of energy in the body

D1 Analyse how two body systems interrelate to perform a named function/ functions.

Key terms

Anabolism: *this is a building and storing process and is sometimes called 'constructive metabolism'*

Catabolism: *the chemical process of breaking down molecules in body cells to release energy*

D1 How is energy supplied to body cells?

When a person eats food, they take in energy. The body, through physical processes and the action of enzymes in the digestive system, starts to break down the food. Enzymes in the digestive system break proteins down into amino acids, fats into fatty acids and carbohydrates into simple sugars (glucose). Sugar, amino acids and fatty acids can all be used as energy sources by body cells. These materials are absorbed from the digestive system into the blood where they are transported by the cardiovascular system to the liver and around the body. Once inside a cell, other enzymes regulate the chemical reactions to metabolise these molecules.

The respiratory system also plays a part because it supplies dissolved oxygen to the cells so that catabolic processes can occur, releasing energy. The cells can use the released energy or store it in body tissues, particularly in the liver, muscles and body fat. When a person consumes too much food, the energy it contains is stored as fat.

Investigate

Using biology or biochemistry textbooks or the internet, find out about the role of ATP (adenosine triphosphate) and ADP (adenosine diphosphate) in energy storage and release. Produce a summary identifying these chemicals and say what each does in the body.

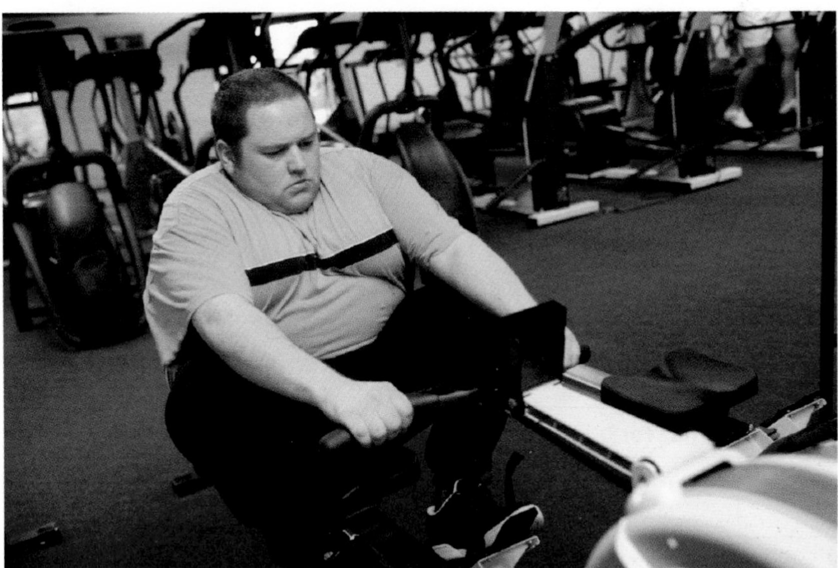

Exercise raises the heart rate and releases energy stored in body tissues.

What do you know?

1. Identify the vital source of energy for the human body.
2. Name the process of converting food into energy.
3. Explain why energy is important for the human body.
4. Name the two types of metabolic process.
5. Where do metabolic processes occur in the body?
6. Using you own words, describe how the digestive system, the cardiovascular system and the respiratory system play a part in metabolism.

The cardiovascular system and the heart

P3 What is the cardiovascular system?

The cardiovascular system consists of the heart, the blood and blood vessels (arteries, veins and capillaries). In basic terms, it is a pumping system; the cardiovascular system's function is to move substances around the body. Blood is the transport medium for the respiratory gases (carbon dioxide and oxygen), food and waste products.

Your assessment criteria:

P3 Outline the gross structure of all the main body systems

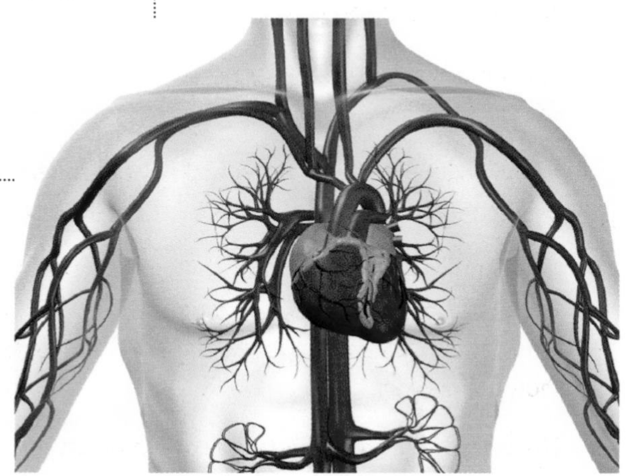

Figure 5.10 Substances carried by the blood.

Substance	Moved from	Moved to	What for?
Oxygen	Lungs	Every cell in the body	For use in respiration
Carbon dioxide	Every cell in the body	Lungs	To expel in exhaled air
Food substances	Gut	Every cell in the body	To be used for energy or to build chemicals
Hormones	Endocrine gland	Target organs	To control the way the organs work
Urea	Liver	Kidneys	To be excreted in urine
Antibodies	Lymph glands	Infected areas	To protect against disease
Heat	Hotter areas	Cooler areas	To equalise temperature across the body

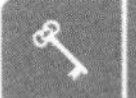

Key terms

Antibodies: *proteins made by the immune system to combat disease*

Structure of the heart

Figure 5.11 shows the structure of the heart. The heart has four chambers joined together in one large block of muscle:

- The heart has an upper area called the atrium and a lower area called the ventricle.

- Because there are two sides to the heart, there are four heart chambers (a right and left atrium, and a right and left ventricle).
- A major blood vessel enters or leaves each chamber.
- The pulmonary artery leaves the right ventricle and takes blood to the lungs.
- The pulmonary veins return the blood (now carrying oxygen) to the heart via the left atrium.
- The aorta is the main artery carrying blood to the body, exiting the left ventricle.
- The vena cava is the main vein bringing blood back from the head and neck (superior vena cava) and the rest of the body (inferior vena cava) to the heart.
- There are valves between the atria and ventricles, known as atrioventricular valves. These ensure that blood flows only one way though the heart.
- The pulmonary artery and aorta also have valves, known as semi-lunar valves, to ensure that blood which is pumped out of the heart doesn't re-enter the ventricles when the heart relaxes between beats.

In a resting adult human, the heart beats roughly 70 times per minute and completes 2.5 million beats in an average lifetime. The heart is located in the thoracic cavity between the lungs and is protected by the rib cage (see page 209).

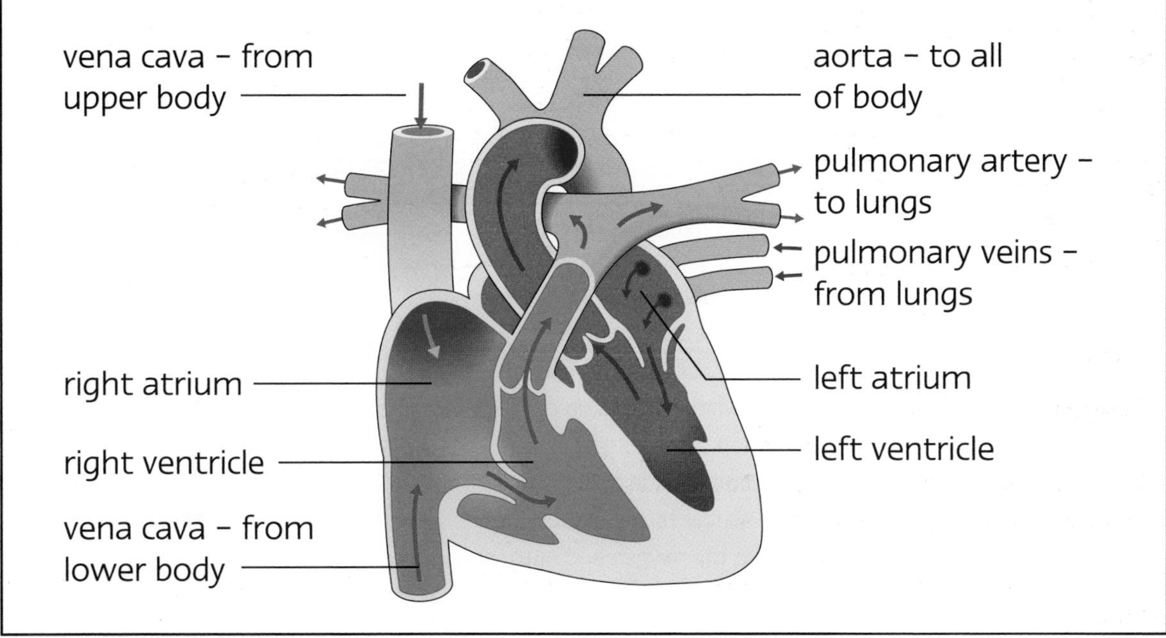

Figure 5.11 The heart.

The cardiac circulation and cycle

P4 Blood circulation through the heart

Figure 5.12 describes the way blood circulates through the heart. Specifically, the right side of the heart pumps blood to the lungs to pick up oxygen. The left side of the heart then pumps the oxygenated blood through the arteries to tissues around the body. Deoxygenated blood then returns to the heart through the body's network of veins. Figure 5.12 shows that:

- the pulmonary artery carries deoxygenated blood from the right ventricle to the lungs; it divides in two (the right and left pulmonary arteries) just outside the heart, so that it can carry blood to both lungs
- blood enters each atrium through pulmonary veins and leaves the heart through arteries in the ventricles
- the aorta is the main artery that takes blood from the left ventricle to the body
- the main vein bringing deoxygenated blood back to the heart from the body via the right atrium is the vena cava.

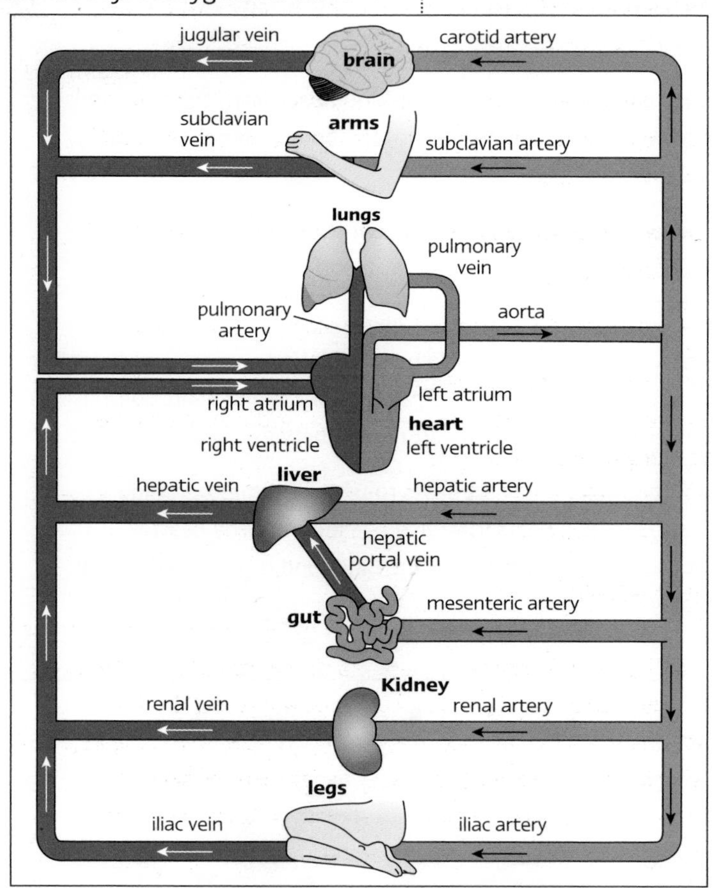

Figure 5.12 Circulation of blood

Because the blood passes through both sides of the heart in one cycle, the heart is said to have **double circulation**. You may also come across the terms **pulmonary circulation** and **systemic circulation**. Pulmonary circulation refers to the circulation of blood to and from the lungs where it picks up oxygen and releases carbon dioxide. Systemic circulation carries blood around the body, releasing oxygen and picking up carbon dioxide for removal. Every organ in the body has an arterial blood supply taking blood to it and a venous supply draining blood away when the oxygen and nutrients in it have been used up.

Your assessment criteria:

P4 Explain the physiology of two named body systems in relation to energy metabolism in the body

Key terms

Double circulation: *the passage of blood first through the lungs (pulmonary circulation) and then through the body (systemic circulation)*

Pulmonary circulation: *circulation of blood between the heart and lungs*

Systemic circulation: *circulation that supplies blood to all parts of the body except the lungs*

The cardiac cycle

The cardiac cycle is a term used to describe what happens every time the heart beats. If the average adult heart beats 70 times per minute at rest, each cardiac cycle lasts only 0.8 seconds. When the heartbeat quickens, the cardiac cycle gets faster too. A number of things happen during a cardiac cycle:

- step 1 – contraction of the atria forces blood into the ventricles
- step 2 – the ventricles fill with blood and force the atrio-ventricular valves to close (so blood doesn't flow back)
- step 3 – the muscular walls of the ventricles contract, increasing pressure on the blood and forcing open the semi-lunar valves in the aorta and pulmonary artery
- step 4 – contraction of the ventricles forces blood into the aorta and pulmonary artery
- step 5 – the ventricles start to relax and the semi-lunar valves close
- step 6 – when the ventricles are relaxed, the atrioventricular valves are pushed open by the blood that has been filling the atria and the cardiac cycle begins again at step 1.

Investigate

Using online or library resources, investigate heart valve disease. Find out about the causes, symptoms and treatment of this heart condition. Present your findings in the form of a leaflet or poster to inform others of your main findings.

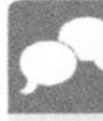

Discuss

What can people do to keep their hearts healthy and functioning well? Identify the strategies that you already use or which you know about and share ideas with a small group of class colleagues. Is there anything else that you could, or think you should do, to protect yourself from heart disease and to have a healthier heart?

Case study

Eddie Jones, a 55-year-old lorry driver, went to his GP complaining that he had been feeling dizzy and light-headed for several weeks. He had also collapsed whilst unloading a delivery, hitting his head in the process. Mr Jones's GP referred him to the cardiology department of his local hospital for urgent investigation. Following a series of tests, including an electrocardiogram (ECG), Eddie Jones was diagnosed as having third-degree atrioventricular (AV) block, a potentially life-threatening bradycardia (slow heart beat). The hospital consultant responsible for his care recommended that Eddie should have a pacemaker fitted urgently.

1. What is happening in Eddie's heart to cause his symptoms?
2. Explain what a pacemaker does when it is implanted in the human body.
3. What might happen to Eddie if he does not have a pacemaker fitted and his condition cannot be treated in another way?

Heartbeat and blood pressure

P4 Organising the heartbeat

All the events described in step 1 to 6 of the cardiac cycle (see page 221) happen in a single heartbeat! As we know, the heart is made up of muscle cells. If the heart's muscle cells contracted and relaxed in an uncoordinated way, the heart would simply quiver like a nervous jelly! This quivering, disorganised contraction is called **fibrillation**. So, how does the heart organise the contraction and relaxation of the muscle cells in different parts of the heart to produce a functional heartbeat?

The contraction of a heartbeat starts off in a small area of the left atrium called the sinoatrial node. This area of specialised cells produces a signal which causes heart muscle cells to contract. The signal passes across the top of the heart, making the atria contract and forcing blood into the ventricles. Another specialised area called the atrioventricular node, near the base of the atrium, picks up the signal and sends it quickly down the bundle of His to the muscles of the ventricles. The signal then causes the muscles of the ventricle wall to contract – this happens slightly after the atria have finished contracting. As the ventricles finish contracting, the sinoatrial node starts the whole process off again.

Your assessment criteria:

P4 Explain the physiology of two named body systems in relation to energy metabolism in the body

Key terms

Fibrillation: *erratic electrical activity of the heart*

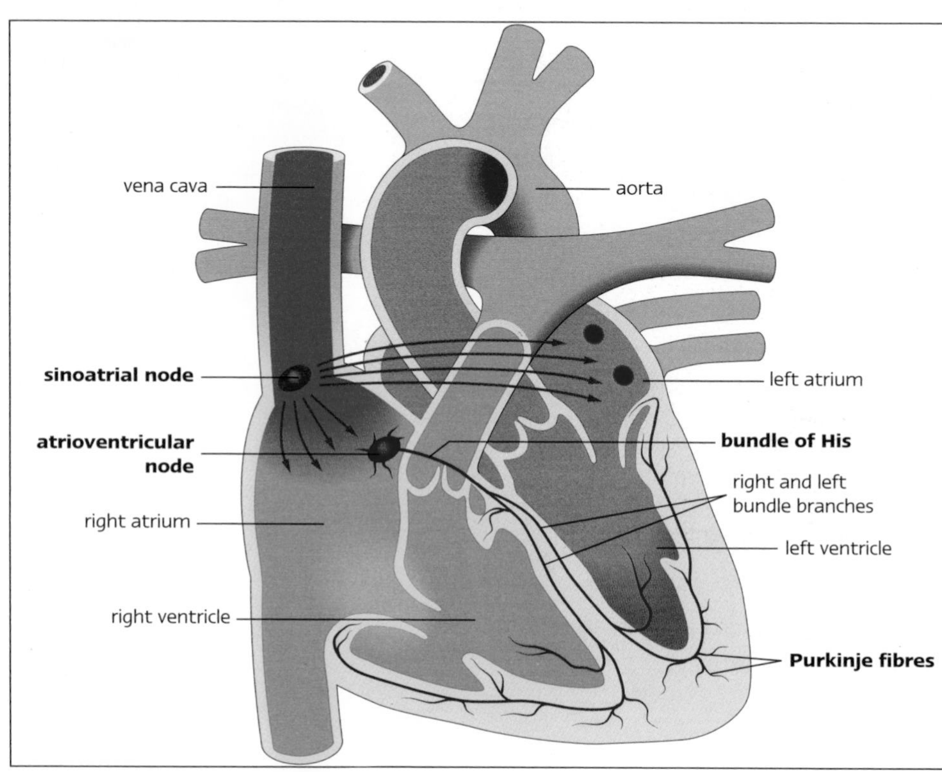

Figure 5.13 Coordinating a heartbeat.

Heart rate and stroke volume

The volume of blood pushed out of a person's heart in 1 minute is called the cardiac output. This is calculated by recording a person's heart rate (the number of beats per minute) and by measuring the stroke volume (the volume of blood pushed out of the left ventricle per minute). On average, a healthy adult has a stroke volume of 70 cm^3 and a heart rate of about 70 beats per minute.

Blood pressure

When a health professional checks your blood pressure, two measurements are made:

1. the force, or pressure, which the blood puts on the walls of an artery when the heart beats; this is known as the **systolic blood pressure**
2. the continuous pressure that the blood puts on the arteries between heart beats; this is known as the **diastolic blood pressure**.

Therefore, a blood pressure reading is recorded as two numbers. The systolic measure comes first, followed by the diastolic measure. On average, a healthy young adult will have a blood pressure reading of 120/80 mm Hg (millimetres of mercury is a unit of measurement of pressure).

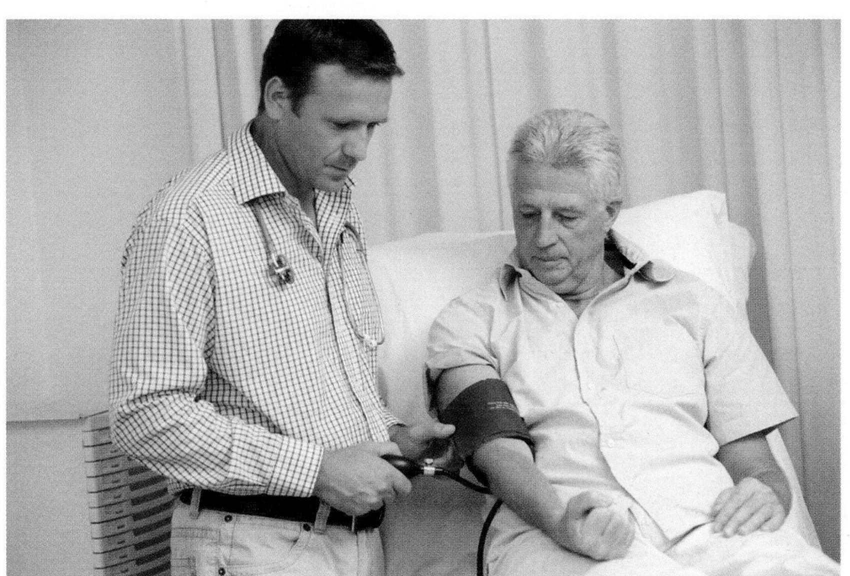

A person's blood pressure is an indicator of their cardiac health.

Reflect

Would you expect a very fit person's stroke volume to be higher or lower than that of an average person? What about their heart rate?

Key terms

Diastolic blood pressure: *the second or bottom figure of a blood pressure reading, showing the minimum pressure in the arteries between beats of the heart*

Systolic blood pressure: *the first figure in a blood pressure reading that indicates the maximum pressure in the arteries when the heart beats*

Blood vessels and blood

P3 P4 Blood vessels

Arteries are the tubes that carry oxygenated blood away from the heart to organs and tissues around the body. Arteries deliver blood to smaller blood vessels called arterioles, which in turn supply **capillaries**. The pulmonary and umbilical arteries are the exceptions to the rule that arteries carry oxygenated blood. The pulmonary artery carries deoxygenated blood from the heart to the lungs where the blood picks up oxygen; during pregnancy, the umbilical artery carries deoxygenated blood from the foetus to the placenta where oxygen transfers from the mother's blood to the foetus's blood.

Veins and smaller venules are the tubes that carry blood from the body back towards the heart. Both arteries and veins can get wider or narrower to control the flow of blood to different organs. When they get wider, or dilate, more blood flows but when they get narrower, or constrict, the blood flow drops. Every major body organ has its own artery and vein.

All the arteries branch off the aorta. When the left ventricle of the heart contracts it pushes a surge of blood into the aorta. The aorta stretches slightly in response to the increase in pressure. When the ventricle is filling with blood, the walls of the aorta spring back and squeeze on the blood. This stretching and contracting helps to smooth out the flow of the blood, but cannot stop the surging completely. Where an artery runs over a bone or near to the surface of the body, you can feel the blood surges through the skin. This is the pulse. Every pulse beat corresponds to a heartbeat.

Capillaries are the smallest blood vessels in the body and have walls that are only one cell thick. Capillaries join arteries to veins. They carry blood into every part of the body and allow food and oxygen to pass from the blood to the body tissues. Waste products pass the other way. No cell in the body is more than 1 mm away from a capillary.

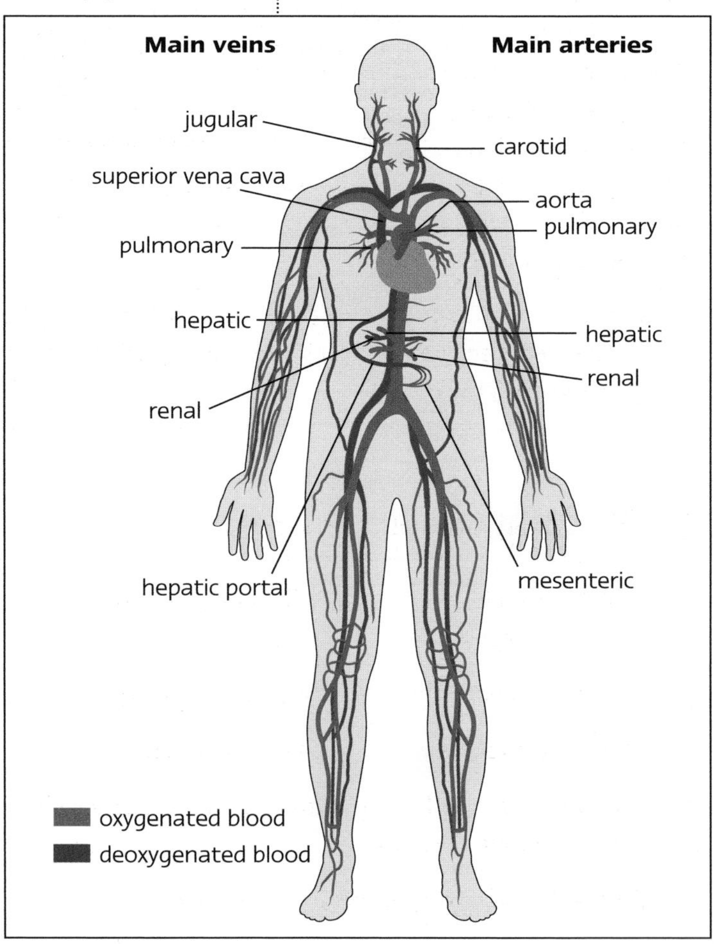

Figure 5.14 Blood supply to the major organs of the body.

Your assessment criteria:

- **P3** Outline the gross structure of all the main body systems
- **P4** Explain the physiology of two named body systems in relation to energy metabolism in the body

Key terms

Capillaries: *the smallest of the body's blood vessels, with a diameter just larger than that of a red blood cell*

The blood

A normal adult male will have roughly 6 litres of blood, comprising about 8 per cent of their total body weight. The blood is a complex mixture of substances with different components doing different jobs. For example, the red cells carry oxygen around the body, while the white cells protect against disease. Figure 5.15 gives the main blood components and their functions.

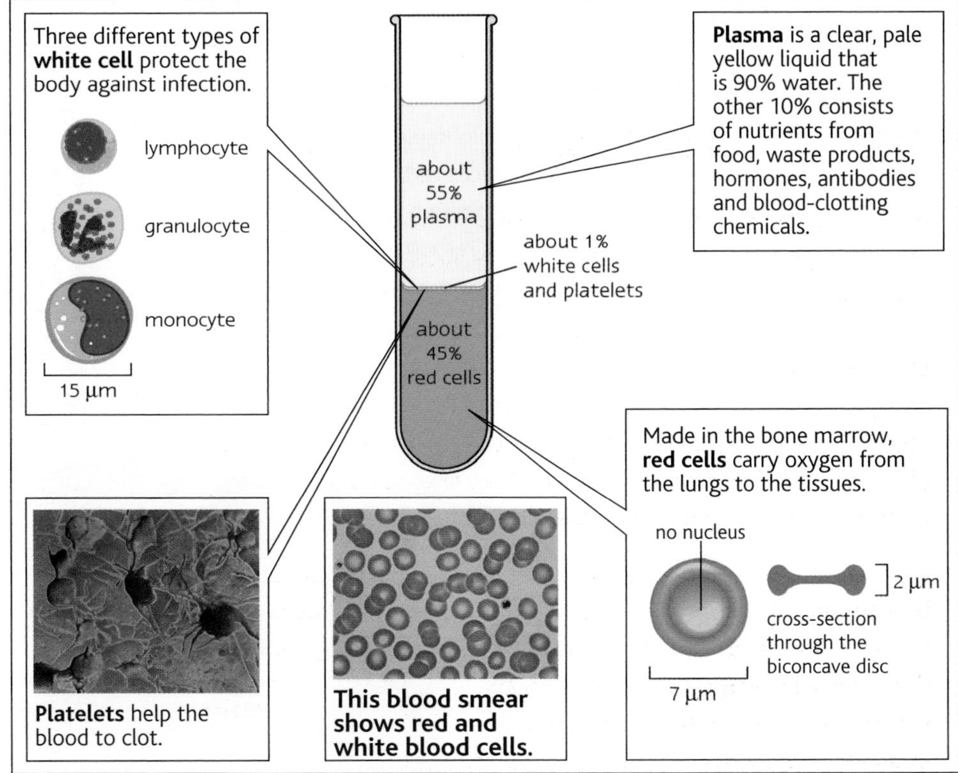
Three different types of **white cell** protect the body against infection.
lymphocyte
granulocyte
monocyte
15 µm
about 55% plasma
about 1% white cells and platelets
about 45% red cells
Plasma is a clear, pale yellow liquid that is 90% water. The other 10% consists of nutrients from food, waste products, hormones, antibodies and blood-clotting chemicals.
Made in the bone marrow, **red cells** carry oxygen from the lungs to the tissues.
no nucleus
2 µm
cross-section through the biconcave disc
7 µm
Platelets help the blood to clot.
This blood smear shows red and white blood cells.

Figure 5.15 Blood components and functions.

The blood is monitored constantly by the body to make sure the level of every single component remains within healthy limits. It is a dynamic system with old components being destroyed at the same rate as replacement parts are made.

As we have seen, no cell in the body is more than 1 mm away from the blood. This means any poisons that get into the blood spread rapidly and dangerously through the body.

What do you know?

1. Identify three physical structures that are part of the cardiovascular system.
2. Describe the purpose of the cardiovascular system.
3. What are the four chambers of the heart called?
4. Using your own words, or by drawing a diagram, explain how blood circulates through the heart.
5. Identify the main components of human blood.
6. Explain how blood is transported to organs and tissues around the body.

The respiratory system: structure and function

Human beings need energy for movement, growth and repair of tissues and to keep body temperature stable. This energy is obtained through **respiration**. Respiration uses glucose and oxygen and produces carbon dioxide, water and energy (as adenosine triphosphate or ATP). Respiration must happen continuously to sustain human life. The respiratory system is responsible the supply of oxygen that keeps this process going, and for removing some waste products.

Your assessment criteria:

P3 Outline the gross structure of all the main body systems

P4 Explain the physiology of two named body systems in relation to energy metabolism in the body

P3 Structure of the respiratory system

The **respiratory system** (the lungs, trachea, nose and mouth, moves air in and out of the lungs, allowing the body to absorb oxygen and remove carbon dioxide. The respiratory system works with the **cardiovascular system** to make sure every cell in the body has a supply of oxygen and can get rid of waste carbon dioxide. Figure 5.17 shows the respiratory organs that make up the respiratory system.

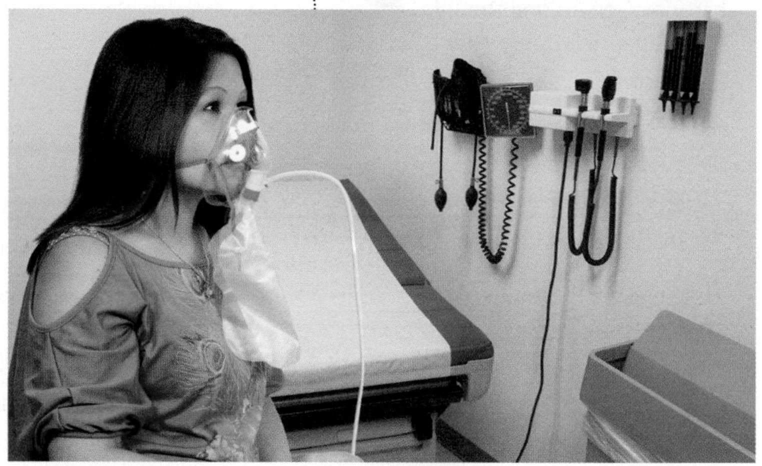

Respiration is essential for life.

P4 The terms 'respiration' and 'breathing'

The term 'respiration' covers:

- 'breathing', the movement of air in and out of the lungs
- **gaseous exchange** in the lungs
- transport of oxygen and carbon dioxide through the blood
- respiration in body cells (cellular respiration).

The process of respiration is illustrated in Figure 5.16.

Key terms

Cardiovascular system: *the organs and tissues involved in circulating blood through the body*

Gaseous exchange: *the exchange of respiratory gases (oxygen and carbon dioxide) by diffusion across the walls of the alveoli in the lungs*

Respiration: *the biological term for breathing, but also the term used to describe the process through which cells obtain chemical energy (cellular respiration)*

Respiratory system: *the organs and body structures that allow respiration to occur in the human body*

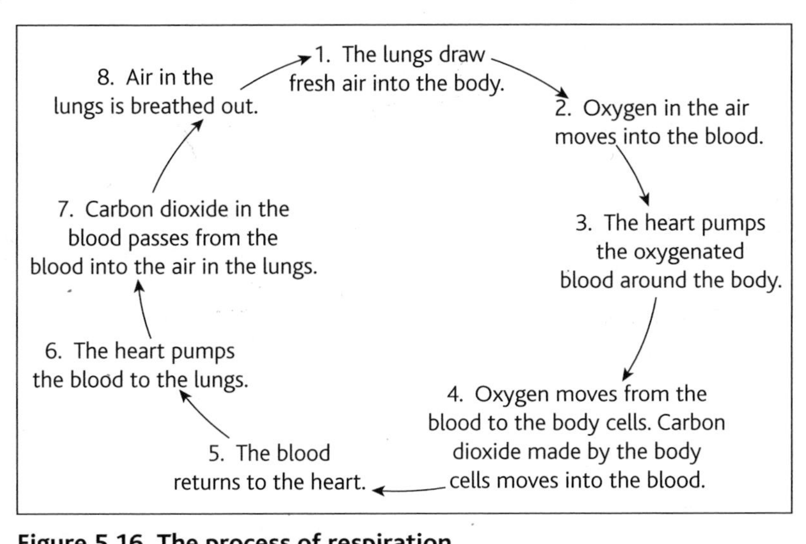

1. The lungs draw fresh air into the body.

5. The blood returns to the heart.
6. The heart pumps the blood to the lungs.

Figure 5.16 The process of respiration.

Investigate

Using the internet or human biology textbooks, find out about the composition of atmospheric air and how this is different from that of exhaled air. Summarise your findings in a table.

P3 P4 The lungs

A typical pair of human lungs weighs just over 1 kg and fits into a space that measures less than 40 cm from top to bottom. However, the lungs have surface area for gaseous exchange of over 80 m^2. For comparison, the skin surface area in the same person is roughly 2 m^2! The enormous surface area in the lungs is produced by 500 million small sacs called alveoli. **Alveoli** (singular = alveolus) are balloon-like swellings on the ends of **bronchioles**, the thinnest tubes in the lungs which carry air directly into the alveoli. The alveoli are made from a thin membrane, covered with tiny blood vessels.

Travelling up from the alveoli, the bronchioles connect to the **bronchi**, rather like the branches on an upside-down tree. The bronchi join together to form the **trachea** (the trunk of the tree), also called the windpipe. Rings of stiff cartilage help to stop the trachea and bronchi being squashed flat by the breathing movements. The ribs and sternum (breast bone) protect the lungs and heart.

Key terms

Alveoli: *small air bags at the end of airways, where oxygen and carbon dioxide move in and out of the blood*

Bronchi: *two airway passages, one to each lung, in the respiratory tract (singular = bronchus)*

Trachea: *the windpipe that connects the larynx to the bronchi*

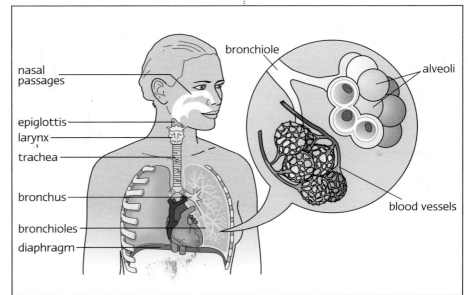

Figure 5.17 The lungs.

The respiratory system: breathing and gas exchange

P3 P4 What causes breathing movements?

The lungs are unable to move on their own as they have no muscle. However, the air in the lungs would soon run out of oxygen if breathing did not happen. Breathing, sometimes also called **ventilation**, is the movement of air into and out of the lungs. The lungs inflate and deflate due to the action of different sets of muscles:

- The external **intercostal muscles** (between the ribs) contract, pulling the ribs upwards and outwards. This pulls on the surface of the lungs (the pleural membranes), sucking air into the lungs.
- When the internal intercostal muscles contract, the ribs are pulled down. This squeezes air out of the lungs.

Your assessment criteria:

P3 Outline the gross structure of all the main body systems

P4 Explain the physiology of two named body systems in relation to energy metabolism in the body

Key terms

Intercostal muscles: *groups of muscles that run between the ribs, helping to form and move the chest wall*

Ventilation: *the process of inhaling and exhaling*

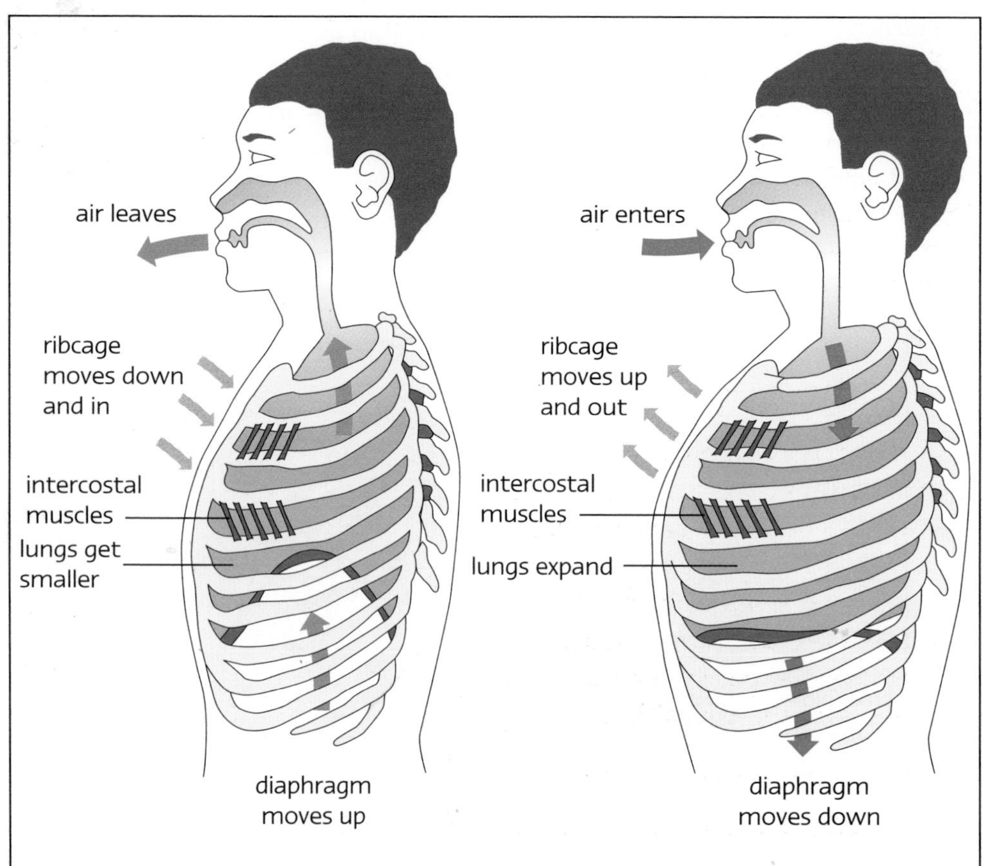

Figure 5.18 Ventilation of the lungs.

Gas exchange

Air enters the body through the nose or mouth. The nose contains fine bones covered with ciliated mucus membrane (epithelial tissue with fine hairs) which warms and moistens the air. The air passes into the throat, where it enters the trachea and then goes into the bronchi. The air then filters through the sub-dividing bronchioles and into the alveoli. This is where gaseous exchange takes place.

The lungs are responsible for exchanging gases (especially oxygen and carbon dioxide) between the blood and the air outside of the body. Oxygen diffuses rapidly through the walls of the alveoli and into the blood, combining with haemoglobin in red blood cells. At the same time, carbon dioxide diffuses out of the blood into the alveoli and back through the air passages until it is breathed out.

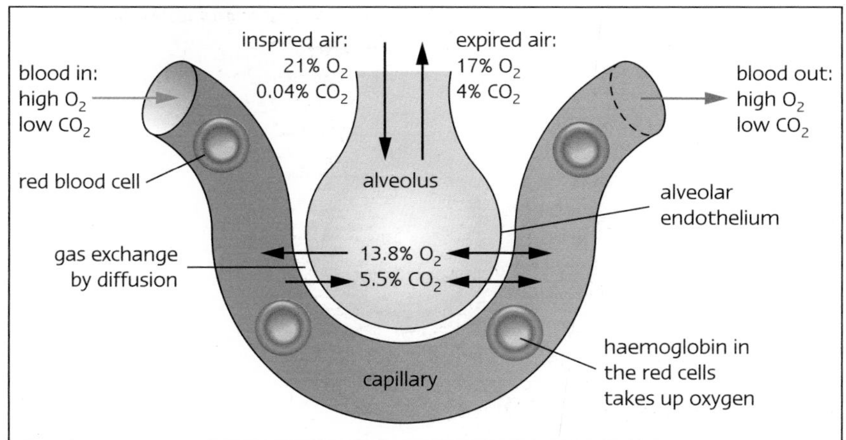

Figure 5.19 Gas exchange at an alveolus.

Case study

Alfie was born prematurely, at only 30 weeks into his mother's pregnancy. Doctors assured Alfie's parents that his internal organs were perfectly formed but that some of them were not yet mature enough to function properly; in particular, Alfie's lungs were immature. One of the paediatricians explained that, because he was premature, the cells in Alfie's alveoli hadn't yet produced a substance called surfactant. This is needed for the alveoli to expand during respiration. As a result, Alfie would need to be given surfactant to overcome this problem.

1. Explain the functions of the alveoli in the respiratory system.
2. What might happen to Alfie if he doesn't receive sufficient surfactant quickly?

The respiratory system: the role of diffusion

P3 P4 Understanding diffusion

Gases move into the blood by **diffusion**. Diffusion is normally quite a slow process, especially if there is a barrier, such as a membrane, between the area of high concentration and the area of low concentration. Figure 5.20 shows some factors that influence the rate of diffusion.

Figure 5.20 Factors that influence the rate of diffusion.

Factor	To speed up diffusion	To slow down diffusion
Barrier	Make the barrier as thin as possible so it is easy for the particles to pass through, e.g. the material of a teabag.	Make the barrier thick or prevent the particles passing through altogether, e.g. the plastic lining of a waterproof jacket.
Surface area	Should be as large as possible to give space for particles to move across, e.g. the exchange surface in a kidney dialysis machine.	Should be as small as possible to give little space for particle movement, e.g. a ball of wet paper dries out much more slowly than the same paper rolled out flat.
Concentrations of diffusing particles	Have the largest possible difference in concentration between the two areas, e.g. wet clothes dry much more quickly on a dry day (even if it is quite cold) than on a wet day.	Diffusion stops if the concentration of particles in both areas is the same, e.g. once a strong smell has filled a room it will not spread any further.

The term 'gaseous exchange' describes the movement of oxygen and carbon dioxide between the air in the lungs and the blood by diffusion. At the moist surface of each alveolus, oxygen dissolves in a thin layer of liquid. The dissolved oxygen then diffuses through the thin membrane of the alveolus into the blood. In the blood, haemoglobin reacts with the oxygen locking it into red blood cells to be carried around the body. Since the blood is always moving, oxygenated blood is continuously carried away from the alveoli. At the same time, deoxygenated red blood cells from the body keep arriving, maintaining a steep concentration gradient for oxygen and encouraging rapid diffusion. The blood that arrives at each alveolus is rich in carbon dioxide. This diffuses out of the blood into the air in the lungs from where it can be breathed out.

Your assessment criteria:

P3 Outline the gross structure of all the main body systems

P4 Explain the physiology of two named body systems in relation to energy metabolism in the body

Key terms

Diffusion: *the spread of molecules from areas of high concentration to areas of low concentration by random movement*

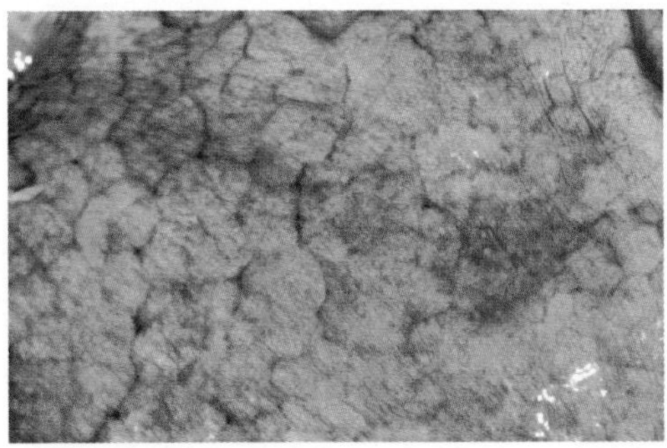
Healthy lung tissue.

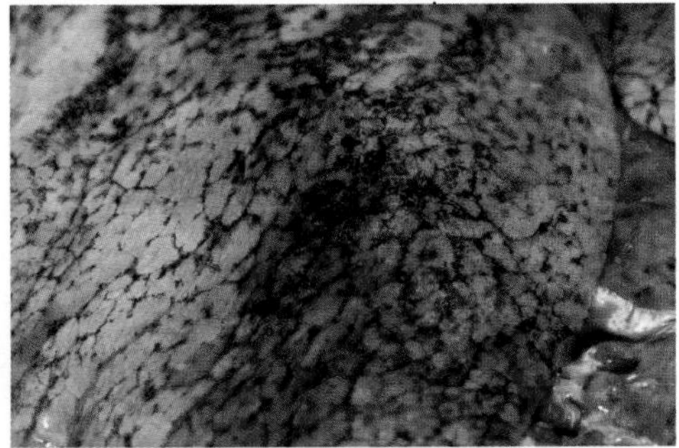
Lung tissue from a smoker.

The effects of smoking on the lungs

Smokers are often breathless because cigarette smoke can cause a disease that destroys the alveoli of the lungs. The loss of alveoli decreases the surface area available for gaseous exchange and less oxygen gets into the blood. The lungs and heart have to work harder to make up for this inefficiency. The strain that results causes early death from lung and heart disease in many smokers.

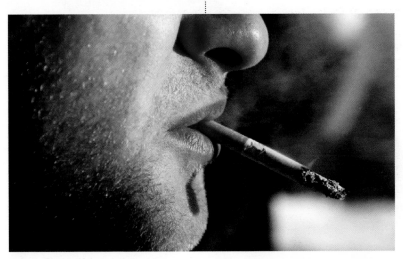
Smoking cigarettes destroys the alveoli and leads directly to lung disease.

What do you know?

1. Identify three physical structures that are part of the respiratory system.
2. Describe the purpose of the respiratory system.
3. Describe how the process of respiration occurs in the body.
4. Describe the physical structure of the lungs.
5. Explain how the lungs work to enable human beings to breathe.
6. What is gaseous exchange and where does it happen in the respiratory system?

Reflect

Do you think that knowledge of what cigarette smoke does to the lungs, and seeing images, would put more people off smoking?

Structure and function of the digestive system

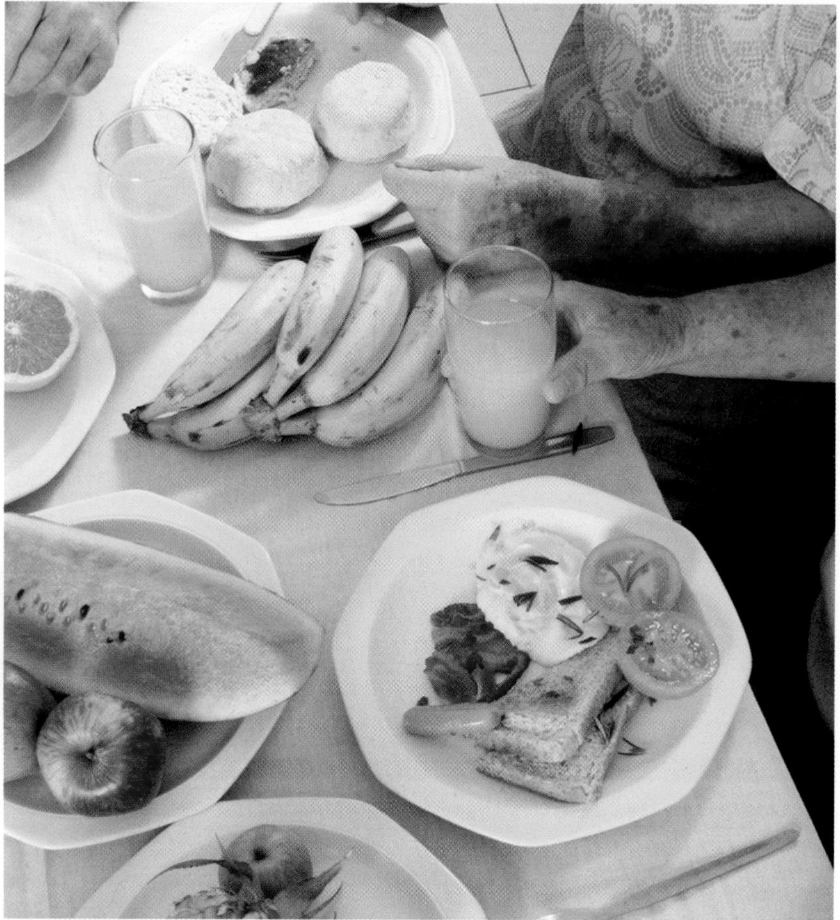

The digestive system processes the food that we eat.

Your assessment criteria:

P3 Outline the gross structure of all the main body systems

P4 Explain the physiology of two named body systems in relation to energy metabolism in the body

Key terms

Absorption: *the process of taking smaller, digested components of food into the bloodstream*

Chemical digestion: *breaking down of food components by enzymes*

Digestion: *the mechanical and chemical breakdown of food into smaller components that can be absorbed into the bloodstream*

Elimination: *the bodily process of discharging waste matter*

Mechanical digestion: *breaking of food into digestible chunks, normally using the teeth and tongue*

P3 The alimentary canal

The digestive system is responsible for the **mechanical** and **chemical digestion**, **absorption** and **elimination** of food materials. The alimentary canal is the main physical structure within the digestive system. Figure 5.21 identifies the various parts of the alimentary canal that make up the digestive system.

Your digestive system is about 9 m long. It extends from your mouth to your anus and most of it is folded and packed neatly inside your abdominal cavity. In a healthy adult, a meal takes between 24 and 72 hours to be fully digested. In this time it will be broken down, processed and absorbed in various ways as it travels through the alimentary canal.

Food begins its digestive journey in the form of large complex molecules of protein, carbohydrate and lipid (fat). In this form, nutrients are unable to pass through the lining of the alimentary canal and cannot deliver the energy the body requires. The process of digestion converts these large molecules into simple soluble molecules that can be absorbed into the bloodstream and distributed to the body's cells to be used in metabolic processes.

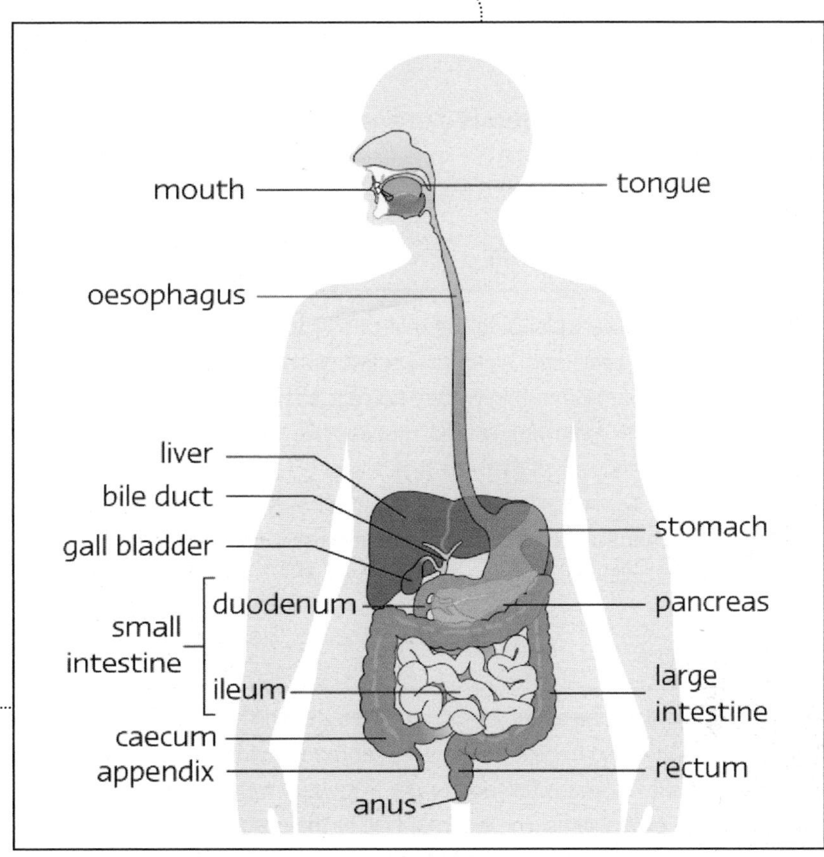

Figure 5.21 The alimentary canal.

P4 The process of digestion

The process of digestion begins when food is first ingested, or taken into the mouth. It is chewed by the action of the teeth and tongue, and softened by saliva. This starts to break down the food. A small ball of food called a bolus is swallowed. This first stage of the digestive process is known as mechanical digestion.

Once mechanical digestion is complete, the food ball goes down the oesophagus to the stomach, travelling partly by gravity and partly by **peristalsis**. When the food reaches the stomach, chemical digestion by enzymes and gastric juices occurs. This partly digested food stays in the stomach for about 5 hours while the enzymes get to work. It is then pushed into the small intestine for further chemical digestion. More enzymes and pancreatic juices continue breaking down the food into components that the body can absorb. This process takes about another 4 hours. Between 7 and 9 hours after the food was first eaten, it will have reached a stage where the nutrients can be extracted. The remaining undigested mass is moved into the large intestine as faeces, which will be eliminated via the anus.

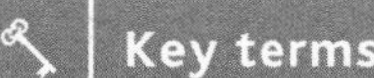

Key terms

Peristalsis: *the wave-like muscle contractions of the alimentary tract that move food along*

Structures and organs of the digestive system

The process of digestion involves a number of different body structures, each with their own particular digestive function.

Your assessment criteria:

P4 Explain the physiology of two named body systems in relation to energy metabolism in the body

P4 The salivary glands

There are three pairs of salivary glands in the oral cavity. Between them these glands secrete between 1 and 1.5 litres of saliva per day. There are two types of saliva. The purpose of thin watery saliva is to wet food. This is done by the tongue during chewing. A thick mucous-like secretion lubricates food particles and causes them to stick together, forming the bolus that is swallowed. As well as lubricating food and cleaning the mouth, saliva also begins the chemical breakdown of food because it contains a digestive enzyme called salivary amylase.

The oesophagus

This is a narrow, muscular tube about 20–30 cm in length which begins at the back of the mouth and transports the bolus of food down to the stomach. It takes about 7 seconds for food to get from your mouth to your stomach via the oesophagus. The external wall of the oesophagus consists of two layers of smooth muscle which contract by peristalsis to move the food along. At the top of the oesophagus is a flap of tissue called the epiglottis. This closes when you swallow to prevent food entering your trachea (windpipe). No digestion actually takes place in the oesophagus because no enzymes are released here.

The stomach

Your stomach is a relatively small pouch made of thick elastic muscles. It is located behind the bottom of your rib cage and under the diaphragm. The purpose of the stomach is to store and help break down food. Once it has entered from the oesophagus, food can remain in the stomach for up to 5 hours. It is churned by the stomach walls to break it into smaller pieces and also to mix it with gastric acid, pepsin and other digestive enzymes, forming a semi-liquid solution known as **chyme**. This is then moved on to the small intestine for further digestion.

Key terms

Chyme: *a semi-liquid mass of partially digested food*

The duodenum

The duodenum is the first, shorter section of the small intestine. Once the milky chyme enters the duodenum, it is mixed with bile from the liver and gall bladder, and pancreatic juice made by the pancreas. The walls of the duodenum also secrete intestinal enzymes that break down proteins, carbohydrates and fats (lipids).

The ileum

The function of the ileum is the absorption of fully digested food components into the circulatory and lymphatic systems. The ileum contains small finger-like structures called villi. These are themselves covered in hair-like microvilli, providing a very large surface area for the absorption of nutrients. Absorbed nutrients are carried in the blood to the liver where the blood is filtered to remove toxins and where the nutrients are processed further. Meanwhile, the remaining food mass is now moved via peristalsis into the colon.

Reflect

Draw a flow chart to show how food moves through the parts of the digestive system. If you can, add in some detail about what happens in each section of the intestines.

The colon

The colon, along with the rectum, is part of the large intestine. The colon is about 1.5 m long. It runs up the right side of the abdomen (ascending colon), goes across the body (traverse colon) and then down the left side of the abdomen (descending colon), until it ends at the anus where faeces are expelled. No enzymes are secreted in the large intestine though some absorption of fluid and nutrients does take place. The large intestine absorbs water from the food bolus and stores faeces until they can be excreted.

The liver

The liver is the largest internal organ in the human body. It is on the right side of the abdominal cavity just below the diaphragm and overlapping the stomach. The liver performs a number of functions including:

- storing iron and some vitamins
- removing drugs and alcohol from the blood
- helping to control levels of glucose in the blood
- producing heat that keeps the body warm
- producing bile salts that break down fat in the small intestines.

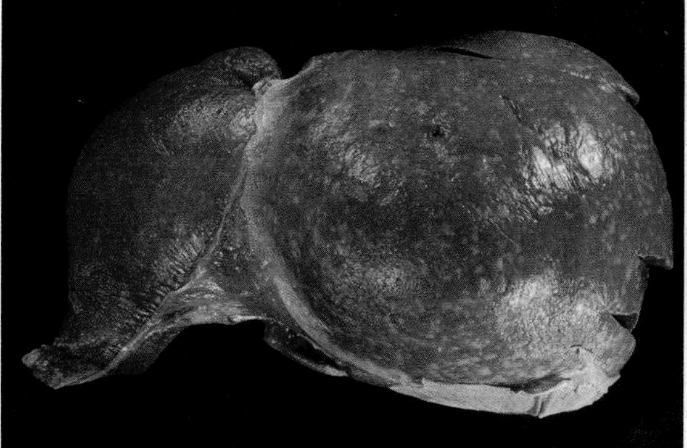

An unhealthy liver.

Bile passes into the duodenum via the bile duct. It emulsifies fats to form tiny globules that can be further broken down by enzymes.

The pancreas

The pancreas is positioned between the intestine and stomach, close to the duodenum. The functions of the pancreas are:

- to produce hormones that control the glucose level in the blood
- to secrete enzymes into the small intestine to help the body to break down and digest food.

The digestive system: peristalsis and chemical digestion

P4 Peristalsis

Peristalsis is the term used to describe the slow muscular movements that move food and chyme down the alimentary canal. The alimentary canal has two sheets of smooth muscle – one running down the tube and the other encircling it – that work in an **antagonistic** way. When the inner circle of muscle contracts behind the bolus of food or chyme, the muscle that runs lengthways relaxes. This has the effect of pushing the material forward. Slow, rhythmic repetitions of this process gradually move the food or chyme through the alimentary canal.

Your assessment criteria:

P4 Explain the physiology of two named body systems in relation to energy metabolism in the body

Key terms

Antagonistic: *acting against or in opposition to something*

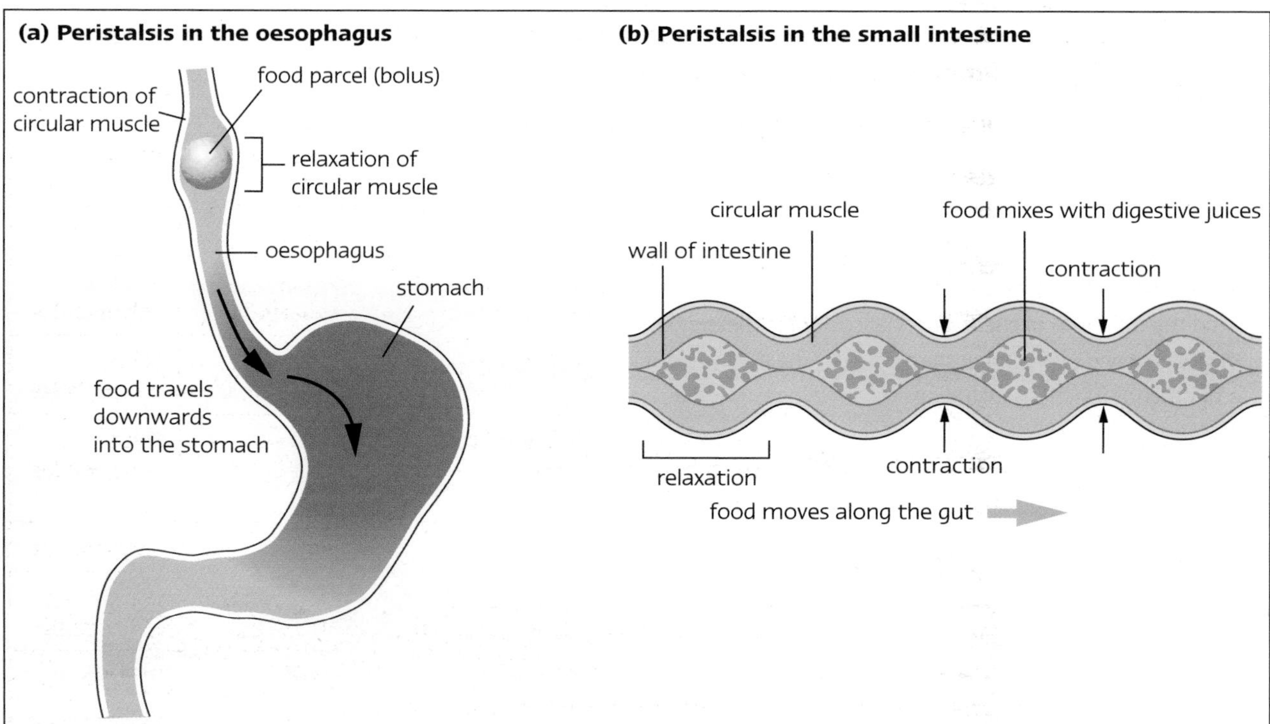

Figure 5.22 How peristalsis works.

Digestive enzymes

Digestive enzymes are produced by the human body to break down complex food molecules such as carbohydrates, proteins and fats into simpler ones. Enzymes act as catalysts. This means that they change the rate of chemical reactions that break down or build up of other chemicals without being changed themselves.

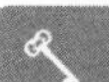

Investigate

Find out why people who have cystic fibrosis have digestive enzyme deficiencies and what effect this has on their physical health and functioning.

Enzymes have very specific actions. Each enzyme acts on a particular type of material, known as a substrate. For example, protease only acts on protein, and lipase only acts on fats (lipids). Figure 5.23 identifies a range of digestive enzymes and their substrates. Figure 5.23 also includes other important information relating to enzyme production and activity. For example, each enzyme:

- is produced in a specific part of the body (site of production)
- has a particular site of activity where it promotes chemical digestion
- requires surroundings with a particular acidity or alkalinity (pH) to work effectively
- acts on a particular food component (substrate)
- produces a particular chemical component of food (product) that can be used by the body.

Figure 5.23 Summary of the main human digestive enzymes.

Secretion	Enzyme produced	Site of production	Site of activity	pH	Substrate	Products
Saliva	Salivary amylase	Salivary glands	Mouth	6.5–7.5	Starch	Maltose
Gastric juice	Pepsin	Stomach	Stomach	2.0	Proteins, polypeptides	Short polypeptides
	Rennin				Caseinogen (milk protein)	Short polypeptides
Pancreatic juice	Trypsin	Secretory cells of the pancreas (acini)	Duodenum	7.0	Proteins, polypeptides	Short polypeptides
	Chymotrypsin				Proteins	polypeptides
	Carboxypeptidase				Polypeptides	Dipeptides, amino acids
	Pancreatic amylase				Starch	Maltose
	Maltase				Maltose	Glucose
	Sucrase				Sucrose	Glucose, fructose
	Lactase				Lactose	Glucose, galactose
	Lipase				Fats and oils	Fatty acids, glycerol

P4 Major products of digestion

The different products of chemical digestion have different roles to play and are used or stored in different ways by the body.

Your assessment criteria:

P4 Explain the physiology of two named body systems in relation to energy metabolism in the body

Figure 5.24 Products of digestion and their roles in the body.

Digestive products	What does the body do with them?
Peptides and amino acids	• Makes enzymes, hormones, plasma proteins. • Carries out cell growth and repair. • Surplus amino acids are broken down in the liver; the nitrogen-containing part is converted into urea by deamination and is excreted by kidneys as urine.
Sugars (glucose)	• Cellular respiration breaks sugars down to release energy. • Surplus carbohydrate is stored in the liver and muscles as glycogen, or is converted into fat and stored under the skin or around organs. • The carbon dioxide and water produced by cellular respiration are removed from the body through breathing, sweating and urination.
Glycerol	• Used for energy or to convert fatty acids into a form that can be stored by the body.
Fatty acids	• Used in cellular respiration to assist metabolic processes. • Excess fat is stored under the skin and around organs.

✓ What do you know?

1. What does the concept of homeostasis refer to?
2. Identify the four main organs involved in homeostasis.
3. Describe how a negative feedback system works.
4. Explain how the heart rate is regulated by nerves and chemoreceptors in the body.
5. Explain how homeostatic mechanisms regulate body temperature.
6. How does the body use a negative feedback system to regulate blood glucose levels?

Case study

Angela Murray is now in her early forties. She has suffered from the potentially life-threatening bowel condition, Crohn's disease, since she was 16 years old. Angela experiences low-level stomach and bowel pain most of the time. She has been through periods where she lives off nutritional drinks and was once unable to eat food for 90 days. In the years before she was diagnosed, Angela had regular episodes of diarrhoea and blood loss, experienced skin rashes, mouth ulcers and persistent stomach pains. However, blood tests showed nothing.

A referral to a consultant led to further tests that identified inflammation of her intestines, ulcers and scarring. Angela says that she always knew that she had a digestive problem because eating had become so painful. According to her consultant, Angela's bowel was in a terrible state. She underwent a food elimination diet, discovering that she was intolerant to dairy products, pineapple, nuts, lamb and caffeine. She has since had surgery to remove part of her large intestine and may require more in the future. Angela now plans her diet very carefully, avoiding all of her problem foods. She also tries to adopt a positive mental approach to life, keeps her stress levels as low as possible and exercises to stay fit.

1. Identify three symptoms of Crohn's disease.
2. Explain how Crohn's disease can affect the structure of an individual's digestive system.
3. Why might a person suffering from Crohn's disease become malnourished?

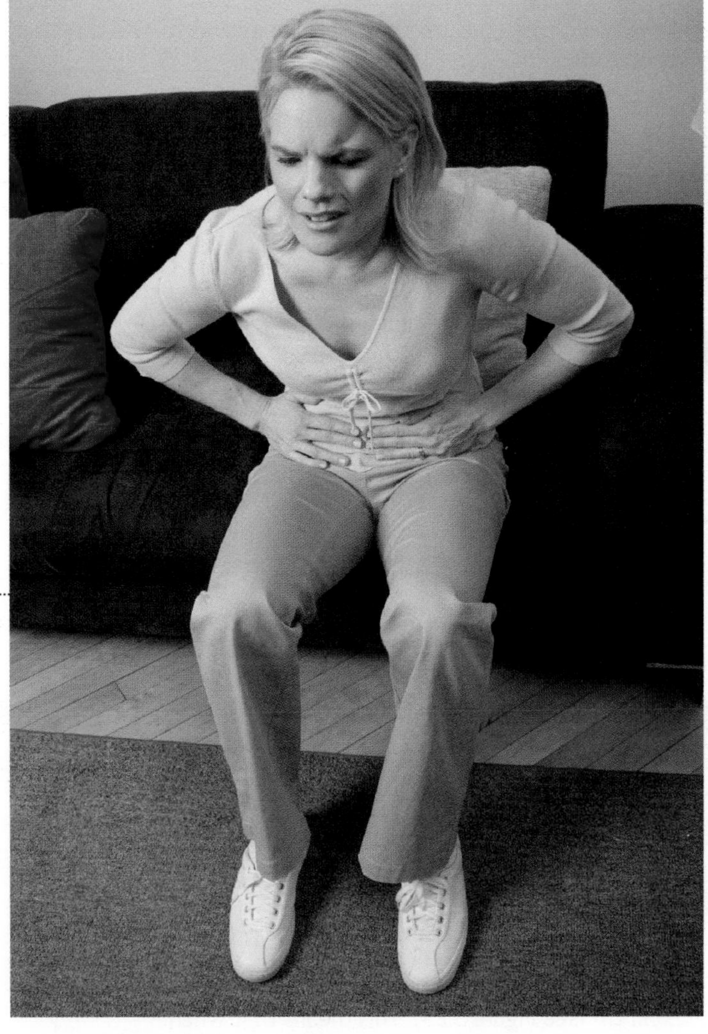

Homeostasis and the human body

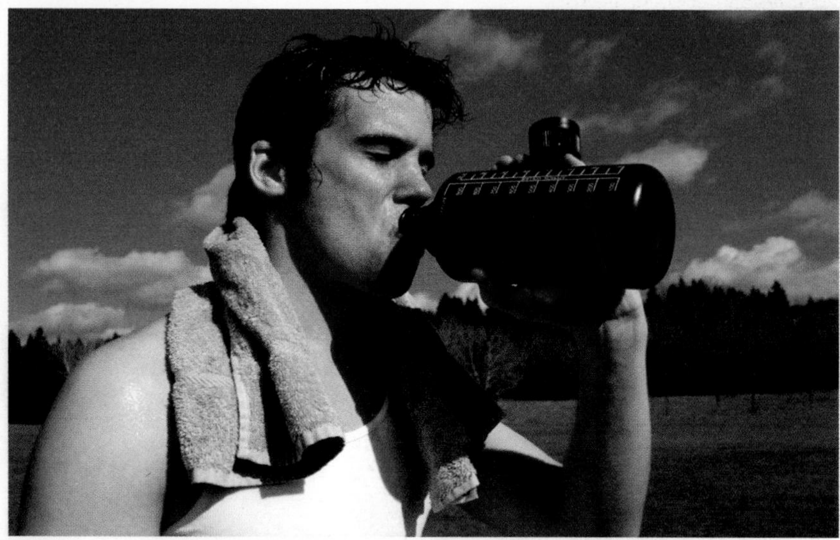

Internal processes ensure that we take action to prevent the body overheating.

Your assessment criteria:

P5 Explain the concept of homeostasis

M2 Discuss the probable homeostatic responses to changes in the internal environment during exercise

P5 What is homeostasis?

The human body has the ability, known as **homeostasis**, to regulate and maintain a stable internal (physiological) environment. This means that the body can respond to changes in the external environment. For example, when the weather is very hot or very cold, homeostatic mechanisms in the body monitor conditions and make adjustments to the way the body functions. The skin, liver, kidneys and brain are the main organs involved in homeostasis:

- The skin acts as a protective barrier to the entry of microbes and viruses, prevents fluid loss and regulates body temperature.
- The liver breaks down toxic substances and carbohydrates.
- The kidneys regulate water levels and excrete waste products, filtering out toxins from the blood.
- The hypothalamus in the brain is the control centre responding to changes that occur in the environment.

Homeostasis works through a **negative feedback system** (see Figure 5.25). This means that when

Key terms

Homeostasis: *maintenance of an optimum internal environment, in this case within the human body*

Negative feedback system: *a body system that monitors a system output, that shuts off once an optimum output level is achieved and turns on if the output level drops below optimium*

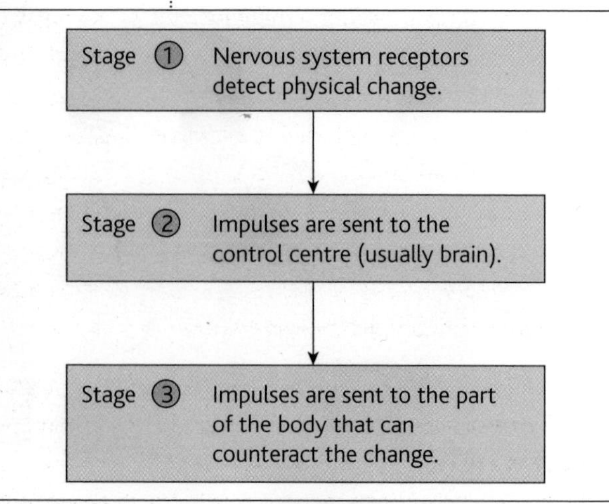

Stage ① Nervous system receptors detect physical change.
Stage ② Impulses are sent to the control centre (usually brain).
Stage ③ Impulses are sent to the part of the body that can counteract the change.

Figure 5.25 A negative feedback system.

changes are detected in the body, systems take action to correct the deviation in order to maintain a constant internal environment.

A range of physiological processes in the body are controlled through homeostasis. These include:

- heart rate
- breathing rate
- body temperature
- blood glucose levels.

P5 M2 Regulating heart rate

As we have seen, the heart muscle ***organises*** the sequence of its own contraction (see page 222). However, two groups of cells in the medulla at the base of the brain control the heart ***rate***. These centres are the:

- cardioacceleratory centre which raises heart rate
- cardioinhibitory centre which lowers heart rate.

Both centres are connected to the sinoatrial node and the atrioventricular node in the heart by nerves from the autonomic nervous system. To lower the heart rate, impulses from the cardioinhibitory system pass down the vagus nerve to the heart. At the sinoatrial and atrioventricular nodes, the nerve secretes a chemical called acetylcholine which acts on the nerve cells in the heart nodes. It inhibits the nodes so that fewer impulses are produced and the heart beats more slowly.

To raise the heart rate, impulses from the cardioacceleratory system pass down a different autonomic nerve to the heart. At the sinoatrial and atrioventricular nodes, the nerve secretes a chemical called noradrenaline which acts on the nerve cells in the heart nodes. Noradrenaline increases the rate at which the nodes produce impulses and the heart rate rises.

So, the nerve centres in the medulla control the heart rate. But what controls the cardiovascular centres in the medulla? Specialised cells called chemoreceptors can measure the amount of a particular chemical in the blood. Chemoreceptors in the carotid sinuses in the neck measure the levels of carbon dioxide and oxygen. If the carbon dioxide level rises or oxygen level falls these cells send impulses along a nerve to the cardiovascular centres in the brain. At first, this seems to increase the breathing rate and, in turn, raises the heart rate. The exact link between the two is not completely understood.

Pressure receptors in the aorta and the carotid sinuses also have an effect on the cardiovascular control centres. A rise in blood pressure detected by the pressure receptors stimulates the cardioinhibitory centre and inhibits the cardioacceleratory centres. This tends to reduce the heart rate.

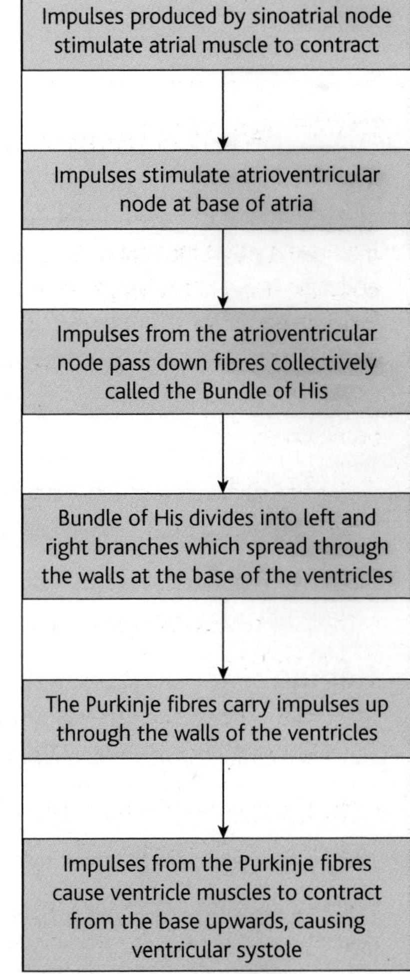

Impulses produced by sinoatrial node stimulate atrial muscle to contract
Impulses stimulate atrioventricular node at base of atria
Impulses from the atrioventricular node pass down fibres collectively called the Bundle of His
Bundle of His divides into left and right branches which spread through the walls at the base of the ventricles
The Purkinje fibres carry impulses up through the walls of the ventricles
Impulses from the Purkinje fibres cause ventricle muscles to contract from the base upwards, causing ventricular systole

Figure 5.26 Control of the heart rate.

P5 M2 Regulating breathing rate

Breathing is controlled by nerve impulses from the brain. A negative feedback system adjusts the rhythm, depth and rate of breathing when receptors in the blood detect changes in the amount of carbon dioxide in the body:

- During exercise or exertion a person will have a high level of carbon dioxide in their bloodstream.
- When resting and relaxed, they will have a low carbon dioxide level.

When the blood carbon dioxide level is high, receptors report this to the brain which sends signals to quicken and deepen the person's breathing rate, so that they breathe out more carbon dioxide and obtain more oxygen.

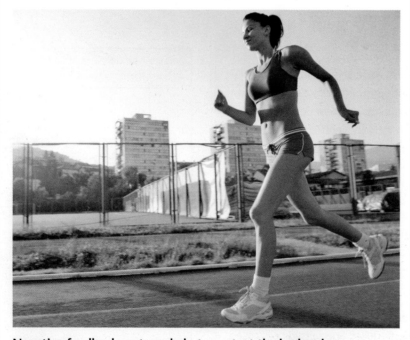

Negative feedback systems help to protect the body when exercising.

Regulating body temperature

Body temperature is controlled through a negative feedback system in which changes in temperature are detected and corrective action is taken to keep the core body temperature constant. This is vital to prevent the body's internal organs overheating. The body will respond to:

- hot conditions by losing heat to keep the core cool
- cold conditions by retaining heat to keep the core warm.

Your assessment criteria:

P5 Explain the concept of homeostasis

M2 Discuss the probable homeostatic responses to changes in the internal environment during exercise

Investigate

Count the number of breaths you take in 1 minute. Now climb a flight of stairs and repeat the count. What happens?

Temperature receptors in the skin and around internal organs detect and report changes in temperature to the brain. The brain then switches on either the body's heat loss or heat retention mechanisms in response.

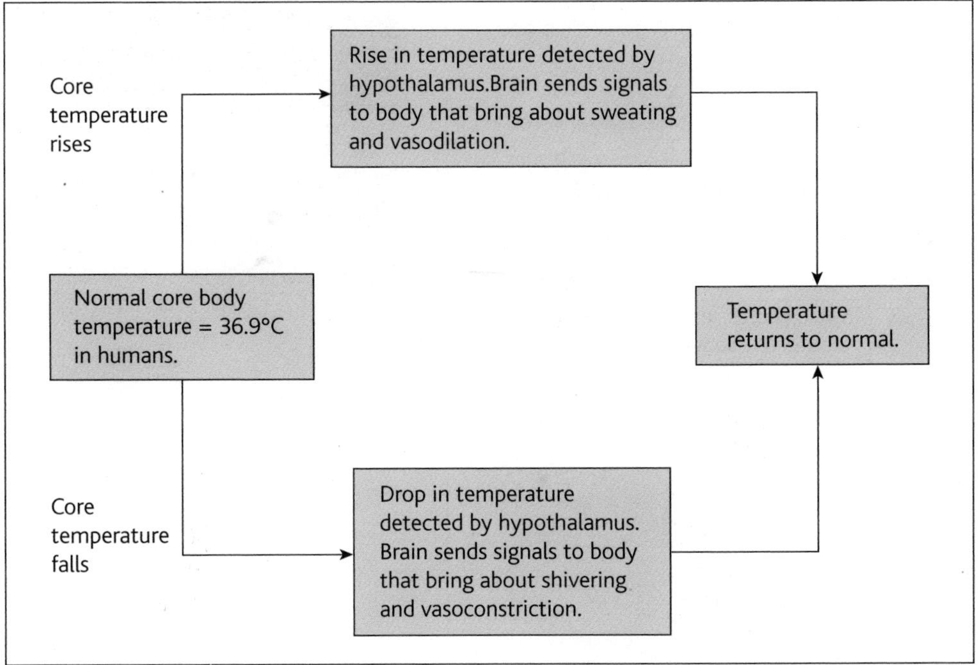

Figure 5.27 Control of body temperature.

Case study

When Lianne, aged 18, went to a birthday party, the weather was dry but a little windy. Lianne was wearing a short-sleeved top and jeans. She decided not to take a coat or a sweater, even though her mum warned her she would get cold. When Lianne left the party, she decided to walk home with a friend. She started feeling cold as soon as she began the 3-mile walk. At first she rubbed her arms, but then noticed she was shivering and that her hands and feet were getting colder and colder. After about 20 minutes' walking Lianne had warmed up a bit, but didn't really feel warm until she was back in bed at home.

1. How did Lianne's body react to the change in temperature when she left the warmth of the party?
2. Explain why Lianne's hands and feet became colder when she first started to walk home.
3. Describe how a negative feedback system worked to control Lianne's body temperature in this situation.

P5 M2 Regulating blood glucose level

The level of glucose in the blood is also controlled by a negative feedback system. The pancreas is the control centre. It monitors how much glucose is in the bloodstream and whether there is sufficient insulin and glucagon to maintain a normal blood sugar level (see Figure 5.28). A person's blood glucose level, and their negative feedback system, is affected by food:

- Shortly after eating a meal, a person will have a high blood sugar level.
- When a person is hungry, they will have a low blood sugar level.

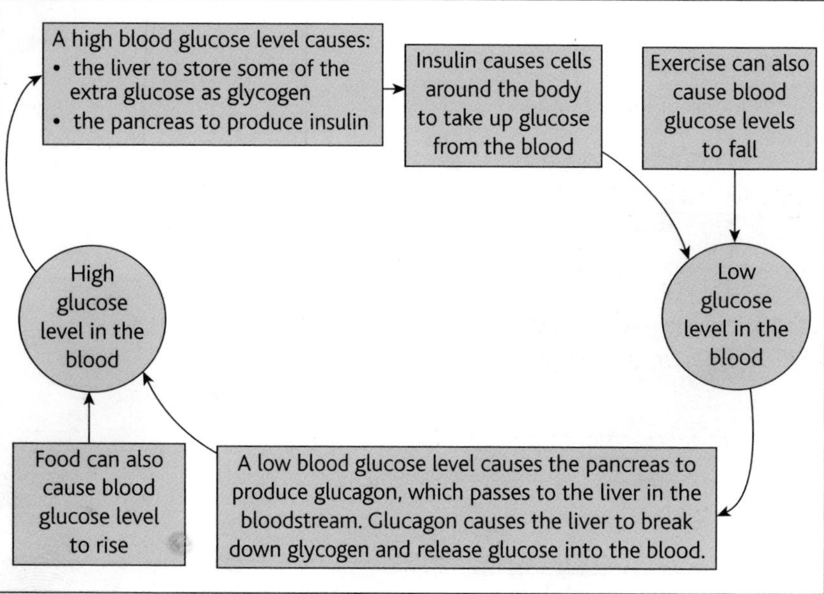

Figure 5.28 A negative feedback loop.

Your assessment criteria:

P5 Explain the concept of homeostasis

M2 Discuss the probable homeostatic responses to changes in the internal environment during exercise

D2 Evaluate the importance of homeostasis in maintaining the healthy functioning of the body

Case study

Andrew hadn't eaten for over 10 hours. He was determined to complete his drive to a holiday cottage in France with as few stops as possible. When he got on the ferry he felt weak and tired, and had poor concentration. Andrew thought he'd better have something to eat as he had another long drive ahead of him when the ferry reached France. After eating a meal and drinking a cup of coffee, Andrew felt much less tired and much more alert. He also bought a sandwich and some chocolate to eat on the next leg of his journey.

1. Give a biological explanation for the way Andrew felt when he arrived at the ferry.
2. How would eating a meal boost Andrew's blood glucose levels?

Reflect

What are your eating habits like? Do you eat regular meals, snack through the day or only eat irregularly? Do you think your blood sugar level stays relatively constant through the day? How will you feel if your blood sugar level has dropped? What should you do to help your body correct it?

D2 Why is homeostasis important?

Homeostatic mechanisms regulate a number of processes in the human body, keeping internal conditions as stable as possible. Homeostasis maintains optimum conditions for cell function by regulating the composition of the surrounding tissue fluid:

- Nutrients and oxygen must be delivered to body cells from the blood, via the tissue fluid.
- Waste products are removed.
- The concentration, temperature and pH of the tissue fluid between cells are kept at optimum levels.

If homeostatic mechanisms break down, the conditions inside the human body can change in ways that prevent self-regulation of important processes. For example:

- failure to control blood glucose levels results from a lack of the hormone insulin, causing Type 1 diabetes
- failure of thermoregulation (temperature control) causes fatal cell damage in cases of both hyperthermia (too hot) or hypothermia (too cold) and, in the case of hypothermia, this damage can stop a person's heart.

What do you know?

1. What does the concept of homeostasis refer to?
2. Identify the three main organs involved in homeostasis.
3. Describe how a negative feedback system works.
4. Explain how the heart rate is regulated by nerves and chemoreceptors in the body.
5. Explain how homeostatic mechanisms regulate body temperature.
6. How does the body use a negative feedback system to regulate blood glucose levels?

Interpreting and presenting physiological data

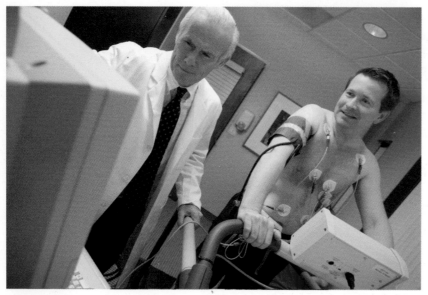

Physiological data can be used to assess a person's health and physical capabilities.

Your assessment criteria:

P6 Follow guidelines to interpret collected data for heart rate, breathing rate and temperature before and after a standard period of exercise

P6 Taking measurements safely

Health practitioners who measure and observe patients for signs of illness are trained to carry out these procedures safely. Most observations require knowledge and experience rather than equipment, and are straightforward and non-hazardous to carry out. Where equipment is used to measure a patient's health, the health care practitioner has a responsibility to:

- use only equipment that they have been trained to use
- check that equipment is in a safe, clean condition
- ensure that they minimise the risk of cross-infection by washing their hands before and after touching the measuring equipment
- carry out the measurement procedure according to local policies and by following the equipment manufacturer's instructions
- dispose safely of any equipment that may be hazardous because it is broken or has become infected.

 **Discuss**

Discuss the reasons why health care practitioners take physiological measurements. What can several measurements made over time tell you about someone's health?

Reliability in measurement

A **reliable** measurement is both **valid** and **accurate**. Imagine you are caring for an older person with a fever. You have been asked to keep a close watch over her progress, so you are measuring the level of sugar in her urine every 30 minutes. Your results could be ***accurate*** but are ***irrelevant*** (not valid). Measuring body temperature would have been much more useful, or ***valid***.

Validity

So, valid measurements are the right measurement made using the correct technique. Blood pressure measures taken through clothing or using the wrong-sized cuff will not be valid. They may appear to be accurate, but will be an accurate measure of the wrong thing!

Accuracy

Accuracy is the precision of a measurement. A clinical thermometer that is only accurate to within 5°C is completely useless! If your thermometer is reading 2.5°C below the correct value, a temperature of 36.5°C on your thermometer could really be a life-threatening temperature of 39°C. Equally, if it is reading only 2.5°C above the real value, your thermometer's 36.5 °C could be masking a case of hypothermia at 34°C!

Test results need to be ***accurate enough*** to allow decisions to be made. Clinical thermometers are accurate to within 0.1°C. So, a temperature of 36.5°C on the thermometer could be anything from 36.45°C to 36.55°C. This is ***accurate enough*** for medical and care purposes. A thermometer could be accurate to 0.01°C but would not provide any more ***useful*** information since treatment decisions are made on temperature changes of 0.5°C or more.

Key terms

Accurate: *near to the true value*

Reliable: *consistent or dependable*

Valid: *whether the chosen measurement actually measures the feature it is intended to measure*

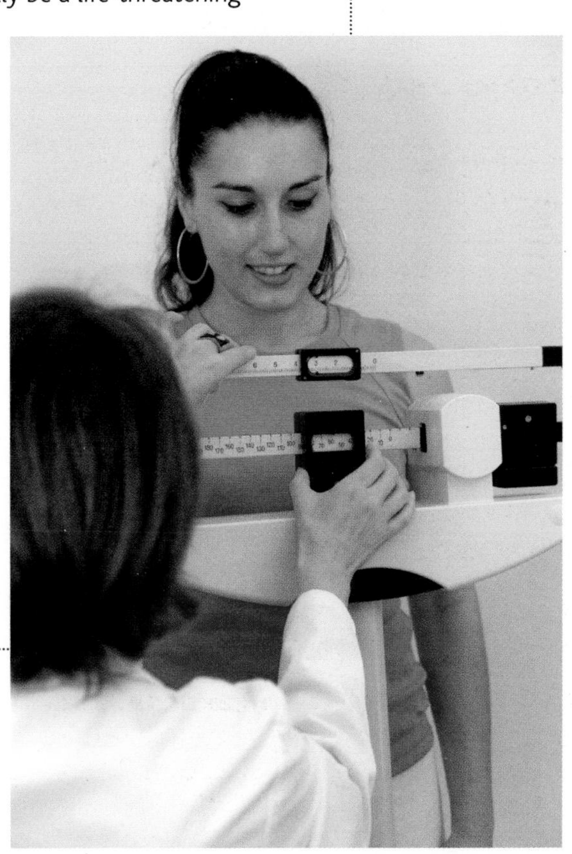

Clinicians often repeat the health measurements they take to ensure their reliability.

P6 Improving reliability

To improve the reliability of your measurements, you need to understand the limitations of the equipment and the test you are using. No piece of equipment is 100 per cent accurate. No test can be ***guaranteed*** to produce a useful result ***every*** time. So, keep your wits about you at all times. Reliable results depend on:

- understanding the test to make sure you are collecting the right information
- accurate equipment
- good technique.

Your assessment criteria:

P6 Follow guidelines to interpret collected data for heart rate, breathing rate and temperature before and after a standard period of exercise

Figure 5.29 Issues that can affect the reliability of test results.

Issue	Questions to ask yourself	Action to take
Readiness of the client	• Are they nervous or worried? • Have they eaten something that will affect the test results? • Are they taking any medicines that will affect the results?	Try to calm the client by talking to them. Ask about any medicines they may be taking or whether they have eaten recently. Find out as much as you can before you even start the test.
Readiness of the equipment	• Does it need to be cleaned? • Does it need to warm up before it can be used? • Are all the bits present?	Check any equipment before you start. Look out for anything that is broken or missing – and leave the equipment so that people who come after you can use it!
Your competence	• Do you know how to use the equipment or perform the test? • Is this a new piece of kit that you have not used before? • Has it been modified since you last used it?	Make sure you know what you are doing before you start. Do not be afraid to ask for help – it is better to do it beforehand than while you have a client with you.

Measuring pulse rate

A person's pulse rate indicates how fast their heart is beating. The pulse, a wave of pressure caused by blood being pumped through the arteries by the heart, can be felt in any artery. For adults, the average (or normal) resting rate is usually between 70 and 80 beats per minute. Babies and young children normally have a faster pulse rate than adults.

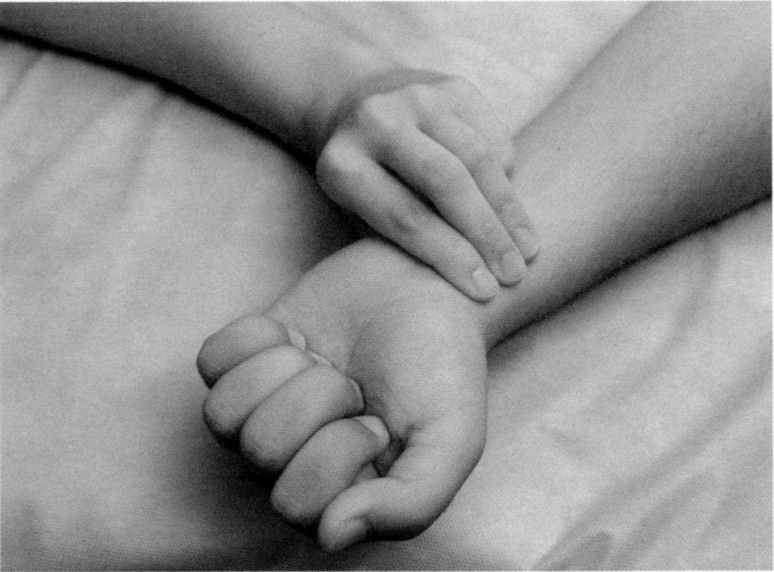

How to take a pulse.

In conscious people, it is usual to take a person's pulse at the **radial artery**, found in the wrist. In unconscious people, the **carotid artery** in the neck may be used. A person's pulse rate increases when they exercise, when they are emotionally upset or if they develop a form of heart or respiratory disease. Unfit people, smokers and overweight people also have a faster resting pulse rate.

Measuring breathing rate

A person's breathing rate is simply the number of times they take a breath per minute. A healthy adult breathing rate is about 16–18 breaths per minute. Babies and children have a faster breathing rate. Breathing rate can be measured by:

- observing and counting the number of times a person's chest rises and falls in a minute
- putting your cheek close to the person's nose and mouth and counting the number of breaths you feel on your cheek.

Key terms

Carotid artery: *the artery felt in the neck below the jawbone*

Radial artery: *the main artery that enters the wrist on the side of the thumb*

Discuss

How might each of the following factors have an impact on an individual's pulse rate?

- *stress*
- *blood loss*
- *drugs*
- *strenuous exercise*
- *age*
- *infection*
- *sleep.*

Investigate

Measure your own (or someone else's) pulse rate using the radial pulse for 1 minute. Compare the resting pulse rate with the pulse rate after some brief exercise.

Investigate

Observe a friend or relative for a few minutes to measure their breathing rate. It's probably best to do this by watching their chest rise and fall, rather than by feeling their breath on your cheek!

P6 Measuring temperature

Normal body temperature is between 36.5°C and 37.2°C, varying throughout the day and depending on activity levels, clothing, **ovulation** and the weather, for example. Regardless of conditions, a thermometer is needed to measure body temperature accurately.

A health practitioner would usually place a thermometer under a person's armpit or in their mouth to record their temperature. Core temperature is measured by placing a thermometer in the person's anus. Specialist equipment such as ear thermometers and thermometers strips placed on the forehead can also be used to measure body temperature, if an individual is too young, too unwell or unable to hold a thermometer in their mouth or under their arm for some other reason.

Interpreting measurement data

Results from tests mean nothing until they have been interpreted. To interpret results properly, you need to understand:

- the significance of the test (what were you looking for?)
- the circumstances in which the test was carried out (was the person resting after a heavy meal?)

To interpret results, practitioners usually consult tables of normal values to see if their result matches healthy values. This means that results have to match the standard way of displaying that sort of data. Modern medical equipment does a great deal of data preparation for you, but you still need to be able to read information in standard formats like tables, charts and graphs.

Measurement data

Data is the information produced by your tests. Data can be:

- a number (e.g. temperature of 36.8°C, a lung volume of 5.7 litres)
- a presence or absence (e.g. sugar is absent in the urine, a pulse is present)
- a class label (e.g. eye colours are blue, the pulse is strong).

Sometimes data must be processed before it can be used. For example, the forced expiratory volume (FEV_1), sometimes called the peak flow rate, must be calculated from raw data supplied by a spirometer.

Data is used, along with our theoretical understanding, to make treatment decisions. The data needs to be clear, easily understood and in the easiest possible format to read in a hurry. Data can be displayed in tables, graphs and charts, or can be reduced to a single representative value, such as an average which could include information from many separate data points.

Your assessment criteria:

P6 Follow guidelines to interpret collected data for heart rate, breathing rate and temperature before and after a standard period of exercise

M3 Present data collected before and after a standard period of exercise with reference to validity

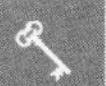 **Key terms**

Ovulation: *the process of releasing an egg or ovum from the ovary*

M3 Using standard units

Medical and care staff use a wide range of different units to measure body functions. The same value given with two different units of measurement could mean very different things. So, it is important always to quote the units for every measurement you make – otherwise the data could be useless or even dangerous.

Figure 5.30 Commonly used units in physiological measurements.

Factor	Commonly used units	Conversion methods
Body temperature	°C (degrees Celsius or degrees centigrade), occasionally °F (degrees Fahrenheit)	• To convert Celsius to Fahrenheit: divide by 5, multiply by 9 and add 32 • To convert Fahrenheit to Celsius: take away 32, divide by 9 and multiply by 5
Body mass	kg (kilograms), occasionally stones and pounds	
Height	centimetres (cm) or metres (m), occasionally feet and inches	• To go from centimetres to inches: multiply by 0.3936 • To convert inches to centimetres: multiply by 2.54
Lung volumes	litres (l), millilitres (ml) or cubic centimetres (cm^3)	• To convert ml to l: divide by 1000 • To convert litres to ml: multiply by 1000
Forced Expiratory Volume (FEV_1)	litres per second (l/s) or millilitres per second (ml/s)	• To convert ml to l: divide by 1000 • To convert litres to ml: multiply by 1000
Blood pressure	millimetres of mercury (mmHg), occasionally quoted in bars	
Pulse rate	beats per minute (bpm)	
Heart rate	beats per minute (bpm)	

Investigate

Practise taking and recording measurements by measuring some of your own physiological data. Refer to Fig 5.30 for some ideas of things you could measure. How many times will you repeat each measurement to get a sufficiently reliable answer? You could draw a table of your results.

M3 Using standard units

Your assessment criteria:

M3 Present data collected before and after a standard period of exercise with reference to validity

Tables

Tables are a useful way to organise data. It is easy to look up a particular value in a table.

Age range	Males Kilocalorie	Females Kilocalorie
0–3 months (formula fed)	545	515
4–6 months	690	645
7–9 months	825	765
10–12 months	920	865
1–3 years	1230	1165
4–6 years	1715	1545
11–14 years	2220	1845
15–18 years	2755	2110
19–59 years	2550	1940
60–64 years	2380	1900
65–74 years	2330	1900
75+ years	2100	1810

Figure 5.31 Using a table format to display data.

Bar charts

Bar charts are used to display results where at least one of the axes shows data that falls into discrete categories (categoric data).

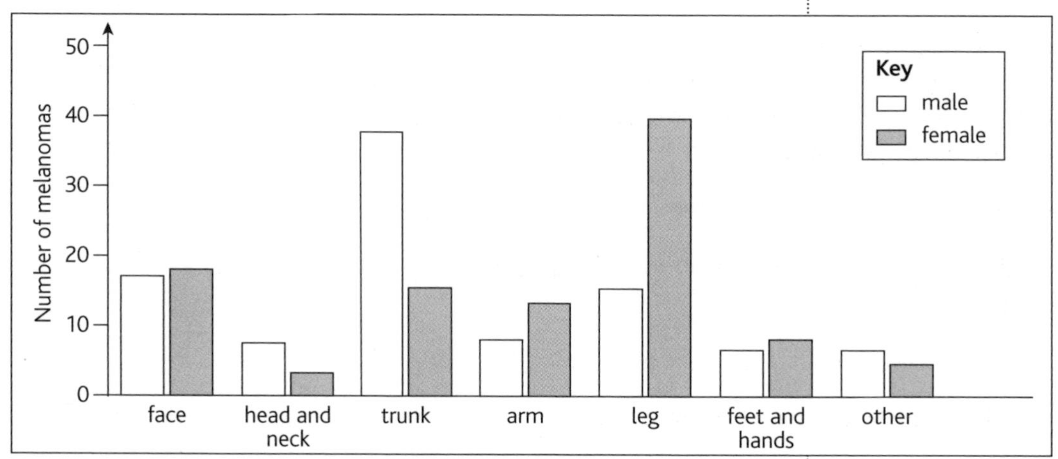

Figure 5.32 Using a bar chart format to display data.

Graphs

Graphs are a way of displaying continuous numerical data. Graphic date is usually easy to interpret. There are also other advantages to drawing graphs:

- extrapolating means we can predict results that are 'off the scale'
- interpolating means we can estimate the result for a test we did not do
- spotting unusual results that are outside the pattern is easy.

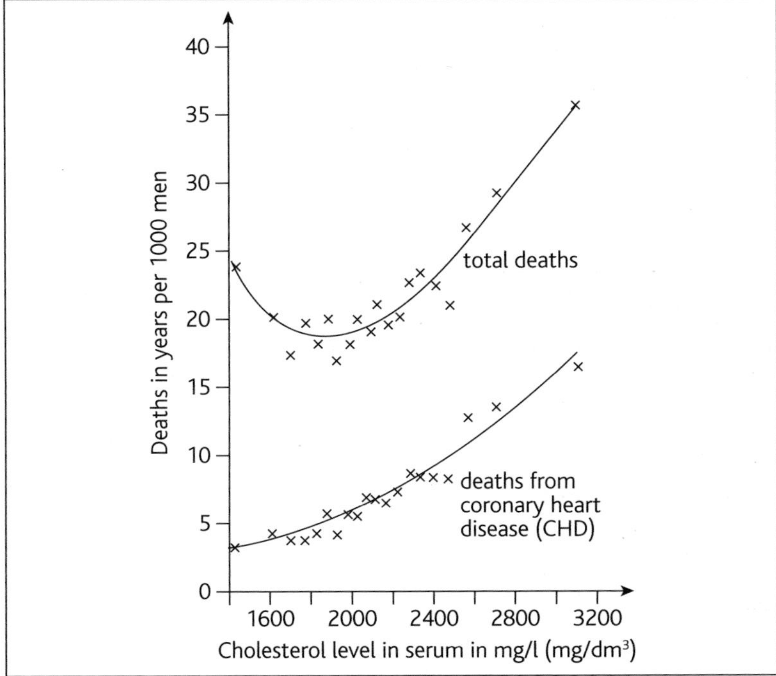

Figure 5.33 The advantages of using graphs to display data.

What do you know?

1. Identify three things a care practitioner should do to ensure they carry out health measurements safely.
2. What is a 'valid' measurement?
3. Explain why health measurements taken in health and social care settings are not always reliable.
4. Which artery is normally used to measure a person's pulse rate?
5. Describe how a child's breathing rate could be measured.
6. What is the best way of presenting categories of data visually?

Assessment checklist

Your learning and level of understanding of this unit will be assessed through assignments given to you and marked by your teacher or tutor. Before you submit your assignment work for assessment you should make sure that you have produced sufficient evidence to achieve the grade you are aiming for.

To pass this unit you will need to present evidence for assessment which demonstrates that you can meet all of the pass criteria for the unit.

Assessment Criteria	Description	✓
P1	Outline the functions of the main cell components.	☐
P2	Outline the structure of the main tissues of the body.	☐
P3	Outline the gross structure of all the main body systems.	☐
P4	Explain the physiology of two named body systems in relation to energy metabolism in the body.	☐
P5	Explain the concept of homeostasis.	☐
P6	Follow guidelines to interpret collected data for heart rate, breathing rate and temperature before and after a standard period of exercise.	☐

You can achieve a merit grade for the unit by presenting evidence that also meets all of the following merit criteria for the unit.

Assessment Criteria	Description	✓
M1	Discuss the role of energy in the body.	☐
M2	Discuss the probable homeostatic responses to changes in the internal environment during exercise.	☐
M3	Present data collected before and after a standard period of exercise with reference to validity.	☐

You can achieve a distinction grade for the unit by presenting evidence that also meets all of the following distinction criteria for the unit.

Assessment Criteria	Description	✓
D1	Analyse how two body systems interrelate to perform a named function/functions.	☐
D2	Evaluate the importance of homeostasis in maintaining the healthy functioning of the body.	☐

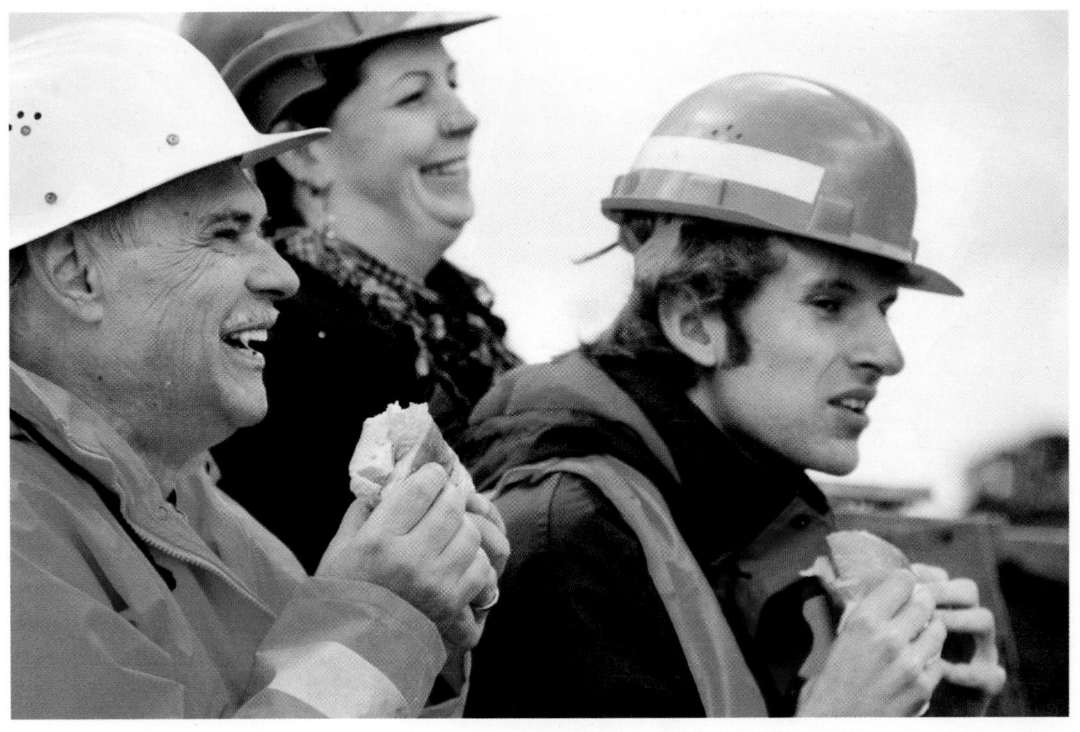

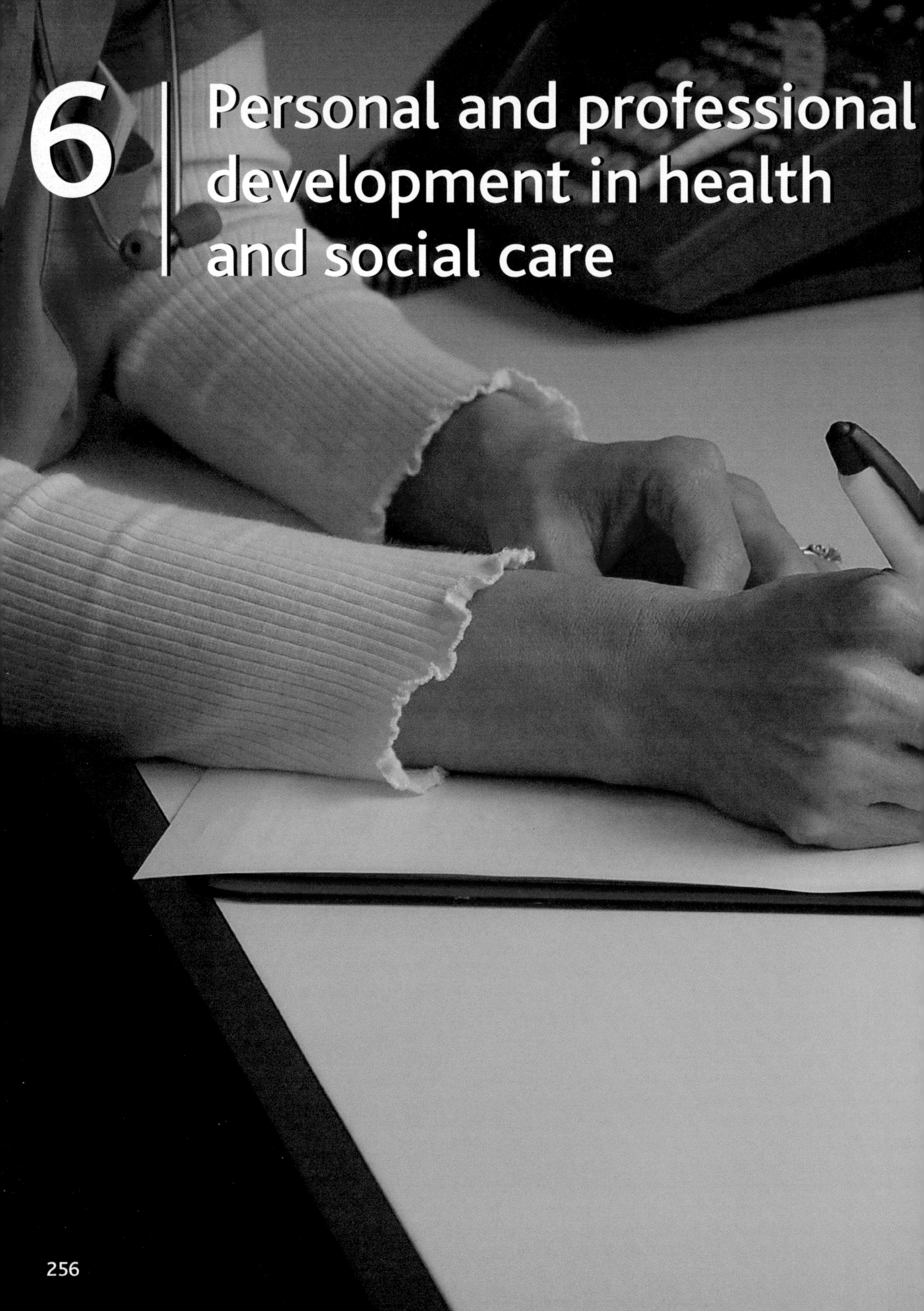

6 Personal and professional development in health and social care

LO1 Understand the learning process

- theories of learning
- influences on learning
- skills for learning
- support for learning
- learning opportunities

LO2 Be able to plan for and monitor own professional development

- review at start of programme
- knowledge
- skills
- practice
- values and beliefs
- career aspirations
- action plan for own development
- consider personal goals

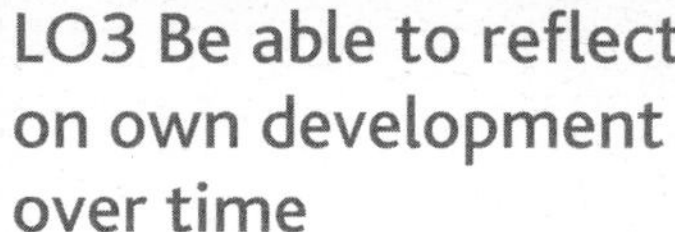

LO3 Be able to reflect on own development over time

- monitor and evaluate plan
- changes
- contexts
- professional development portfolio
- relevant evidence
- support for development
- reflect on own development

LO4 Know service provision in the health or social care sectors

- provision of services
- local health or social care
- health and social care workers

What is learning?

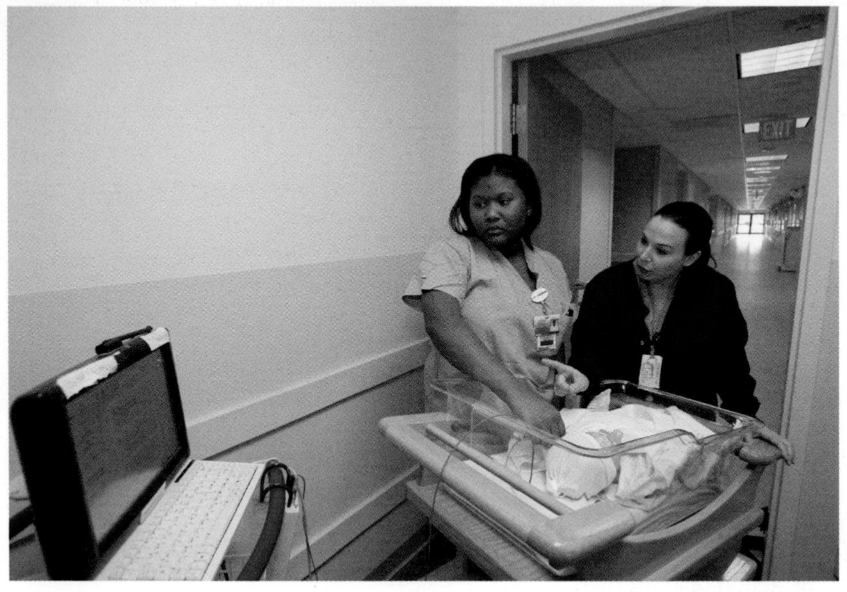

Care practitioners learn a great deal from experience in practice settings.

Your assessment criteria:

P1 Explain key influences on the personal learning processes of individuals

P1 Formal and informal learning

Learning involves acquiring knowledge and skills, and understanding abstract concepts. Beginning at birth, progressing through infancy, childhood and adolescence into adulthood and old age, learning is a lifelong process. A person's learning is partly facilitated through schooling, but also develops through **informal learning**.

Key terms

Informal learning: *learning from events or situations that occur in everyday life or which arise unexpectedly in the workplace*

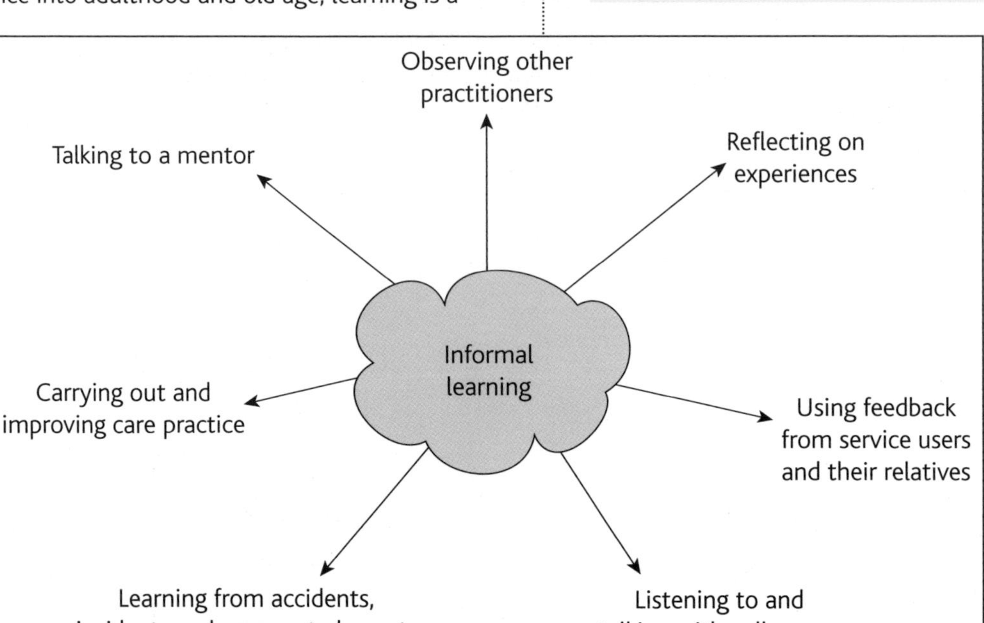

Figure 6.1 Ways of learning informally.

Health and social care workers are expected to learn through both **formal learning**, such as training, and informal learning opportunities – observing and talking to colleagues, interacting with people who use services and their own everyday experiences.

Promoting your learning and development

You can improve your current learning and development by:

- understanding how you learn
- reviewing and understanding what you have learnt (formally and informally) up to this point
- setting goals for your own achievement and development
- reflecting on your progress and the extent to which you are achieving your career and personal development goals.

The learning and development of health and social care workers tends to occur in three phases:

1. a pre-qualification phase of personal and professional development
2. a qualifying phase in which vocational training is undertaken
3. a post-qualification phase known as continuing professional development (CPD).

As someone at the beginning of this learning and development process, you need to be aware of the range of formal and informal learning opportunities open to you. As your career develops you will benefit from many different experiences, as you apply theories and knowledge in practice. Ultimately the goal of your learning and development is for you to become a more effective care practitioner.

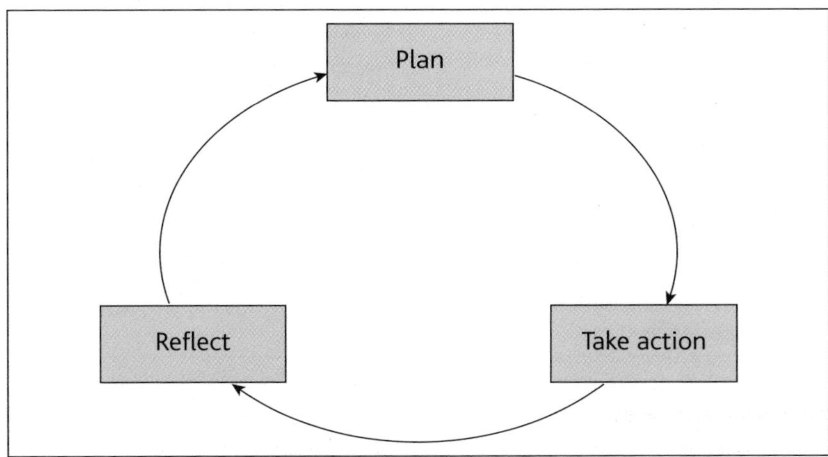

Figure 6.2 A learning and development process.

Key terms

Formal learning: *learning in a structured and planned way, such as at school or college*

Reflect

Have you ever thought about how you learn best? Are there some situations or ways of working that seem to suit you better than others?

Kolb's theory of learning

Theories provide systematic and formal models of how people learn; here we are thinking about how adults learn. Kolb's (1984) experiential learning cycle theory and Honey and Mumford's (1982) learning styles theory are two well-known theories of adult learning.

Your assessment criteria:

P1 Explain key influences on the personal learning processes of individuals

P1 The experiential learning cycle

Kolb argued that, during adolescence and early adulthood, individuals develop a preference for how they process information and make sense of experience. Kolb developed the **experiential** learning cycle to explain this. Kolb argued that learning occurs when an individual follows each stage in the sequence (see Figures 6.3 and 6.4).

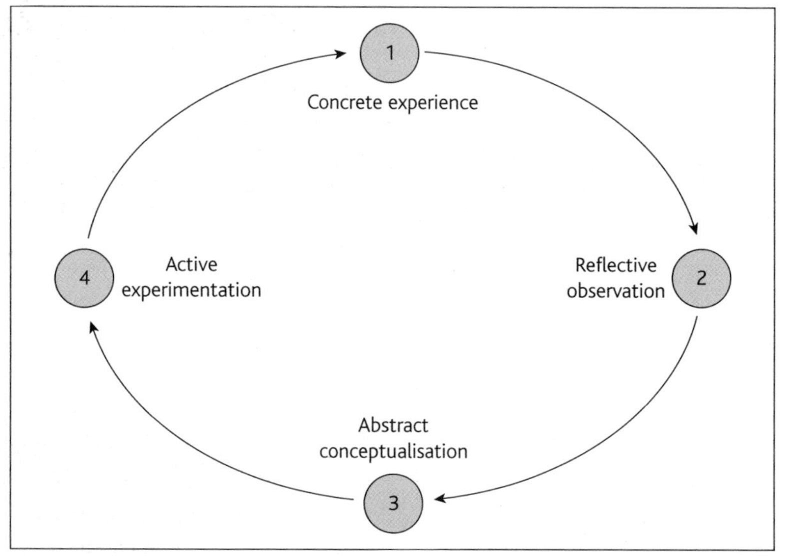

Figure 6.3 Kolb's experiential learning cycle.

Key terms

Experiential: *based on a person's experience*

Theories: *a set of concepts that claim to explain something*

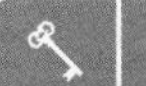

Key terms

Conceptualisation: *creation or development of an idea or explanation*

Figure 6.4 Kolb's stages of the experiential learning cycle.

Stage	What happens at this stage?
Concrete experience	An individual does something, such as carrying out a task or participating in an activity.
Reflective observation	The individual reviews or reflects on what they did (or on what happened) during the concrete experience stage.
Abstract **conceptualisation**	Information about concrete experience is used to reorganise thoughts into a new order and to make sense of experience.
Active experimentation	When the individual repeats the original activity, they try out new skills or knowledge by doing it differently.

Case study

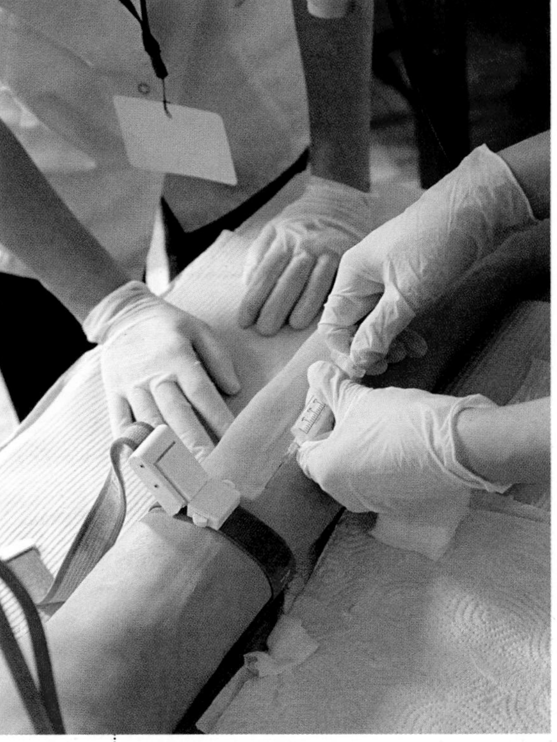

Christina is a first-year student nurse. She is currently on placement, learning through experience, on a medical ward in a large teaching hospital. Anna is Christina's mentor. Today Christina is going to learn how to give an insulin injection to a patient. Christina knows why some people with diabetes require insulin injections, but she has never given an injection to anyone. She has, however, observed Anna giving a couple of injections. When the time comes to give the patient the injection, Christina is nervous but remembers the technique Anna has shown her. In particular, Christina remembers to talk to the patient while she is giving the injection – just like Anna did. Christina feels proud of herself afterwards and remarks to Anna that, 'It's not quite like in the textbook, is it?'

1. What was the concrete experience in the learning experience described above?
2. How did Christina use reflection to learn informally from Anna?
3. How, according to Kolb, is Christina likely to develop her practical skills as a result of this learning experience?

Criticisms of Kolb's theory

Kolb's learning cycle theory is widely used in care, education and workplace learning settings, because it helps to explain the stages of learning. However, it has been criticised because it:

- doesn't take into account learning that happens through feedback from others, concentrating only on learning through individual reflection
- suggests that individuals need to follow the stages of the learning cycle in sequence for learning to occur; this isn't always the case.

Your own learning approach or style may be similar to that described by Kolb. However, it is also clear that people approach learning situations in a variety of different ways. This has resulted in other theories being developed that take this into account.

Discuss

Share ideas and experiences about skills that you learnt when you were younger (for example, skipping, riding a bike, reading, handwriting, dancing, cooking). Does Kolb's experiential learning cycle help to explain how your skills improved over time?

Honey and Mumford's theory of learning

P1 The learning styles theory

Honey and Mumford (1982) developed a learning styles theory. They identified four learning style preferences:

- Reflector
- Theorist
- Activist
- Pragmatist.

Each learning style is linked to preferred learning situations and has particular associated characteristics (see Figure 6.5).

Your assessment criteria:

P1 Explain key influences on the personal learning processes of individuals

Figure 6.5 Honey and Mumford's preferred learning styles.

Learning style	Preferred features of learning situations	Associated characteristics
Reflector	• observational learning • enough time to think • opportunities to analyse • completion of tasks to own deadline	• likes to be an observer or to assist rather than be the person in charge • able to take a range of views or approaches into account • makes decisions after weighing up a situation and collecting a range of information
Theorist	• complex, theoretically challenging tasks • abstract ideas • investigative tasks • structured, purposeful tasks	• likes to gain knowledge or new insights • tends to be a logical thinker • can seem emotionally detached, treating problems as intellectual challenges
Activist	• new and unusual situations and experiences • collaboration with others • difficult tasks • team working	• needs to feel directly involved but may dominate • may lose interest or get bored with routine tasks • doesn't always think before acting
Pragmatist	• links between theory and practice • making a difference in a practical way • trying things out • working with role models and mentors	• seeks and feels reassured by feedback from others • prefers to get on with tasks rather than discuss them • wants to feel useful

Preferred learning styles are usually identified through the completion of a questionnaire. The outcome for most people is that they use a mix of learning styles but have a preference or a leaning towards one or two particular styles. Knowledge of your preferred learning style or styles will enable you to work in ways that are helpful to your learning and to avoid situations that are not. Planning your learning around your preferred style may be beneficial, but bear in mind that you also need to be able to adapt to situations you face in the workplace. Being flexible will help both your personal and professional development.

Reflect

Which of the learning styles outlined by Honey and Mumford seem to fit with your own preferred way of learning? You should be able to locate a learning styles questionnaire based on Honey and Mumford's theory by searching the internet. Try this to see if it confirms your own views about your preferred learning style(s).

Influences on learning

As we have seen, a person's learning style influences their learning and development. However, a range of other factors affect this too (see Figure 6.6).

You need to be aware of the range of influences that affect your own learning and that of others. Learning can be supported or promoted more effectively if you take these factors into account. A person's previous experiences of learning are particularly important when you are trying to teach them something or help them to develop a new skill. Aspirations, motivation and personal priorities also have a significant effect on the extent to which a person commits, or is able to commit, themselves to learning and development.

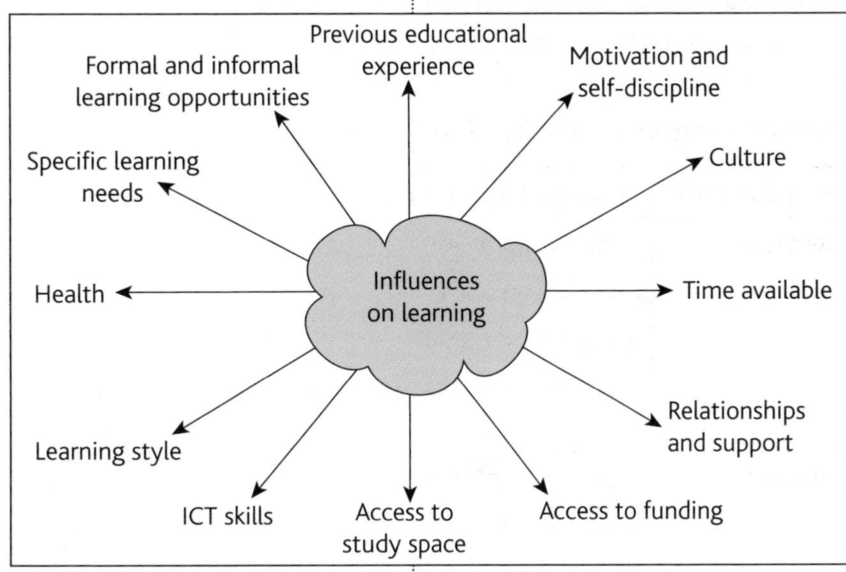

Figure 6.6 Influences on learning.

What do you know?

1. Identify two ways in which health and social care practitioners learn and develop.
2. Describe the three main phases of learning and development that health and social care practitioners can experience.
3. How, according to Kolb, do adults use experience to learn and develop?
4. Name the four different learning styles identified by Honey and Mumford.
5. Describe the learning situations that a pragmatist is likely to prefer.
6. Explain how your own learning and development has been influenced by a range of different factors.

Functional and research skills

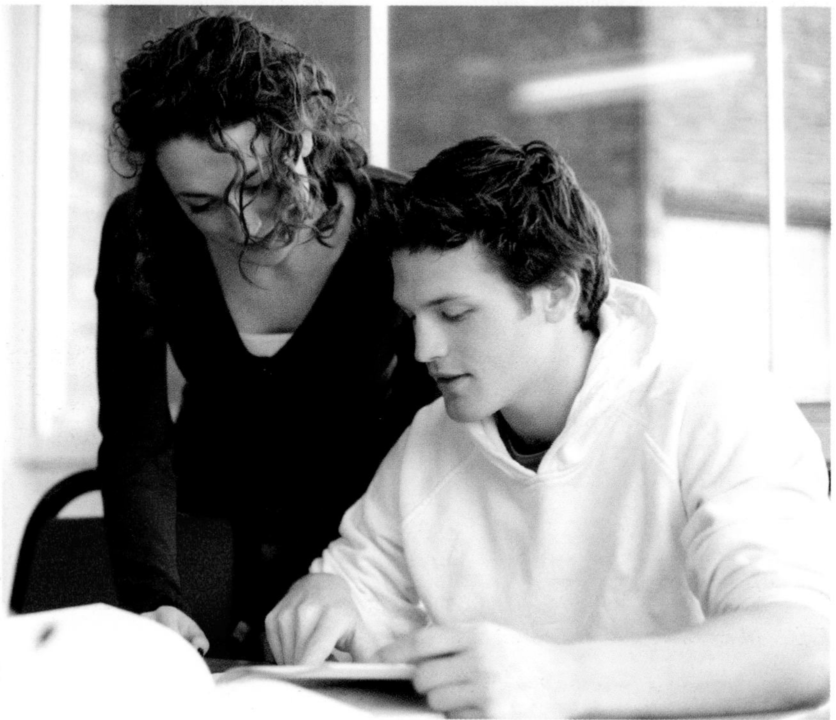

Literacy and numeracy skills are essential for health and social care work.

The extent to which an individual is able to learn and develop depends partly, but significantly, on the skills they have developed (or are able to develop) for learning. Different learning situations require different skills. For example, BTEC courses require different learning skills – and perhaps a different learning style – to traditional academic GCE A level courses. Assessing your knowledge and skills at the beginning of a period of personal development and learning is an important first step in producing a personal development plan.

P1 Developing your functional skills

Functional skills or key skills cover the literacy, numeracy and information and computer technology (ICT) skills that are needed for everyday life, as well as in the workplace. **Literacy** skills involve the use of written and spoken language. They include reading and writing skills, and the ability to hold conversations. These skills are as important for daily life, as they are in health and social care work.

Numeracy skills involve the use of numerical information. Reading charts, calculating dosages or explaining financial issues to people can be important aspects of health and social care work. ICT skills are

Your assessment criteria:

P1 Explain key influences on the personal learning processes of individuals

Reflect

What do you think is the difference, in terms of learning skills and approach, between studying for a BTEC National award and GCE A levels? What skills do you have that will help you to complete your BTEC course successfully?

Key terms

Functional skills: *the literacy, numeracy and ICT skills needed for everyday living*

Literacy: *the ability to read and write*

Numeracy: *skills with numbers*

increasingly important in everyday life as people use computers to shop online, keep in touch with friends and relatives, and communicate via email, text messaging and other digital means. Using this range of skills will be an important part of your BTEC studies.

Developing research skills

Research skills are needed to obtain, make sense of and use information and numerical data. This may be an important part of your BTEC National course and of your subsequent health and social care training. A summary of research skills is shown in Figure 6.7.

Health and social care practitioners benefit from developing research skills. These skills improve a practitioner's ability to assess and use different sources of evidence in their care practice.

Reflect

How do you use ICT skills in your everyday life?

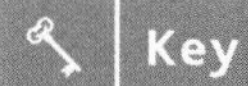

Key terms

Plagiarism: *copying and passing off someone else's work as your own*

Figure 6.7 A summary of research skills.

Research skill	Things you might do
Observation	• learn from informal and experiential situations • gather information systematically for research purposes • learn about routines and procedures
Questioning	• focus your attention on a particular aspect of a situation or on a particular topic, issue or problem
Use of the internet	• assess the validity or accuracy of the huge array of information that is available on the internet • establish reliability of the source before relying on it yourself
Using secondary sources	• access books, journals and newspapers that contain a range of qualitative and quantitative information • use these as a resource, always avoiding plagiarism • establish validity and reliability of the source
Using feedback	• accept valuable verbal and written feedback on your performance • use negative or critical feedback to make positive improvements • be open-minded and willing to adjust your approach, accepting that using constructive criticism is helpful
Reflection	• accept feedback and be self-critical • honestly appraise your own skills, abilities and performance • embrace self-development

Making the most of learning opportunities

P1 M1 D1 Support for learning

In order to make the most of the learning opportunities that arise, most learners will require some type of support during their development. Learners can be supported in a number of different ways (see Figure 6.8). The relevance and usefulness of each form of support depends on an individual's particular development needs at a particular time.

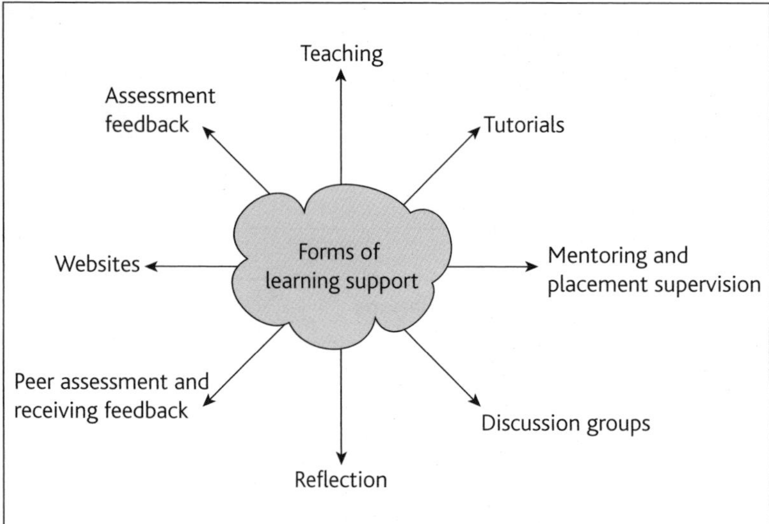

Figure 6.8 Forms of support for learning.

You will probably use and benefit from several forms of support during your course. Written feedback, informal guidance on how to improve your performance and help with specific learning needs are forms of support that address weaknesses and help to improve skills.

It is important to know how you can access different sources of support and to seek help and guidance when you need it. Asking for support is a sign of maturity; tutors and workplace supervisors will view any such request in a positive light, not as a sign of incompetence or lack of ability. It is always best to make the most of the different sources of support that exist.

Using learning opportunities

Opportunities to acquire and apply new knowledge or to develop new skills can occur at any time. Being aware of learning opportunities that arise and making the most of them is an important developmental skill. In particular, a lot of informal learning happens when you spend

Your assessment criteria:

P1 Explain key influences on the personal learning processes of individuals

M1 Assess the impact of key influences on the personal learning processes on own learning

D1 Evaluate how personal learning and development may benefit others

Discuss

Find out about the kinds of support and guidance that your tutor, work placement supervisor or mentor can provide. Can your peers support you? Think about the different kinds of support and guidance you might expect from each of these people. Share your ideas with class colleagues and make a note of the good ideas that arise.

time with care practitioners and service users in care settings. Formal learning occurs in a more structured and organised way; tutors, **mentors** and supervisors may guide and support formal learning in classroom or workshop situations. You will tend to learn from informal opportunities by acting (carrying out tasks) and then reflecting on your performance later. Being aware of Kolb's cycle of learning will help you to make the most of the various learning opportunities you encounter.

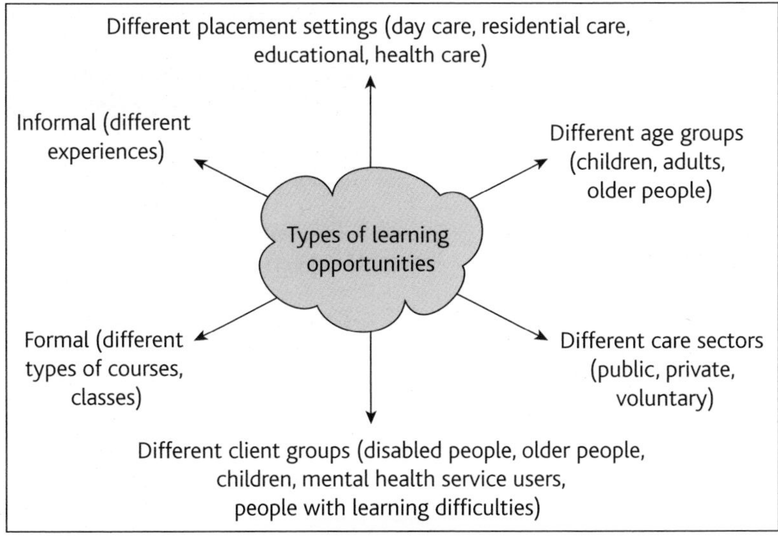

Figure 6.9 Types of learning opportunity.

Key terms

Mentors: *experienced and knowledgeable people who provide supportive, developmental relationships*

What do you know?

1. Identify two types of literacy skill that are needed for health and social care work.
2. Describe a care situation in which a care practitioner may need to use numeracy skills.
3. Explain what research skills are and say why they are useful to health and social care practitioners.
4. What is ***plagiarism*** and why should this be avoided, especially during your BTEC National programme?
5. Identify four different sources or forms of support that you could access as part of your BTEC programme.
6. Explain the difference between formal and informal learning opportunities, giving an example of each.

Reflecting on your development

P2 Reviewing your skills and abilities

Planning for and monitoring your own development requires you to:

- assess your skills and abilities at the beginning of your course
- develop your understanding of the knowledge and skills needed to work in the areas of care that interest you
- create a plan that will enable you to progress from where you are now to the point you would like to be
- from time to time, assess your progress in relation to the plan.

Finding your baseline

The first step in your professional development journey is to work out where you are now. That is, you need to establish a **baseline** set of achievements or abilities – a place to start. Essentially this involves identifying what you can do and what you have achieved up to this point in your life and care career.

Identifying a skills gap

Having found your baseline, the next step is to compare your current knowledge, skills, achievements and level of practical competence to those expected of health and social care practitioners: the **benchmark standards** of the profession. The purpose of this is to identify where there are gaps between what *you* can do now and what a competent health and social care practitioner can do. The size of the gap between what you know and can do and what is expected shows you how much you need to develop. You will use a **personal development plan** to bridge this gap. Pages 272 to 275 contain guidance on how to identify the skills that a professional uses and that you might need to plan to develop.

Your assessment criteria:

P2 Assess own knowledge, skills, practice, values, beliefs and career aspirations at the start of the programme

Key terms

Baseline: *the starting point or point at which something is first measured*

Benchmark standards: *established standards of practice*

Personal development plan: *an action plan designed to improve a person's knowledge, skills and performance*

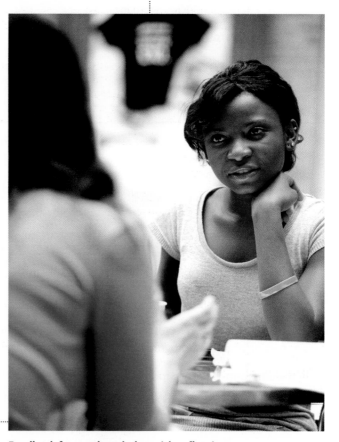

Feedback from others helps with reflection.

Conducting a personal review

Figure 6.10 shows some of the questions you can ask to reflect on your position in preparation for devising a personal development plan (see page 278).

You will need to be as objective and as honest as possible when reviewing your current knowledge, skills, achievements and level of practical competence. For each claim that you make, try to ensure that you can provide clear supporting evidence (such as exam results, school reports, feedback from others, tasks completed on work experience and specific examples of what you have done). It is a mistake to exaggerate or overestimate your current position as this will result in an unrealistic personal development plan.

Figure 6.10 Questions for a personal review.

Area of plan	Questions to ask
Your strengths now (your baseline)	• What can you do well right now (perhaps communicating, working with others, creative or craft skills, practical care skills)? • What personal qualities do you have that will help you in health and social care work (kind, caring, empathetic, practical, calm)? • What skills do you have that will help you study for your BTEC award (functional, research, organisational and interpersonal skills)? • What kinds of relevant formal and informal learning have you undertaken to date?
Your developmental needs (your skills gaps)	• Are there gaps in your knowledge and understanding? • Are there any skills and abilities that you think you need to develop to be a more effective *student*? • Are there any skills and abilities that you think you need to develop to be a more effective *care practitioner*? • What gaps exist in your practical experience of care work?
Plan for development (plan to fill your skills gap)	• Can you identify some goals, timescales and deadlines that would help you to meet your development needs? • What kind of actions do you need to take to achieve these goals?

Key terms

Objective: *factual and free of bias*

Skill: *something you can do well, usually as a result of training and practice*

Reflect

What have you achieved in your life so far? What are you capable of at this point in your health and social care career? Think about your:

- *knowledge and skills (including qualifications)*
- *care experience*
- *personal values and beliefs*
- *career aspirations*
- *self-awareness.*

Make a note of your thoughts. You will be able to use your notes later when you write a personal development plan (see page 278).

Reflect

What kinds of objective evidence can you use to show what you know or what you can do at this point?

Thinking about careers in health and social care

In order to identify your skills and knowledge gap, you will need to do some research into the skills used by professionals in different areas of health and social care.

Your assessment criteria:

P2 Assess own knowledge, skills, practice, values, beliefs and career aspirations at the start of the programme

P2 Assessing your knowledge and understanding

Knowledge is information acquired through studying and experience – in essence, what you know. Your understanding of health and social care-related knowledge is demonstrated through your ability to use this knowledge in real-life situations. Figure 6.11 identifies a number of different sources of knowledge that you may have benefited from already or could use to promote your development and learning in future. You will need different knowledge and understanding depending on the career pathway that you choose.

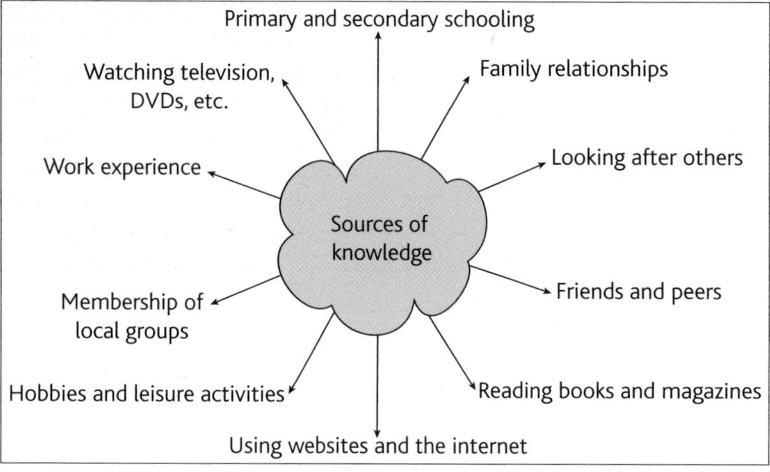

Figure 6.11 Sources of knowledge.

Key terms

Knowledge: *what a person knows*

Reflect

How many of the sources shown in Figure 6.11 have provided you with information and guidance on possible careers in health and social care?

Understanding potential careers

Knowing about the potential career pathways that you could take when you complete your BTEC National award will help to focus your personal and professional development plan so that you concentrate on acquiring the most useful knowledge, understanding and skills.

Your career aspirations may be quite general at the start of your BTEC National course (such as 'nursing', 'social work' or 'work with children'). However, it is useful to find out more about potential careers so that you know about the specific requirements for entry.

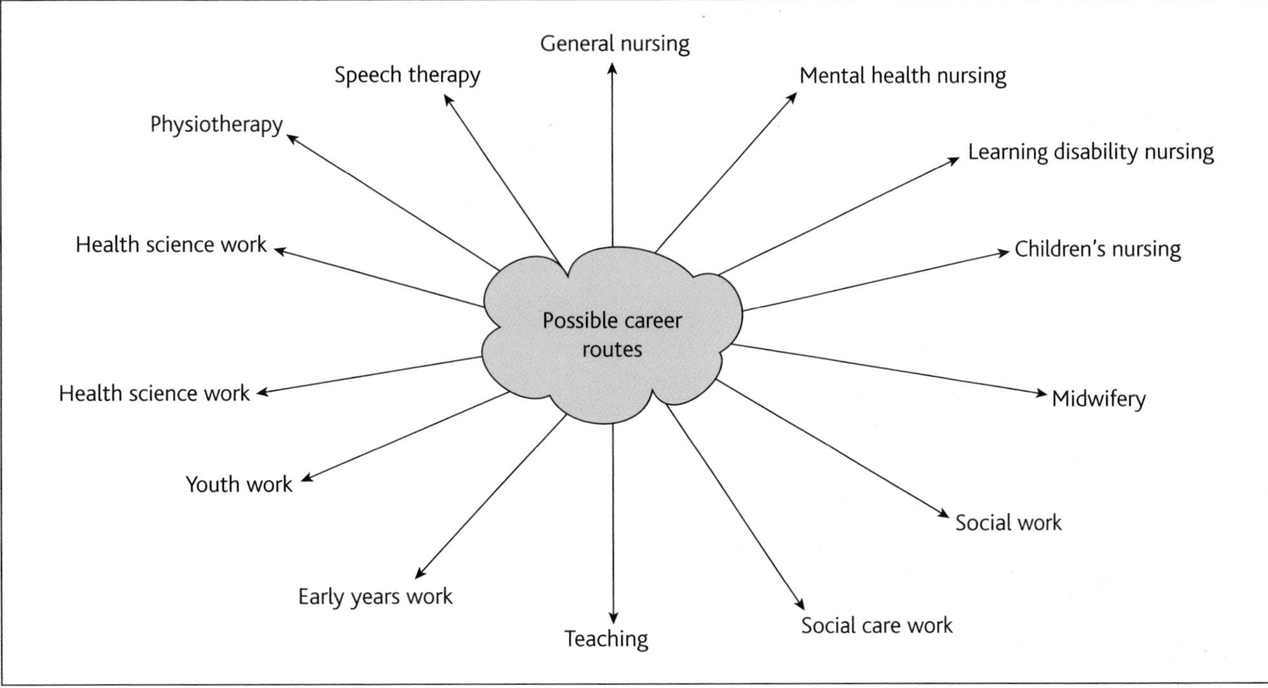

Figure 6.12 What can you do next?

Using placements to find out about careers

It is a good idea to use your work placements and any part-time work opportunities to try out different areas of care work before making major decisions about which direction to take. Undertaking different types of work placement, for example, will enable you to compare and contrast different approaches to care work in different settings. Try to get a sense of where you feel most comfortable working. For example:

- Which type of care setting do you prefer?
- Do you like working with a particular age group, or particular type of service user?
- Which health and social care sector (public, private, voluntary , see page 288) would you like to work in?

Reflecting on your career aspirations should help you to develop some goals to aim for during your BTEC National programme. Finding out now about entry qualifications and required experience, and the skills and standards of practice involved in particular areas of care work will also help you when applying for courses and job roles in the future.

However, it is worth bearing in mind that your career aspirations may change while you are studying and gaining more experience, so it is best to keep your options open. You will need to be realistic, practical and prepared to work hard to achieve your goals.

Reflect

Which areas of health and social care are you interested in working in? How much do you actually know about these areas? What could you do over the next 12 months to increase your knowledge and understanding of potential careers in these areas?

Identifying skills needed in care work

P2 Finding out about skills for different career paths

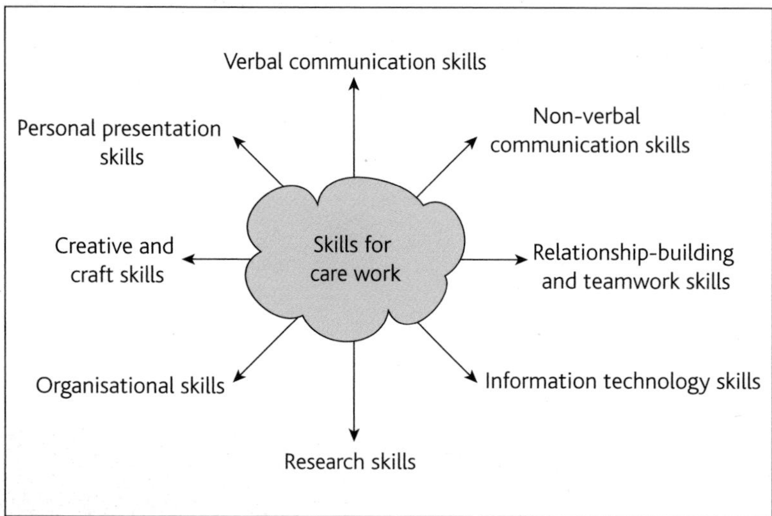

Figure 6.13 Skills needed for care work.

At this point in your life, you will have developed and be able to use a range of physical, intellectual and social skills. You now need to develop the specific communication, research and personal skills that are needed for training and work in the health and social care sector. Health and social care practitioners require a range of language, teamwork, technical, research and personal skills to deliver effective care.

You are probably also aware that health and social care students need effective reading and writing skills to succeed in BTEC National Health and Social Care programmes! It is important to find out about the kinds of skills that colleges, universities, private training providers and care employers expect people to have at different stages of their care careers. You can do this by:

- obtaining job descriptions for care vacancies (look at the ***desirable*** and ***essential*** criteria)
- using careers services and information resources to gain background information on entry requirements and expected skills
- talking to and observing health and social care practitioners while you are on work placement.

Your assessment criteria:

P2 Assess own knowledge, skills, practice, values, beliefs and career aspirations at the start of the programme

 **Reflect**

What three skills do you think an effective health or social care practitioner should have?

Developing skills for working with others

People generally work in teams in health and social care settings. Care practitioners also need to be able to interact with people using services, and with their relatives and friends. As a result, effective communication skills are an important part of care work (see Unit 1). To work effectively with others you will need to:

- have a good understanding of your own knowledge, skills and experience and know how to apply these in teamwork situations
- understand the knowledge, skills and experience of your colleagues and know how they contribute to the team's work
- be supportive and respectful of others
- be able to judge the extent to which team members are achieving their shared goals
- be able to evaluate your own contribution to the team's work.

People who are good at working with others tend to be flexible in their approach and adaptable to the needs of others.

Reflect

Are your teamwork skills good? Are you comfortable working with others on joint tasks or do you find this difficult? Think about previous experiences of teamwork. Identify positive contributions that you made and aspects of the experience you would like to improve on.

Developing technical skills

Health and social care practitioners have to use a number of different forms of technology in their care practice. ICT (information and computer technology) skills are now a core part of health and social care work, for example. People working in busy, modern care settings need to be familiar with word processing and spreadsheet software. Report-writing, updating computer-based records, and sending and receiving emails are everyday tasks for many care practitioners. You will probably have opportunities to develop ICT skills as part of your BTEC programme. You will need them to complete coursework assignments and to write letters and reports, for example.

Teamworking skills are needed in all areas of care work.

Obtaining training in the use of specialist diagnostic or treatment equipment may also help your career development, depending on the area of care work you go into. You may see practitioners using specialist equipment to record health measures (blood pressure, weight, temperature, blood glucose levels, for example) or have the opportunity do this yourself while on work placement. It is good to have a go at using equipment whenever you have the opportunity. However, you should always work under supervision and be trained in the correct procedures. Ensure that you have permission from your supervisor and the client before you undertake any activity.

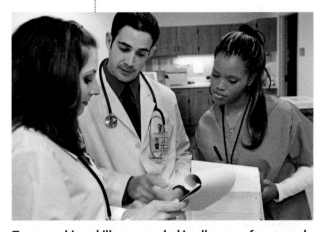

Discuss

What kinds of technology have you seen care practitioners using in your placement setting? Share examples with class colleagues and discuss the skills needed to operate the equipment you saw being used.

P2 Developing research skills

You probably have some basic skills and experience in using research skills to:

- observe health and social care practice
- obtain information in face-to-face situations
- obtain information from text and other online sources
- analyse your findings and present them in the form of graphs, tables and charts.

Previous courses may have enabled you to develop some research skills; you can build on them now and extend your abilities. Identifying, collecting, analysing and using primary and secondary data can be a part of many different care jobs. Developing your research skills and your confidence in data handling will be beneficial to your study and future training, and when you begin work as a health or social care practitioner.

Your assessment criteria:

P2 Assess own knowledge, skills, practice, values, beliefs and career aspirations at the start of the programme

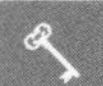

Key terms

Dress code: *a set of rules specifying the correct way to dress*

Developing personal and organisational skills

Personal skills involve the use of personality and temperament in positive ways, but also include an individual's organisational abilities and the way that they present themselves to others. Being well organised is important in health and social care settings; people who use care services and colleagues need to know you are a reliable and efficient practitioner. The way that you dress and use your non-verbal communication skills to present yourself makes an impression. Presenting yourself in a positive and credible way will inspire others to have confidence in you, seeing you as a professional. In some care settings, you will be required to follow a **dress code** or to wear a uniform in order to project a professional image.

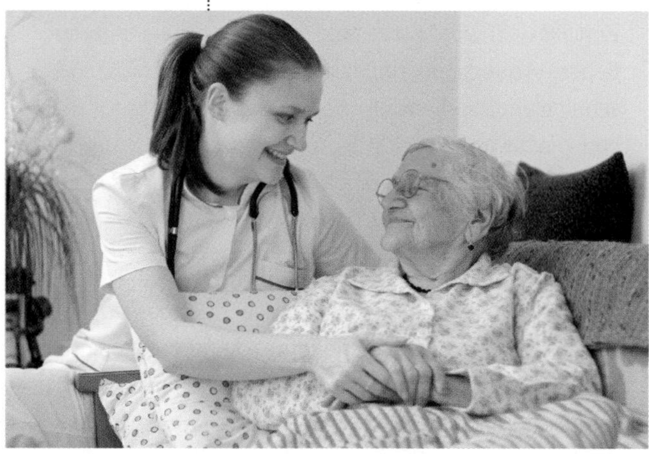

Professionalism is vital in care practice.

Developing your professionalism

What health and social care workers do at work is known as their *practice*. The precise nature of a person's care practice depends on the type of setting they work in and their work role. To work at a professional level, you will need to:

- demonstrate the skills expected of others performing the same work role
- achieve the same standards of good practice as those performing the same role

- use and demonstrate care values
- communicate effectively with others
- support and contribute to teamwork
- work within the legal framework of care
- accept responsibilities
- acknowledge the limits of your own abilities and competence.

Key terms

Beliefs: *knowledge-based convictions that affect how people view the world and respond to others*

Values: *moral beliefs that affect the way people think and behave*

Developing appropriate beliefs and values

Your own **values** and **beliefs** should fit comfortably with those of your health and social care sector. This may mean that you have to reflect on your personal beliefs and values; consider whether they are appropriate for care work and ask whether you are always supportive of others. It is important that you are empathetic and non-judgemental, and that you are able to accept diversity and difference, for example. In this context, you will have to develop your knowledge of relevant legislation, codes of practice and the organisational policies and procedures that establish the minimum standards for care practice and that guide the behaviour of care practitioners.

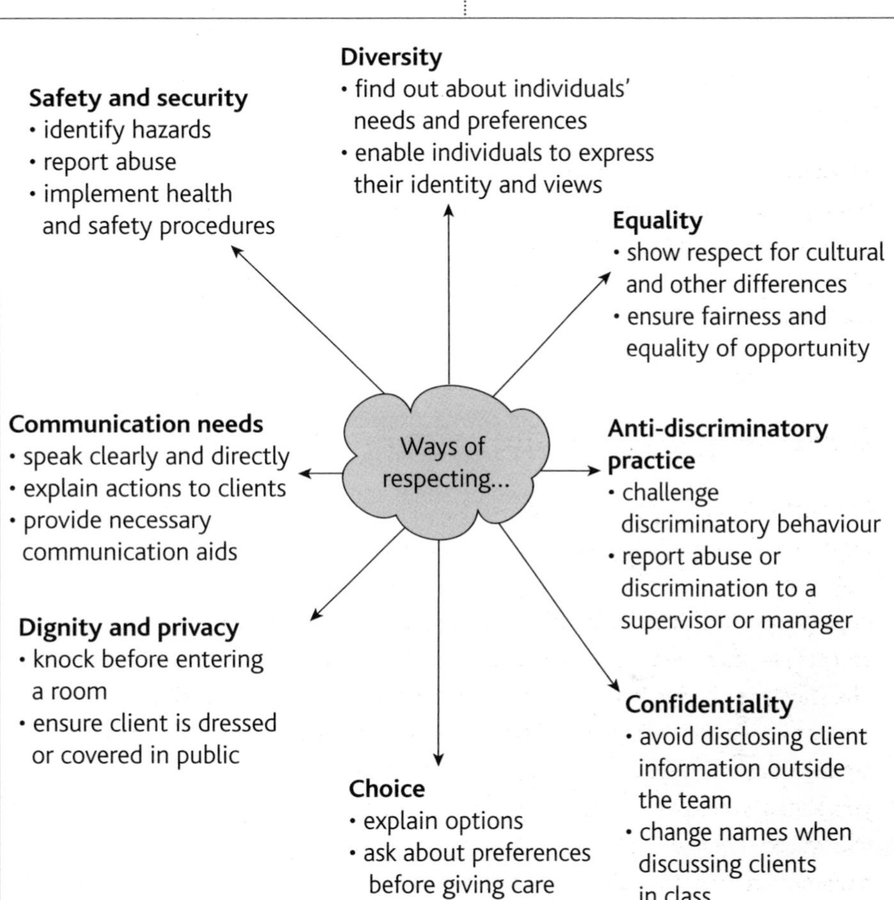
Ways of respecting...
Safety and security
• identify hazards
• report abuse
• implement health and safety procedures
Diversity
• find out about individuals' needs and preferences
• enable individuals to express their identity and views
Equality
• show respect for cultural and other differences
• ensure fairness and equality of opportunity
Communication needs
• speak clearly and directly
• explain actions to clients
• provide necessary communication aids
Anti-discriminatory practice
• challenge discriminatory behaviour
• report abuse or discrimination to a supervisor or manager
Dignity and privacy
• knock before entering a room
• ensure client is dressed or covered in public
Confidentiality
• avoid disclosing client information outside the team
• change names when discussing clients in class
Choice
• explain options
• ask about preferences before giving care

Figure 6.14 How to use care values.

A care practitioner's values and beliefs affect they way they provide care for others (see Unit 2). It is important to recognise and accept other people's values and beliefs, and to avoid imposing your own. Remember that care values should be written into the policies and procedures used in the care settings where you work. Following them will ensure that you demonstrate good practice and high standards of professional conduct.

Acknowledging your limitations

P2 Recognising personal responsibilities and limitations

Working at a professional level and presenting a professional image are important goals for all care practitioners. However, as a student starting out as a care practitioner, it is vitally important to work within the boundaries of your own competence.

Of course, this applies to all care practitioners, but people at the beginning of their care career are sometimes tempted to overstate their competence, perhaps because they are afraid of admitting they don't know something or can't do something.

It is better to be honest about your abilities, gradually increasing your workplace skills and responsibilities over time. Never put yourself and other people in situations where mistakes might be made. Taking responsibility for yourself and your own actions is an important part of developing professionally – and of growing up in general! As such, you need to learn to recognise your own personal and professional limits to protect yourself and others.

Your assessment criteria:

P2 Assess own knowledge, skills, practice, values, beliefs and career aspirations at the start of the programme

Reflect

Have you ever been asked perform care-related tasks that you didn't feel confident about or were not trained to do? How did you deal with these situations?

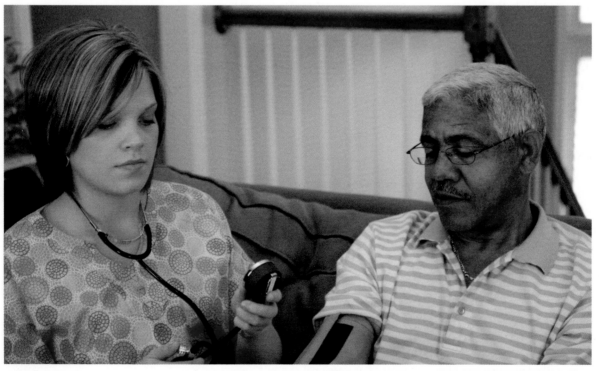

You should not try to take a person's blood pressure unless you have been trained to perform this task.

Case study

Jenna started working as a childminder 6 months ago. She currently cares for three children after school and wants to take on more during the day, to build her career and make more money. Jenna has been given her annual inspection date by Ofsted and is keen to receive a high rating. She believes that this will make the parents who currently use her services feel confident enough to recommend her to other parents.

Jenna has never looked after babies or toddlers but is going to say that she can – she knows that many new mothers are under pressure to return to work. She thinks that she could manage a couple of younger children, as well as the three she currently looks after. Jenna has been advised she must fill in a self-assessment evaluation online. After looking at the questions, she has decided that there is nothing to stop her from exaggerating her experience and performance a bit so that she looks more impressive to parents and the Ofsted inspectors.

1. What concerns, if any, do you have about Jenna's approach to childminding?
2. Would you be happy to leave a young child in Jenna's care?
3. Why is it important that Jenna recognises the limitations of her own experience and skills?

Reflect

Whose health and safety do over-confident care practitioners put at risk? What might be the consequences of this?

What do you know?

1. What does the term ***baseline*** refer to in relation to a personal development plan?
2. Identify three things you should reflect on at the start of your personal development planning.
3. How could you find out about the skills and entry requirements of the care roles that interest you?
4. Identify four different types of skill needed by health and social care practitioners.
5. Describe the qualities and skills a care practitioner needs to work effectively with others.
6. Explain why personal and organisations skills are important in care practice.

Producing and monitoring a professional development plan

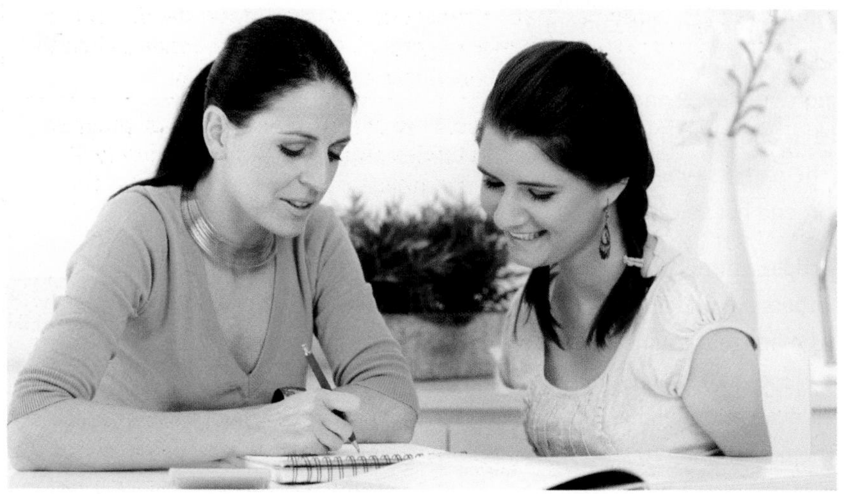

A professional development plan should focus on your individual learning needs.

Your assessment criteria:

P3 Produce an action plan for self-development and achievement of own personal goals

P3 Plan for your own development

As we have seen, carrying out a self-assessment to establish a baseline understanding of your knowledge, skills and achievements is the first step in creating a personal development plan. Once you are aware of the knowledge, skills or other aspects of practice that you need to focus on, you will be able to set some short-term and long-term **goals**. The goals that you set should enable you to develop and achieve the standards expected for your career path in health and social care work.

To plan for your development you need to:

- set goals and **targets**
- produce an action plan to work towards achieving your personal goals
- implement the plan.

Key terms

Goal: *an endpoint to aim for*

Target: *a specific measure of achievement*

Goals and targets

A goal is the destination point in a development journey; targets are specific standards to achieve. For example, you may set a goal of passing this unit with a target of achieving a merit grade. As part of your personal development planning, you should identify goals that complete your knowledge and skills gaps. Your targets will address specific development needs. You should also identify the actions that you will have to take to achieve your goals and targets.

Reflect

Do you have any particular goals relating to your BTEC course? How do these address your development needs?

Figure 6.15 Examples of goals.

Focus of goal	Example of short-term goal	Example of long-term goal
Knowledge	To obtain information about job vacancies at my local nursery by the end of next week.	To know about and understand the differences between general, paediatric and mental health nursing roles by the end of Unit 6.
Skills	To talk clearly and confidently when answering the phone during next work placement.	To report my observations of clients' progress and activities objectively and confidently at team meetings by the end of my final work placement.

Prioritising

Prioritising is an important part of the goal and target-setting process. You will need to establish priorities because some goals and targets are more important than others, and some are easier to achieve than others. Prioritising goals and targets involves putting the most important first and allocating more time, effort and other resources to achieving them, before focusing on less important or relatively minor goals.

Timescales

It is a good idea to work out the sequence in which you plan to tackle your personal development goals (some will be higher priority than others; some will depend on others being completed first) and to set a realistic deadline for each one.

Your timescales and deadlines may be challenging but must always be achievable. Most of your goals for the personal development plan you are about to create will be relatively short term (looking up to 6 months ahead). However, you could set longer-term goals (perhaps 18 months away) linked to your career progression too.

Reflect

Can you think of any particular development goals that you would like to achieve over the next 6 months? Consider the goals you want to achieve in relation to your knowledge, skills, practice, values, beliefs and career aspirations, for example.

Developing an action plan

The action plan that you create to promote your personal development plan should specify a range of goals and targets, being quite specific about how you intend to achieve them. Remember that your action plan is a way of addressing your self-assessed needs and of progressing towards becoming an effective care practitioner.

P3 Setting personal goals

The goals that you set should be stated in a way that allows you to measure your progress. To help you set helpful goals, you should ensure that they are SMART:

- Specific (What, specifically, will I achieve?)
- Measurable (How will I measure it?)
- Achievable (Is it something I am capable of doing?)
- Relevant (Is it directly related to my personal and professional development?)
- Timely (What is my deadline?)

Examples of goals that are SMART, as well as some goals that don't fit these criteria, are presented in Figure 6.16 below.

Goals that are broken down into small steps are less daunting and more achievable than huge, challenging and ambitious goals. When writing your action plan, remember to build in sufficient time and some flexibility in terms of when and how you will achieve each goal. When you have produced your action plan you will have a detailed list of actions that you need to undertake to achieve your goals. You will need to monitor the plan, adjust it as you go along and ensure that you are making progress.

Your assessment criteria:

P3 Produce an action plan for self-development and achievement of own personal goals

P4 Produce evidence of own progress against action plan over the duration of the programme

Reflect

Think about your own development needs and what you would like to achieve during your BTEC National Health and Social Care course. Jot down some ideas that you could develop into SMART goals in a plan like Figure 6.16. You might want to create a similar template so that you can have a go at creating a trial personal development plan.

Discuss

In a small group discuss the goals presented in Figure 6.16. Identify which ones are SMART (and the reasons why) and which are not.

Figure 6.16 An example of a personal development plan (2011–13).

Goals	Actions	Deadline for completion	Review notes	Date completed
1. I want to become a more effective communicator.	• Talk more in class – don't be so shy. • Volunteer to do class presentations. • Be more outgoing in placement setting this year.	30.03.11		
2. I want to get a job working in a care setting in the summer holidays to improve my care practice.	• Identify local care providers who have part-time and temporary work roles. • Create a CV and letter of application and send to local organisations. • Practise and improve my interview technique at college.	30.06.11		
3. I want to do well in my BTEC National course.	• Plan study time each week. • Attend all classes and contribute in class. • Complete all assignments on time.	30.12.11		
4. I want to find out about careers in nursing so that I can apply for a university course next year.	• Find out about entry qualifications and course providers. • Research job roles and career pathways in different areas of nursing.	30.09.12		

P4 Monitoring and evaluating your plan

Your action plan is a working document and it should be subject to revision as you make progress, and respond to changing circumstances and new opportunities. It should guide your activities as you implement the plans that will help you achieve your goals. It will form the basis of your self-evaluation as you monitor your progress against your plans. This involves setting review dates to ask questions about your progress (see Figure 6.17).

Figure 6.17 Questions to ask when reviewing progress.

Aspect of review	Question to ask
Reviewing progress against action plan	What have I done?
Reviewing progress against timescales	Did I meet the deadline?
Recording progress and achievements to date	What have I achieved?
Identifying what to do next	What is my next priority?
Changing goals or adjusting your targets	Do I need to set new goals or change existing ones?

Few personal development plans are completed smoothly and without change. Typically, they are amended to cope with changes in circumstances, goals and responsibilities, for example. However, throughout the planned period of development, the implementation of each action point should to be monitored carefully to ensure that you keep making progress towards your goals.

What do you know?

1. Identify two stages or aspects of personal development planning that occur after a baseline has been established.
2. What are personal development goals?
3. Explain why prioritising is an important part of personal development planning.
4. Identify the five features of SMART goals.
5. Describe two ways of monitoring a personal development plan.
6. Explain why it is important to evaluate a personal development plan and what this involves.

Assessing and evaluating your professional development

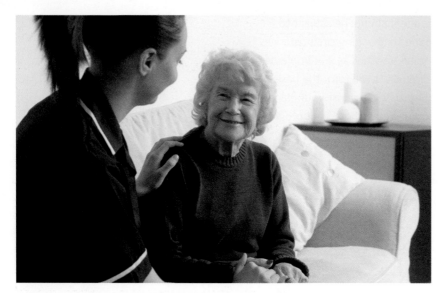

Being compassionate and reflective are important elements of care work.

Your assessment criteria:

P5 Reflect on own personal and professional development

P5 Reflection

As we have seen, your personal development plan should contain some review dates. These are the points at which you **assess** progress made towards your goals and you **evaluate** your professional development. Reflecting on what you can do now and on what you know now in comparison to your baseline point is the key to this process.

Kolb proposed that adults learn a great deal by reflecting on their experiences (see page 260). **Reflection** is important in health and social care practice because it helps care practitioners to:

- develop their judgement
- make sense of complex, confusing situations
- develop self-assessment and self-criticism skills
- improve thinking skills
- develop the ability to see situations from a range of perspectives
- separate their personal feelings from their professional role
- develop problem-solving skills.

Health and social care practitioners often face uncertain and challenging situations in their day-to-day care practice; a reflective approach is helpful in dealing with the unexpected. Learning from reflection during

Key terms

Assess: *make a judgement about the extent to which something has been achieved*

Evaluate: *draw conclusions about something*

Reflection: *this involves thinking about our actions, feelings or experiences to gain further understanding and insight*

your BTEC National course should help you to understand yourself better as a person and as a student. It should also help you to make better informed career choices and to see where you would best fit into the health and social care sector.

Techniques to aid reflection

How do health and social care practitioners reflect on their development and practice? Typically they use techniques such as:

- questioning to explore and consider an issue
- talking through issues with others in an open-minded and inquisitive way
- writing their thoughts and feelings down in a reflective diary or journal.

You could use any (or all) of these techniques to assess your progress and evaluate your professional development plan.

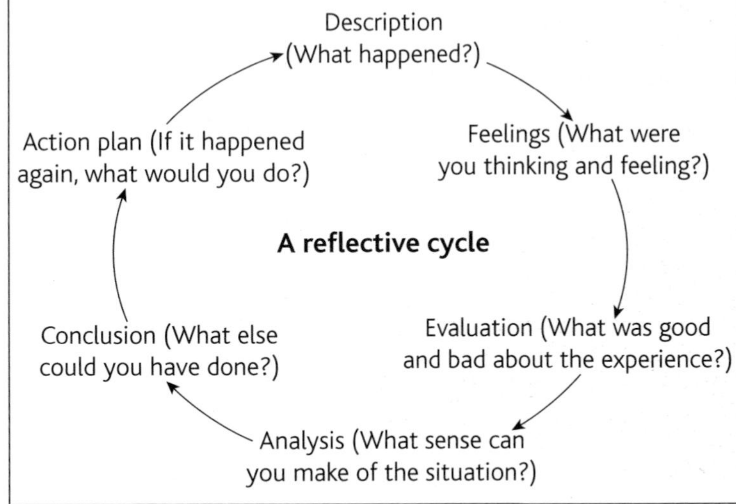
Description (What happened?)
Feelings (What were you thinking and feeling?)
A reflective cycle
Evaluation (What was good and bad about the experience?)
Analysis (What sense can you make of the situation?)
Conclusion (What else could you have done?)
Action plan (If it happened again, what would you do?)

Figure 6.18 Reflective questions.

Case study

Kelly is an experienced classroom assistant; she has worked in a primary school for 3 years, mainly with children aged between 9 and 10 years. At the start of term, she moved to work in the reception class with 4-year-old children. Kelly struggled to adapt to the different ways of working in the reception class. At first she felt overwhelmed by the amount of practical help that the younger children needed. She wasn't used to helping children with coats and shoes, and didn't always notice when they needed to use the toilet. This led to several accidents and Kelly became cross and impatient with some of the children. Jane, the class teacher, asked Kelly to reflect a bit more on her approach to her new role. Kelly wrote down her thoughts and feelings a couple of times a week. This really seemed to help as Kelly became more aware of the children's needs and realised that her role should involve providing more hands-on physical assistance. As a result, Kelly felt much happier in her new job and became a more effective team member.

1. did Kelly need to do in order to reflect on her work role and practice?
2. What do you think were the benefits for Kelly of becoming a more reflective practitioner?
3. How do you think others may have benefited from Kelly's ability to reflect on her practice?

Discuss

In pairs or with a small group of class colleagues, discuss the techniques that you each use to reflect on your development and care practice.

- *Do you make time to think about what you have achieved?*
- *Do you write a reflective diary or journal?*
- *Are there any particular people with whom you feel comfortable discussing your progress?*

Creating a professional development portfolio

P5 Collecting evidence

You have to provide evidence for your end of unit assessment – evidence of your personal development planning and progress over the duration of the course. In practical terms this means that you will need to record and store evidence of your progress, reflections and achievements. The conventional way of doing this is to create a professional development portfolio.

An effective, well-organised portfolio might include:

- a practice diary or reflective journal detailing what you have done on placement and your reflections on this
- witness statements or signed records from supervisors and senior care workers to demonstrate your progress
- information about any training or development events you have attended
- your personal development plan and interim reviews.

Your professional development portfolio could be paper-based and ring-bound, or an ePortfolio. Your tutor may advise on the usual format used in your centre, or may allow you to choose your own format. Whatever format you use, your professional development portfolio should contain all the evidence required to complete Unit 6. The portfolio structure could include:

- a contents list, mapped against relevant assessment criteria or against aspects of your personal development plan
- evidence in the form of authenticated documents (e.g. witness or tutor statements and signatures), as well as examples of any written work
- a personal progress section that includes your personal development plan, monitoring and review notes on the plan, and your reflective diary
- an evaluative discussion of your achievements (focusing on the PDP goals)
- a list of the kinds of support that you have accessed during the course of the programme.

Your assessment criteria:

P5 Reflect on own personal and professional development

M2 Assess how the action plan has helped support own development over the duration of the programme

Investigate

Find out from your tutor what portfolio format you should use to record and collect evidence of your learning and development. If you have a free choice, try to obtain examples of portfolio formats used by successful students in previous years.

M2 Relevant evidence

Your professional development portfolio should contain sufficient relevant evidence to show that you have met the assessment criteria for Unit 6 *and* that you have achieved (or made progress towards) your PDP goals. This could include both formal and informal evidence that records your knowledge and abilities.

Figure 6.19 Examples of formal and informal evidence.

Type of evidence	Examples
Formal evidence	• assignments • reflective reports • witness statements • UCAS forms
Informal evidence	• notes on feedback received • notes of your own reflections • a reflective diary or journal of placement activity and experiences

Remember, each piece of evidence that goes into your professional development portfolio should demonstrate how you have met the assessment criteria for this unit or that you have achieved a PDP goal.

Reflect

Do you have examples of these types of evidence that you could include in your professional development portfolio?

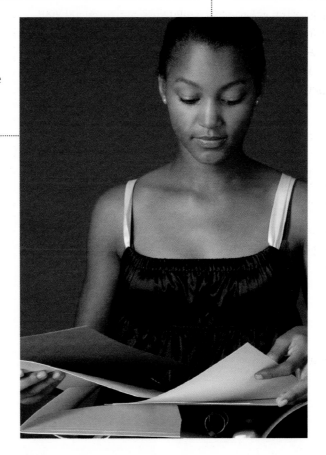

M2 M3 Producing a reflective diary or journal

A reflective diary or journal is a record of your own experiences on placement, in a format that you prefer. Bear in mind that any information you record and store electronically should be protected by a password, so that the confidentiality of others is protected.

Your reflective diary is the place to record all of the relevant development activities you take part in, especially those that are placement-related. Your reflective diary is a good place to:

- write about the ways in which you are – or sometimes are not – making progress in achieving your personal development plan goals
- explore the links between the theory-based learning you have experienced in college and the realities of care practice on work placements.

You should update your diary regularly so that you have an ongoing record of what you have done and how you have been developing. Writing a reflective diary should improve your self-awareness and ability to think about the ways in which you provide care. Writing in your diary regularly, ideally soon after taking part in activities, is a really good way of capturing accurately the details of developmental activities and your feelings about them. Remember to date the entries in your personal diary as this will help you to see your development over time. It is important to know that your diary cannot be totally confidential. Your tutor may ask to see it from time to time to monitor your learning and development for example, so bear this in mind when writing your entries.

M2 Support for your development

A number of different types of support should be available (see page 266) to promote your personal and professional development during your BTEC National programme. On work placement your supervisor will be a key source of support when you are putting your college-based learning into practice. This will support your practice learning and improve the quality of your care skills. Reflecting on how well you can apply theory to practice is a good way of assessing your progress.

Your assessment criteria:

- **P4** Produce evidence of own progress against action plan over the duration of the programme
- **M2** Assess how the action plan has helped support own development over the duration of the programme
- **M3** Use three examples to examine links between theory and practice
- **D2** Evaluate own development over the duration of the programme

Reflect

Who are the key people in school or college and in your placement setting who are willing and able to support your personal and professional development?

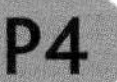

P4 M2 D2 Achievement of personal goals

Ultimately, you will be required to evaluate the extent to which you have met the goals you set as part of your personal development planning. Being as objective and honest as possible, you will need to reflect on the different ways in which you have made progress towards each goal. It is equally important to acknowledge goals that you have not been able to achieve. This may be because your goals or ability to meet them changed or because your priorities shifted over the year. Where this does happen, you should acknowledge and record changes, and update your personal development plan accordingly.

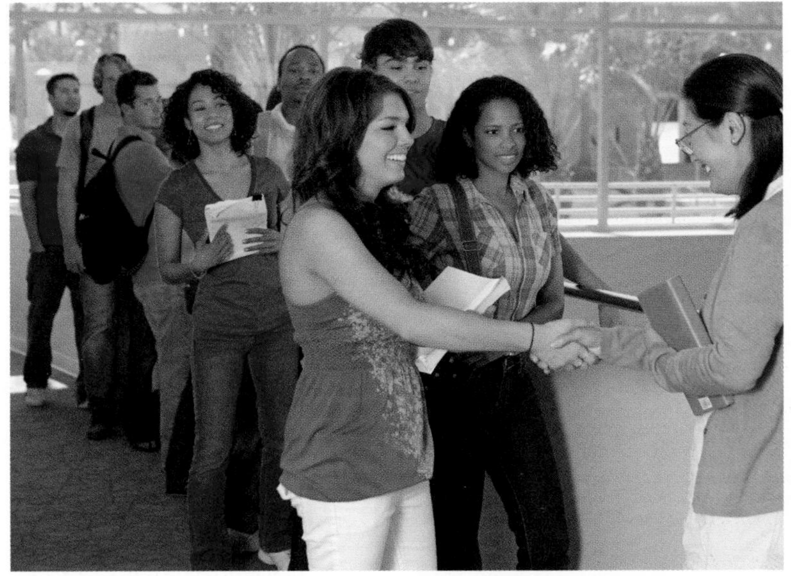

What do you know?

1. What does the term *assess* mean?
2. When should you evaluate your personal development plan?
3. Explain how developing reflective skills can improve an individual's care practice.
4. Identify three techniques that can be used to aid reflection.
5. Describe the purpose and contents of a personal development portfolio.
6. What is the purpose or value of completing a reflective diary or journal?

Health and social care services by sector

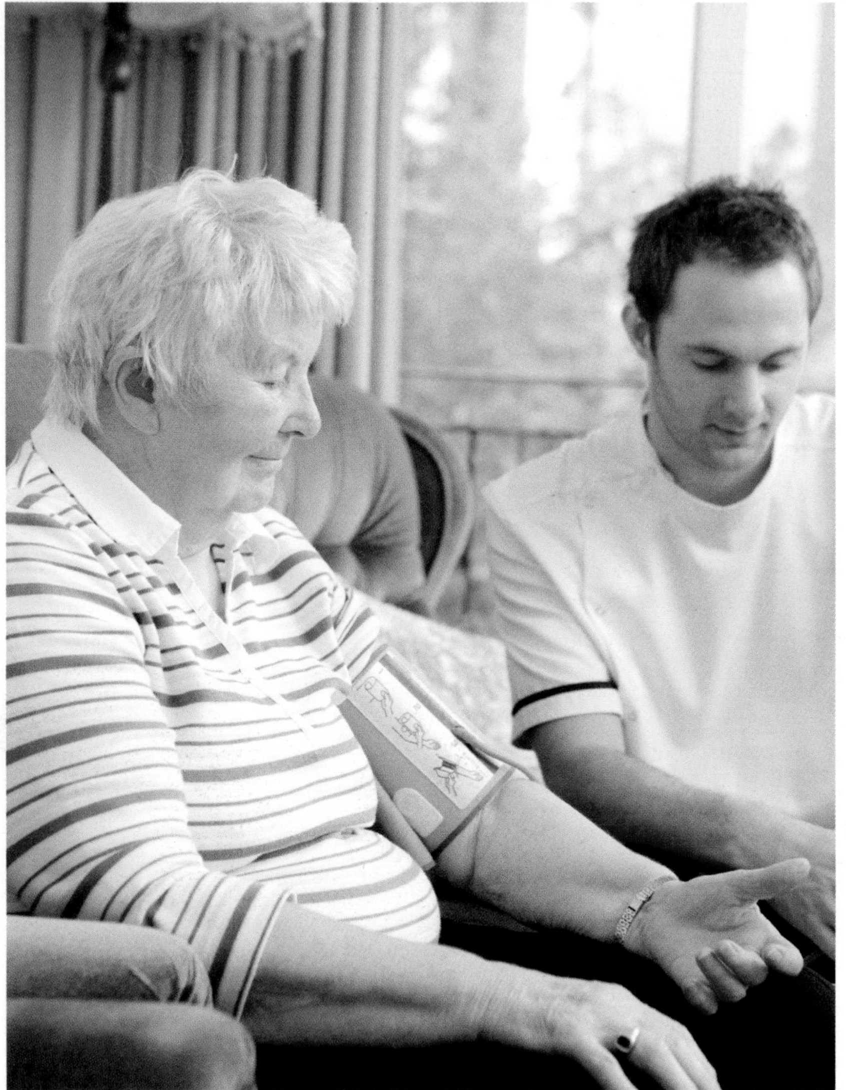

Care work with older people occurs in a variety of different settings.

Your assessment criteria:

P6 Describe one local health or social care provider identifying its place in national provision

P6 Forms of service provision

You probably know about a number of health, social care and early years services in your local area; there may be a hospital, health centre, family GP service, a nursery or a residential home near to where you live. One way of understanding how care services are provided is to look at how they are organised into **statutory**, **voluntary**, **private** and **informal** care sectors.

Key terms

Informal care sector: *relatives, friends and neighbours who provide physical care and emotional support on an unpaid basis*

Private sector: *this consists of care businesses and practitioners who charge for their services*

Statutory sector: *the public sector, fulfilling the government's legal (statutory) obligation to provide care*

Voluntary sector: *this consists of registered charities and not-for-profit organisations*

Reflect

Make a list of all the health and social care services you can remember using. Do you know which of these were provided by statutory (public), private or voluntary sector organisations?

The statutory or public sector

The government is responsible for controlling and running the part of the care system known as the statutory or public sector (see also page 290). This part of the care system includes organisations such as the National Health Service (NHS) and Local Authority-run care services. These organisations provide a lot of health, social care and early years services throughout the United Kingdom. By law, the government has to provide some types of care services. The laws that set out these duties are also known as 'statutes' – this is where the term ***statutory*** comes from.

The private sector

The private sector is made up of care ***businesses***, such as private hospitals, high street pharmacists and private nurseries, as well as self-employed care practitioners, such as childminders, counsellors and osteopaths, for example. Private sector organisations and self-employed practitioners usually charge people a fee for the health, social care or early years services that they provide. These care providers work to make a profit, as well as to meet service users' care needs. In the United Kingdom, the private sector offers fewer services, has fewer organisations and fewer service users than either the statutory or voluntary sector. Private sector organisations focus more on health and early years services than on social care. Many of the services that are provided in the private sector cannot easily be obtained in the statutory system and are specialist, non-emergency services. Day care nurseries and osteopathy services are examples.

The voluntary care sector

The care system in the United Kingdom includes a large voluntary sector. The voluntary care sector is made up of organisations that provide their care services on a charitable basis. Voluntary sector care organisations are independent of government; they don't have a legal duty to provide care service but do it voluntarily. The sector is also called 'voluntary' because many of the organisations have workers who are unpaid volunteers. Voluntary organisations provide a large range of non-profit making social care and early years services in the United Kingdom. *MENCAP* is an example of a voluntary sector organisation that recruits volunteers to work with people who have learning disabilities.

Key terms

Local Authority: *a local council, responsible for social care provision in an area*

National Health Service: *the organisation that provides government-funded public health care services throughout the UK*

Public sector: *this consists of statutory or government-funded health and social care services*

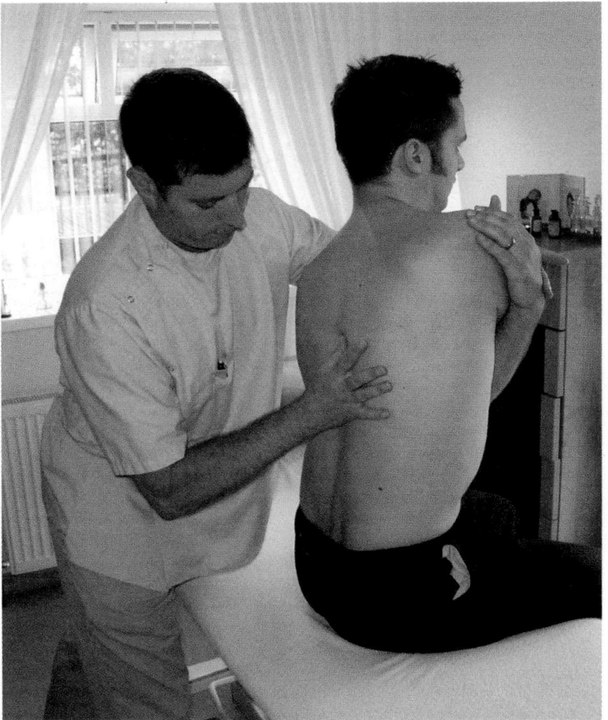

Osteopaths typically work in the private sector.

Public sector health care provision

P6 Public sector funding in the UK

The strategic planning and funding of public health and social care services in the United Kingdom is the responsibility of central government, specifically the Department of Health based in London. The Department of Health obtains funding for health and social care services from the Treasury. Some of this funding is then allocated to the Welsh Assembly, the Northern Ireland Assembly and the Scottish Parliament so that health and social care services can be provided in each of the home nations of the UK.

Public health care services

Statutory health care services first became available in the UK in 1948 when the National Health Service (NHS) was founded. The NHS was launched to tackle widespread problems of ill-health and to provide free services for all in the United Kingdom.

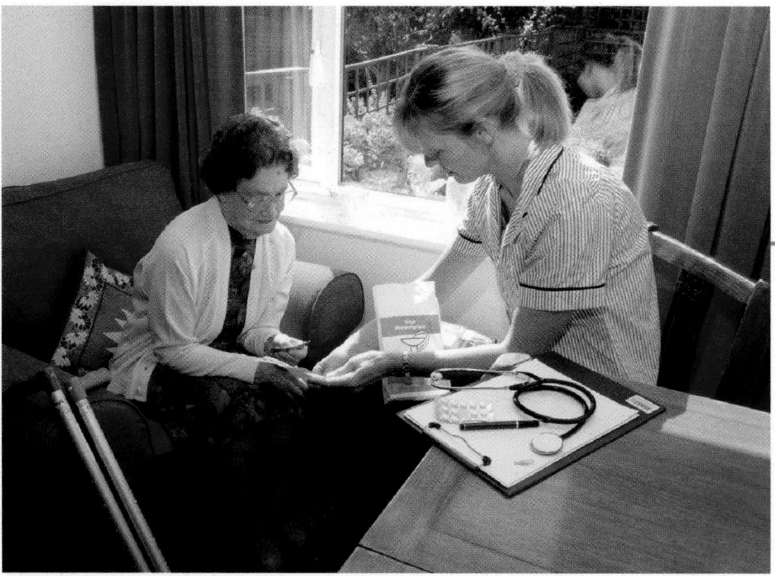

Health care work may involve teaching people to deliver aspects of their own care.

Government politicians and civil servants make decisions about how statutory health care services should be organised and paid for throughout the country. The politician who has overall responsibility for this is called the **Secretary of State for Health**. England, Wales, Scotland and Northern Ireland each have different Secretaries of State for Health. They are each responsible for planning and making decisions about NHS services in their country (see Figure 6.20).

Your assessment criteria:

P6 Describe one local health or social care provider identifying its place in national provision

 Key terms

Secretary of State for Health: *the government politician responsible for health and social care provision and policy*

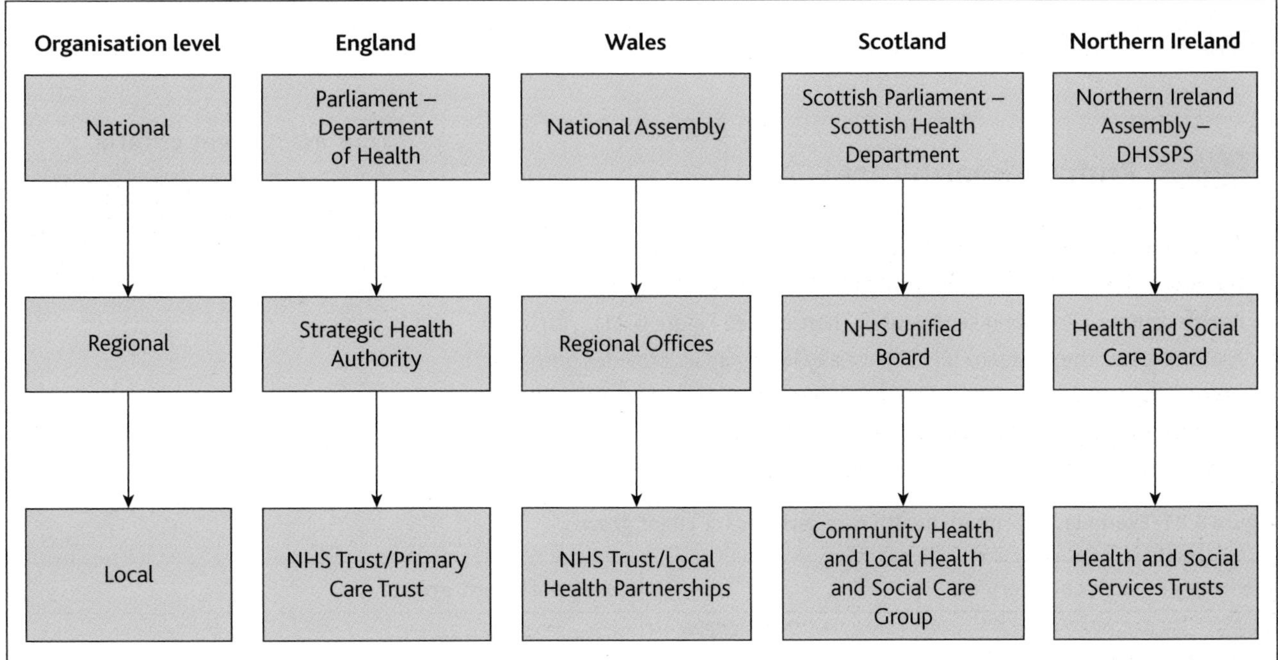

Figure 6.20 National and local health care structures.

The government funds most hospitals, GP practices and community health services in the United Kingdom. The actual planning and monitoring of local statutory health care services is carried out by regional bodies. These are called strategic health authorities in England, regional offices in Wales, NHS unified boards in Scotland, and health and social care boards in Northern Ireland (see Figure 6.20).

Types of NHS provider

Most of us will use public health care services at some point in our lives. We might need emergency hospital care or, more likely, have a less severe illness and go to our GP (family doctor) for help. The public or statutory health care services that we use will be provided by an **NHS Trust** organisation. Every area of the UK has an NHS Trust that takes responsibility for providing statutory health care in their locality. NHS Trust organisations provide three main types of health care service for people of all ages:

- **primary** health care services
- **secondary** health care services
- **tertiary** health care services (see page 292–3).

Reflect

Which national and local care structures apply to your area of the UK? Do you know how each part of the national and local structure contributes to the delivery of services?

Key terms

NHS Trust: *a statutory organisation that provides health care services to the public through hospitals and community health services*

Primary, secondary and tertiary health care services: *different levels of health care provision*

Primary, secondary and tertiary health care provision

P6 Primary health care

Primary health care involves assessment, diagnosis and non-emergency treatment services for all client groups in community settings, such as health centres, clinics and service users' homes (see Figure 6.21). A primary health care team (PHCT), usually led by a GP, provides primary care services. Other team members include practice nurses, district nurses, community psychiatric nurses and health visitors.

Your assessment criteria:

P6 Describe one local health or social care provider identifying its place in national provision

Figure 6.21 Examples of primary health care services for client groups.

Primary health care service	Example client group
Immunisation	Babies and children
Health visitor services	Babies
Health assessment and treatment	All client groups
'Flu vaccination	Older people and other vulnerable groups
Health promotion	All client groups
Referral to secondary services	All client groups
Family planning and contraception	Adolescents and adults

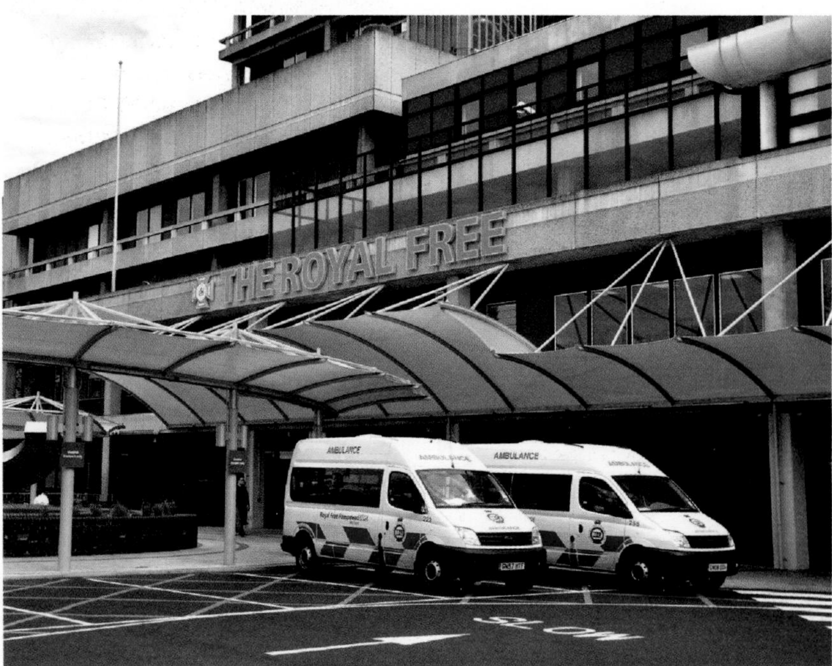

Secondary health care, such as emergency care, is provided in NHS Trust hospitals.

Reflect

What type of events or situations can result in people needing urgent care or specialist treatment from secondary health care services?

Secondary health care

Specialist types of care and treatment that are provided in a hospital or a specialist clinic are known as secondary care (see Figure 6.22). Most secondary health care is provided by NHS Trust hospitals. For example, large general hospitals usually have an accident and emergency department that deals with life-threatening and more minor injuries, a surgical department that deals with operations and a maternity unit that deals with childbirth. All of these departments provide specialised health care services.

Figure 6.22 Examples of secondary health care services for client groups.

Secondary health care service	Example client group
Midwifery	Pregnant women
Surgery	All client groups
Radiography (X-rays and other scans)	All client groups
Occupational therapy	All client groups
Psychiatric services	All client groups
Physiotherapy	All client groups
Paediatrics	Babies and children
Accident and emergency care	All client groups

Tertiary health care

Tertiary care services provide extremely specialised forms of care, often through regional centres of excellence. These tend to specialise in rare, complex and difficult-to-treat conditions or end-of-life care. Stoke Mandeville Hospital near Aylesbury provides tertiary care services at the National Spinal Injuries Centre.

Regulation of care

The Care Quality Commission (CQC) is the main **regulator** of health and adult social care provision in England. The CQC monitors standards of care in provider organisations, carrying out regular inspections to check that national minimum standards are being achieved.

The practice standards of health and social care professionals are regulated by a range of professional regulatory bodies including the Nursing and Midwifery Council, the General Social Care Council and the Health Professions Council. The work of these bodies is overseen by the Council for Healthcare Regulatory Excellence (www.chre.org.uk).

Investigate

Using information available through the internet, leaflets or booklets produced by your local NHS Trust, investigate the services offered by your nearest NHS Trust hospital. What kinds of specialist care and treatment are provided for children? Does the hospital specialise in any other kinds of health care service? Summarise your findings in either a poster or a leaflet.

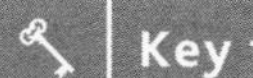

Key terms

***Regulator:** organisation responsible for monitoring the standards of care practice and service provision*

Employment in health and social care

P7 Health and social care workers

There is a wide range of work roles in the health, social care and early years services. These include:

- **direct care workers** – doctors, nurses, community nurses, health visitors, midwives, health care assistants, portage workers, child development workers, early years practitioners, family support workers, occupational therapists and teachers
- **indirect care workers** – practice managers, medical receptionists, school reception staff and catering staff.

Areas of care work

Jobs in health, social care and early years can also be grouped into a number of different areas of work. People working in:

- *health care roles* usually deal with individuals who have physical and medical problems, such as a disease, injury or acute illness
- *social care roles* usually deal with people who are vulnerable and who have care needs that result from social, emotional or financial difficulties
- *early years roles* are usually employed in child care and early education services for children under the age of 8 years.

Some service users have a combination of health, social care or early developmental problems, requiring more than one type of care. For example, a community psychiatric nurse who works with people experiencing mental health problems may need to offer his or her clients both health and social care.

Information about career pathways, training and qualifications required for entry into different areas of care work can be found on specialist websites such as www.nhscareers.co.uk. Many health and social care careers now require degree level qualifications. Details of these, and entry requirements for courses, can be found on the UCAS website at www.ucas.com/students/coursesearch.

Your assessment criteria:

P7 Describe the roles, responsibilities and career pathways of three health or social care workers

Key terms

Direct care workers: *care practitioners who give care directly to service users*

Indirect care workers: *support staff employed by the care organisations to carry out administrative and other tasks*

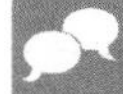

Discuss

In a small group identify examples of work roles related to health care, social care and early years work. Share what you know about the types of work activity each role involves.

Partnership working

Health and social care organisations, or agencies, work together by setting up integrated services. These use multidisciplinary teams in which staff from a range of separate services work in a collaborative way to meet the needs of a particular client group. Community mental health care, child protection and drug and alcohol services usually involve inter-agency working.

Multidisciplinary teams are very common in health and social care settings. They provide a way of pooling resources and expertise and are an efficient means of reducing duplication or overlap of service provision. Effective multidisciplinary teams should be able to provide a comprehensive range of care that meets even the most complex needs of individuals.

Workforce development

Workforce development in the health and social care sector is planned and supported by a number of sector skills councils (SSCs). These include:

- Skills for Care and Development (social care SSC)
- Skills for Health (health care SSC)

Each of these sector skills councils can also provide information on careers and qualifications in different areas of health and social care..

What do you know?

1. Identify three different forms of health and social care provision.
2. Describe examples of primary and secondary health care provided by the public sector.
3. Explain how standards of care provision are regulated in the United Kingdom.
4. Describe three main types of health and social care worker roles.
5. Explain why health and social care organisations often provide care services through multidisciplinary team arrangements.

Assessment checklist

Your learning and level of understanding of this unit will be assessed through assignments given to you and marked by your teacher or tutor. Before you submit your assignment work for assessment you should make sure that you have produced sufficient evidence to achieve the grade you are aiming for.

To pass this unit you will need to present evidence for assessment which demonstrates that you can meet all of the pass criteria for the unit.

Assessment Criteria	Description	✓
P1	Explain key influences on the personal learning processes of individuals	☐
P2	Assess own knowledge, skills, practice, values, beliefs and career aspirations at the start of the programme	☐
P3	Produce an action plan for self-development and achievement of own personal goals	☐
P4	Produce evidence of own progress against action plan over the duration of the programme	☐
P5	Reflect on own personal and professional development	☐
P6	Describe one local health or social care provider identifying its place in national provision	☐
P7	Describe the roles, responsibilities and career pathways of three health or social care workers	☐

You can achieve a merit grade for the unit by presenting evidence that also meets all of the following merit criteria for the unit.

Assessment Criteria	Description	✓
M1	Assess the impact of key influences on the personal learning processes on own learning	☐
M2	Assess how the action plan has helped support own development over the duration of the programme	☐
M3	Use three examples to examine links between theory and practice	☐

You can achieve a distinction grade for the unit by presenting evidence that also meets all of the following distinction criteria for the unit.

Assessment Criteria	Description	✓
D1	Evaluate how personal learning and development may benefit others	☐
D2	Evaluate own development over the duration of the programme	☐

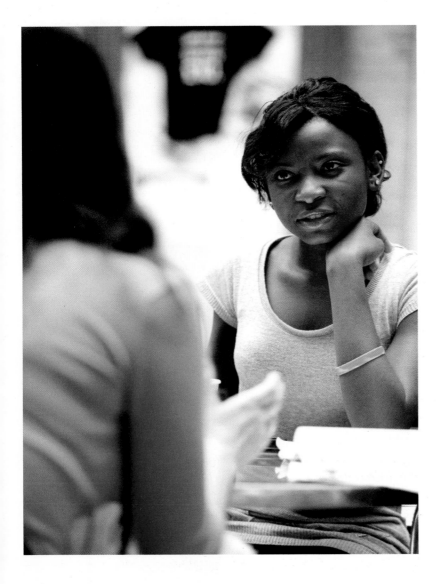

References

Honey, P. and Mumford, A. (1982) *The Manual of Learning Styles*, Maidenhead, Peter Honey

Kolb, D.A. (1984) *Experiential Learning*, Englewood Cliffs, Prentice Hall

7 Sociological perspectives in health and social care

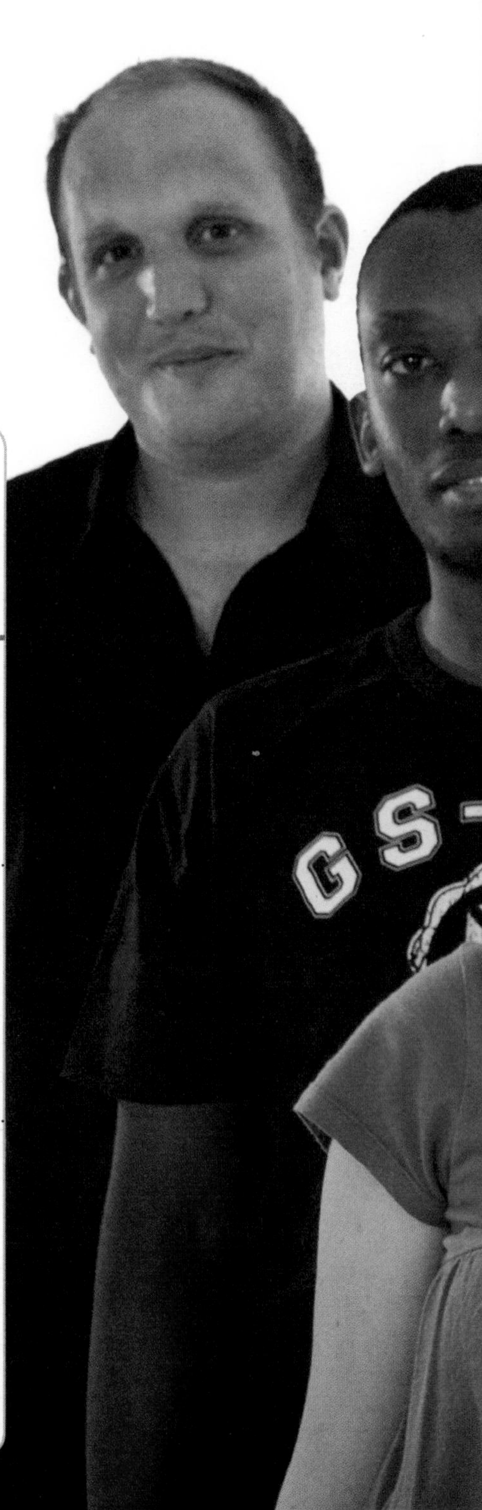

LO1 Understand sociological perspectives

- terminology (social structures, social diversity, socialisation)
- principal perspectives (functionalism, Marxism, feminism, interactionism, collectivism, postmodernism, New Right)

LO2 Understand sociological approaches to health and social care

- application to health and social care (concepts of health and ill health, patterns and trends among different social groups)
- understanding different concepts of health and ill health (concepts of health, models of health, ill health, the sick role, the clinical iceberg)
- understanding patterns and trends in health and illness among different social groupings (measurement of health, difficulties in measuring health, patterns and trends, sociological explanations)

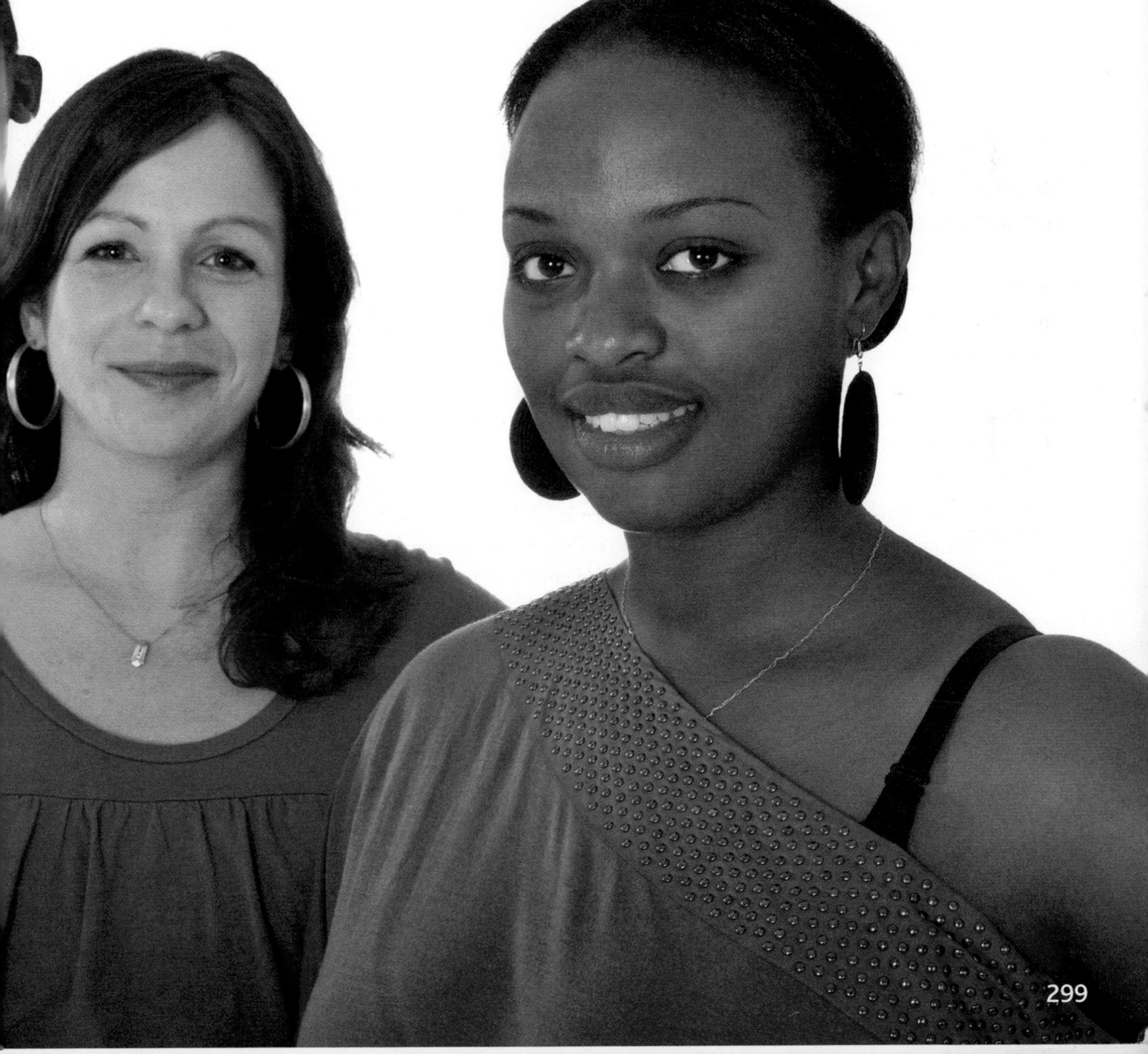

Social structures

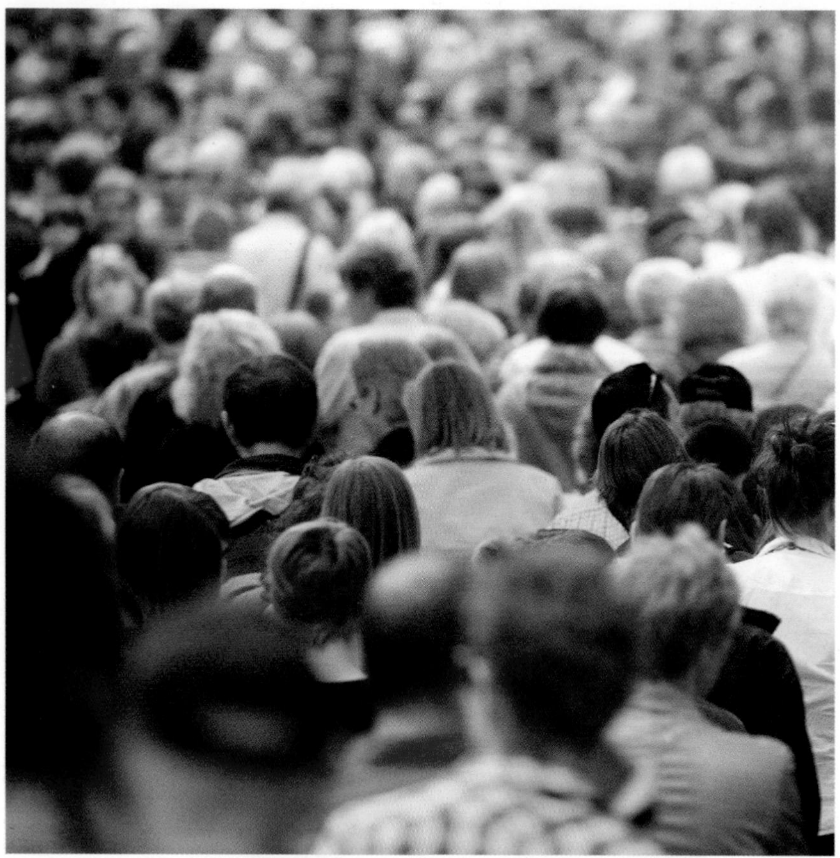

Your assessment criteria:

P1 Explain the principal sociological perspectives

Sociologists study human societies. The term 'sociology' has Latin and Greek origins and means 'reasoning about the social'. Auguste Comte (1798–1857), a French philosopher who lived through the upheavals of the French Revolution, is often given credit for coining the term 'sociology'. The early nineteenth-century period in which sociology emerged was an era of massive social change. From its earliest days, sociology has focused on:

- identifying and describing **social structures** and processes
- describing the effects and patterns of social change
- explaining the relationship between the individual and collective 'society'.

Sociology is now studied by all health and social care professionals as part of their initial training. This gives care professionals a better understanding of the circumstances people live in, and greater awareness of the pressures and factors that influence people's experiences of health and wellbeing.

Sociologists use a number of different concepts, such as social structure, **social diversity** and socialisation, to describe and explain the nature of society and how individuals become a part of it.

Key terms

Social diversity: *this term refers to the range of social differences in a population of people*

Social structure: *an organised pattern of social behaviour and the social institutions within society*

P1 A structured society?

Some sociologists think about and describe 'society' as consisting of a number of connected **social institutions** that organise and structure society (see Figure 7.1). These social institutions are often described as the 'building blocks' of society. From this perspective, each of these institutions has a specific role to play in society and must play it effectively for society to work efficiently. The family, the education system, the legal system and health and social care services are all examples of important social institutions that affect the structure of contemporary society. Though all of these institutions are continually developing and changing, they are also relatively permanent features of society. They each have a history of their own, will survive the death of the people who are currently part of them and provide a way of meeting a particular shared need in society.

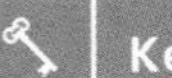

Key terms

Social institutions: *the organised social arrangements that are found in all societies*

Reflect

Can you think of reasons why the family is often described as the foundation or a 'building block' of society? Think about the function(s) it performs for society as a whole.

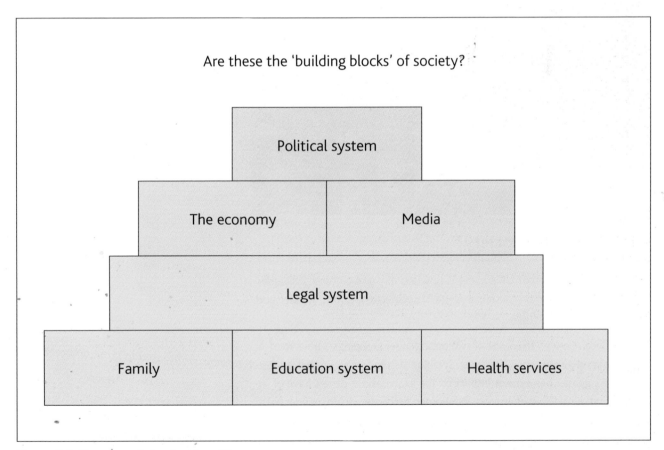

Are these the 'building blocks' of society?

	Political system	
The economy		Media
	Legal system	
Family	Education system	Health services

Figure 7.1 How is society structured?

Social diversity

P1 What is social diversity?

In some ways human beings have the same needs and share many qualities, abilities and interests because we all belong to the same species (*Homo sapiens*). However, sociologists recognise that society is also very diverse in many ways. There are lots of differences between the people who make up the UK population. Sociologists are particularly interested in the 'differences that make a difference' to people's lives. For sociologists, these differences include **gender**, **ethnicity**, **social class**, age, **culture** and locality. Sociological research shows that each of these social factors can have an impact on the life chances, health experiences and social opportunities of individuals and groups in society.

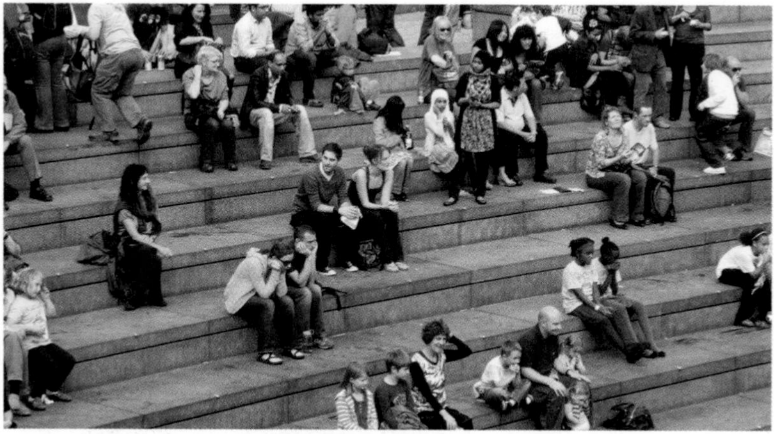

How diverse is society?

Sociologists claim that UK society is now socially and culturally diverse. Within the population there is a range of social class, ethnic, gender and age groups, for example.

Society can be seen to consist of two basic gender groupings – boys/men (males) and girls/women (females). Sociologists tend to argue that a person's gender has a major impact on the expectations others have of them, on our behaviour as men and women (because we 'do' gender as well as 'have' it), and ultimately on the life chances and opportunities of men and women as a population group. The key point sociologists are making is that gender is a difference that makes a difference within society.

Age is often seen to be a neutral fact or feature of the population. It's seen by many people as just a way of summarising how long a person has been alive. However, sociologists argue that there is an 'age

Your assessment criteria:

P1 Explain the principal sociological perspectives

Key terms

Culture: *the language, beliefs, norms, values, customs and practices that make up the 'way of life' of a society or a sub-group within it*

Ethnicity: *the shared culture of a social group that gives its members a sense of identity distinct from that of other groups*

Gender: *culturally created differences between men and women that are learnt through socialisation*

Social class: *a system consisting of broad groups of people (classes) who have a similar economic situation and status (occupation, income/wealth)*

Reflect

Can you think of any ways in which your gender makes, or has made, a difference to your health experience or your experience of care services?

hierarchy' in society and that the way in which society is organised and operates in response to ideas about age leads to the creation of distinct 'age groups' within society. These ideas and the way in which people are placed into age groupings have a big impact on the ways in which health and social care professionals work and the ways services are organised. The current age structure of the UK population is described in Figure 7.2.

Investigate

Using statistical sources, such as the Office for National Statistics website (www.ons.gov.uk), investigate the ethnic diversity of contemporary UK society. How do sociologists classify different ethnic groups and how ethnically diverse is UK society at the moment?

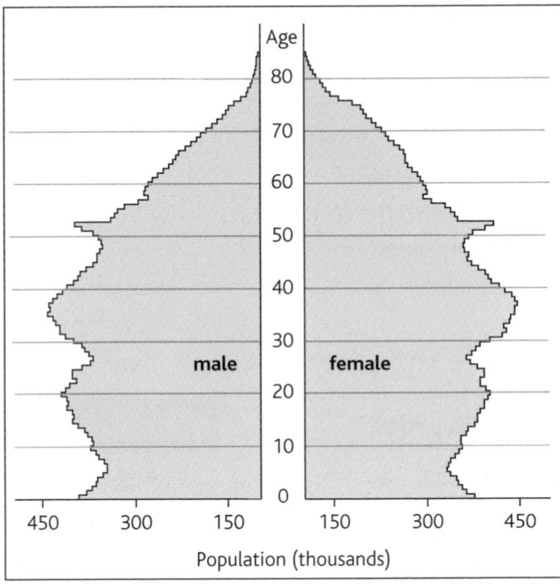

Figure 7.2 The age structure of society (Office for National Statistics, 2010).

Case study

Two Rivers NHS Trust provides mental health services for people of all ages. The Chief Executive of the Trust has recently commissioned research into the mental health care needs of the local population. The findings of the study have identified four distinct age groups consisting of people with shared mental health needs:

- infants and children
- people of working age
- young people
- older people.

The Chief Executive of Two Rivers NHS Trust is now putting together a proposal to reorganise the Trust into these four age-related departments.

1. What age ranges would you expect each of the groups above to cover?
2. Can you think of any advantages of organising services into age-related departments?
3. What might be the drawbacks or disadvantages of organising services into age-related departments?

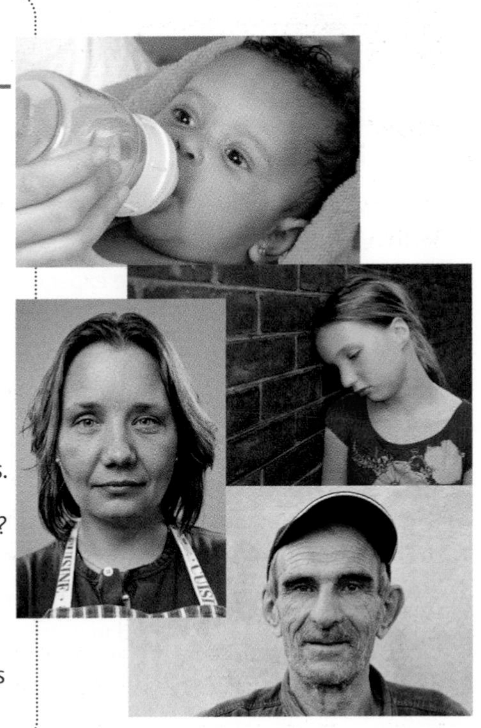

Social class

P1 What is social class?

Social class is a form of social stratification that is found in modern developed societies. Social classes are groups of people who have a similar economic position (type of job, income and status) and often a similar lifestyle, education and shared attitudes and values. Until 2001, the social classification system used to identify and record an individual's social class was the Registrar-General's scale. Statistics based on this scale were developed from census records that held details of the occupation of the ***male*** head of each household in the UK. The scale consisted of six social classes (see Figure 7.3) that were organised into a hierarchy linking occupations to social status.

Figure 7.3 Registrar-General's Social Class Scale.

Social class	Types of occupation
Class 1 – Professional occupations	Lawyers, doctors
Class 2 – Intermediate occupations	Executives, shopkeepers
Class 3N – Skilled, non-manual occupations	Clerks, policemen
Class 3M – Skilled, manual occupations	Electricians, coal miners
Class 4 – Partly skilled occupations	Farm workers, bus drivers
Class 5 – Unskilled	Labourers, cleaners

At the beginning of the twenty-first century, the Registrar-General's scale was felt to be out of date. A new scale, the National Statistics Socio-economic Classification (NS-SEC), was developed for use in the 2001 census. The NS-SEC scale expanded the classification system to reflect the growth of middle-class occupations, the changing nature of work and changes to the status of different jobs in the twenty-first century. There are now eight major social classes in the NS-SEC scale (see Figure 7.4).

Sociologists recognise that social class is not as important in the way that people define themselves as it used to be in the first half of the twentieth century. However, the UK is far from a 'classless' society – class does still have an impact on an individual's life chances and opportunities. This is explained in more detail later in the unit.

Your assessment criteria:

P1 Explain the principal sociological perspectives

Discuss

1. *Which of these categories does your father fit into?*
2. *Is there a gender bias in this scale?*

Figure 7.4 The National Statistics Socio-economic Classification (2001).

Social class	Types of jobs included
Higher managerial and professional occupations	Doctors, lawyers, dentists, professors, professional engineers
Lower managerial and professional occupations	School teachers, nurses, journalists, actors, police sergeants
Intermediate occupations	Airline cabin crew, secretaries, photographers, firefighters, auxiliary nurses
Small employers and own account workers	Self-employed builders, hairdressers, fishermen, car dealers and shop owners
Lower supervisory and technical occupations	Train drivers, employed artisans, foremen, supervisors
Semi-routine occupations	Shop assistants, postal workers, security guards
Routine occupations	Bus drivers, waiting staff, cleaners, car park attendants, refuse collectors
Never worked or long-term unemployed	Students, people not classifiable, occupations not stated

Reflect

How do you define your own, or your family's, social class? Do you aspire to be in a different social class?

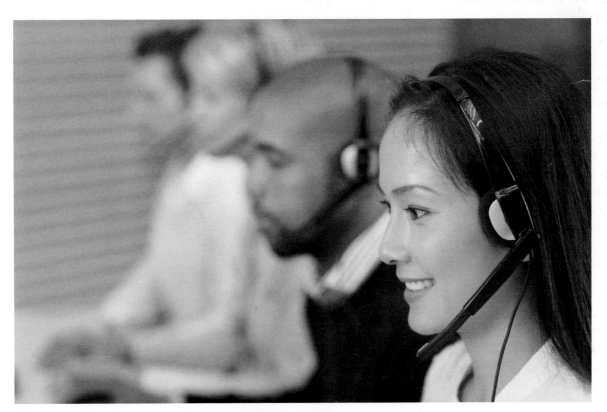

Where do call centre workers fit into the NS-SEC scale?

Socialisation

P1 What is socialisation?

Social institutions like the family and the education system give UK society its general shape, character and structure. UK society is relatively well ordered, law-abiding and cohesive. This is because most members of UK society are quite co-operative and share many attitudes, values and beliefs about the way people ought to behave and relate to one another. But how does this happen? How do all of the different individuals who make up society know how to behave and fit in to society? Sociologists use the concept of **socialisation** to explain this.

Primary socialisation occurs in the family during a child's early years. Children learn (or 'catch') social attitudes, values and acceptable ways of behaving from observing, and being informally educated by, parents, siblings and other significant relatives. However, sociologists also recognise that socialisation is a lifelong process. It continues during adolescence and adulthood into middle and old age.

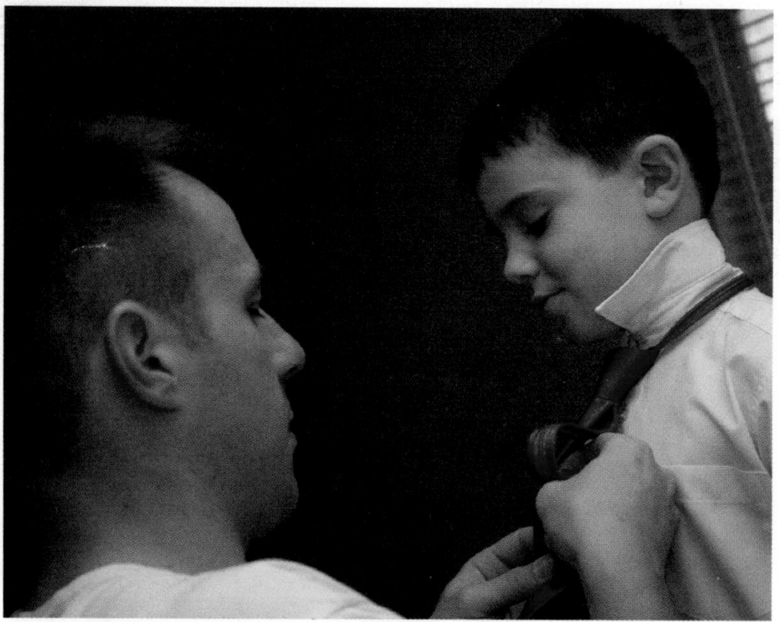

Secondary socialisation occurs outside of the family. Friends and peers, school mates, work colleagues, the media, role models, religious leaders and influential people such as teachers and employers are all agents of secondary socialisation.

Your assessment criteria:

P1 Explain the principal sociological perspectives

Key terms

Primary socialisation: *socialisation within the family during early childhood*

Secondary socialisation: *socialisation outside the family, which occurs throughout life*

Socialisation: *the process through which individuals learn the roles, norms and culture of a social group or society*

Discuss

With a small group of classmates, share your memories of how your parents influenced the way you behaved towards others during early childhood. You could discuss how you were taught to 'be polite' or to 'have good table manners' or any other aspect of socialisation that was important in your family.

How does socialisation affect us?

Sociologists argue that it is through socialisation processes that we all learn how to become members of society. We are born without any sense or knowledge of culture or of the **values** or **norms** of society. Culture, values and norms are transmitted to us though primary socialisation and then secondary socialisation. This enables us to relate to, fit in with and understand other members of society. Socialisation also plays a key part in forming an individual's identity. Many aspects of identity are formed through our particular experiences of family, friends, school, the mass media and the workplace, for example. We are affected by the way others see us and the way we define ourselves in these contexts, identifying with some groups or institutions and not others. In this way our sense of 'who' we are is shaped by and is also a response to lots of socialisation influences. As a result, we learn how to perform certain **roles** – as brother/sister, student, employee, for example – and also acquire and take into account the **status** of these roles when relating to others.

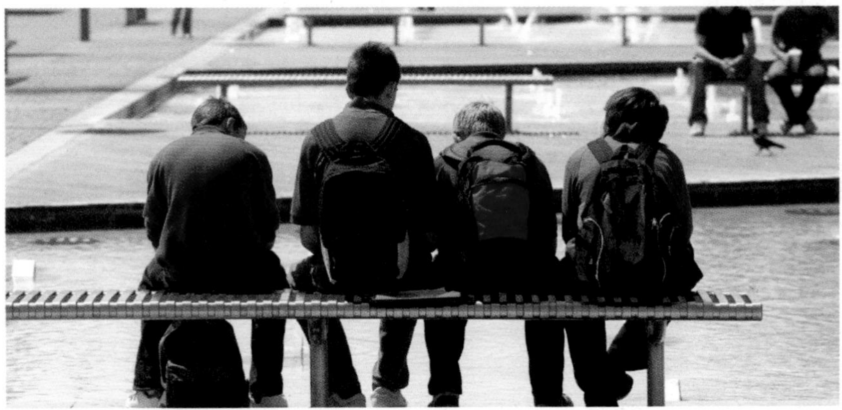

Some socialisation will take place at school.

What do you know?

1. In general terms, what do sociologists study?
2. Identify two examples of social institutions and describe their main functions for society.
3. In what ways is UK society socially and culturally diverse?
4. Describe the age structure of contemporary UK society.
5. What does the concept of socialisation refer to?
6. Explain how socialisation processes affect individuals in society.

Reflect

Can you think of any individuals, institutions or organisations that have had a significant socialising influence on the way your identity has developed?

Key terms

Norms: *social rules that define correct behaviour in society or a social group*

Roles: *patterns of behaviour expected from people in different positions in society*

Status: *the prestige or importance a person has in the eyes of other members of a social group or society*

Values: *moral principles*

Reflect

List all of the social roles that you play, identifying what you think others expect of you in each of these roles. What kind of status does each of these roles have? Think about the ways in which you have been socialised to perform each of these roles.

Functionalist and Marxist perspectives

Functionalism and **Marxism** are sociological perspectives that see society as structures with interconnected parts. Both of these perspectives focus on the structural features of society, but take a different approach to what makes society 'tick'. Functionalists opt for a consensus view, believing that the structure of society is designed to achieve harmony and agreement between people. Marxists opt for a conflict view, emphasising social differences and the conflicting interests and values of different groups in society.

Your assessment criteria:

P1 Explain the principal sociological perspectives

Key terms

Functionalism: *a sociological perspective that explains society in terms of interlinked social structures that perform important roles for society as a whole*

Marxism: *a perspective that sees the economy as the basis of society, and social class conflict as an inevitable and ongoing feature of social life*

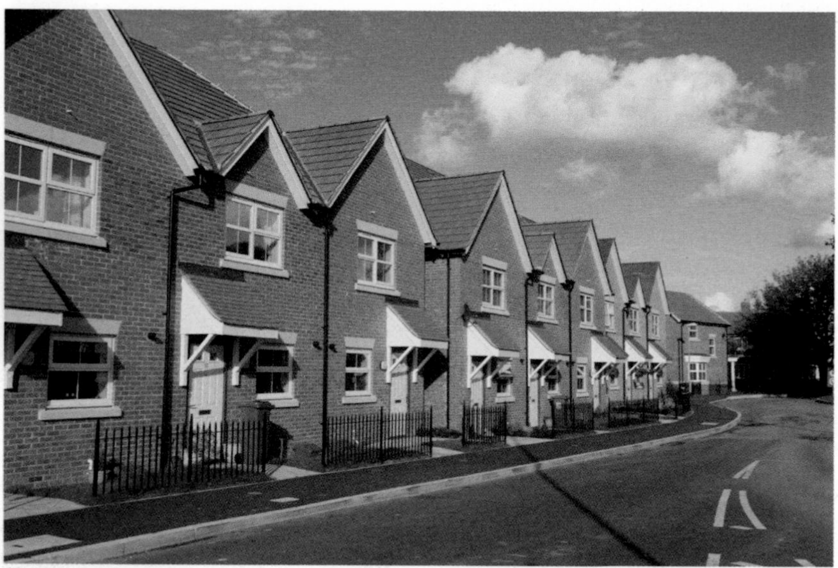

Functionalists present a harmonious view of society.

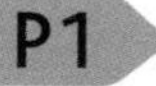

P1 The functionalist perspective

The functionalist perspective is based on the idea that societies are complete systems and that the parts within them cannot be understood in isolation from each other. The functionalist perspective uses a biological metaphor to describe this. Just as the heart, lungs and brain work together to maintain human life, so the family, education system and the law (for example) work together to maintain society. Where the human body consists of interdependent organs, society consists of interdependent social institutions. Each social institution has a particular function or contribution to make to society as a whole. Each social institution must function effectively and link with others appropriately in order for society to work as it should. Functionalists typically referred to society as a 'social system' to express this idea of an interlinked, interdependent network of social institutions.

Reflect

How do you view contemporary society? Do you think it is characterised more by consensus and harmony or by differences and conflict?

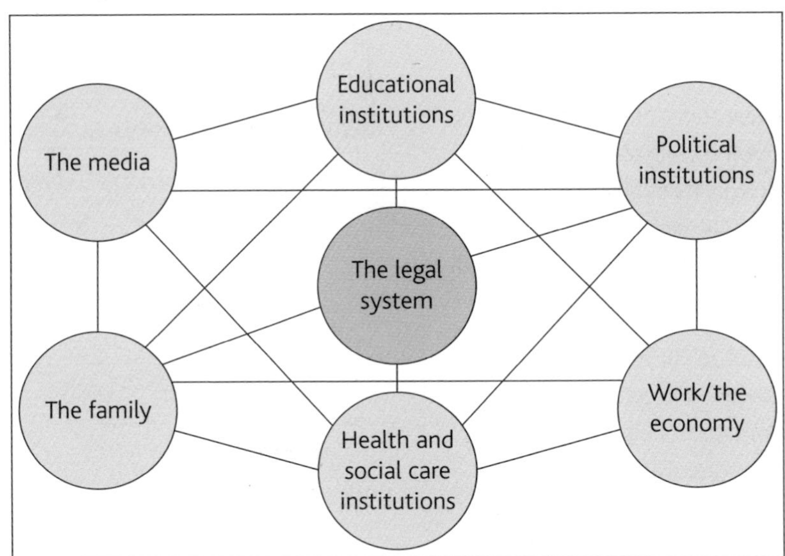

Figure 7.5 Society is a social system of connected institutions.

Functionalism and the family

Talcott Parsons (1902–1979) was an American sociologist who developed important aspects of the functionalist perspective in the mid-twentieth century. He believed that social institutions, like the family, had the role of socialising people to behave in acceptable ways so that order was maintained in society. Functionalists see the family as a key social institution in society. G.P. Murdock (1949) produced a classic functionalist study of the family in which he claimed that every known society, from large, developed societies to small hunter-gatherer tribal societies, contained some form of 'family' institution. Murdock identified four key functions of the family in each of these societies:

1. a sexual function, where the family is seen as the approved context or site for the expression of sexual behaviour
2. a reproductive function, where the family is seen as the best, most stable site or context for producing and rearing children
3. a socialisation function, where the family is given the main responsibility for teaching children how to behave in society
4. an economic function, where the family is given the responsibility for providing its members with food, shelter and financial security.

Parsons (1951) also saw the family as pivotal in society, arguing that its basic functions were:

- the primary socialisation of children
- stabilisation of adult personalities (looking after and nurturing adults, especially the male breadwinner).

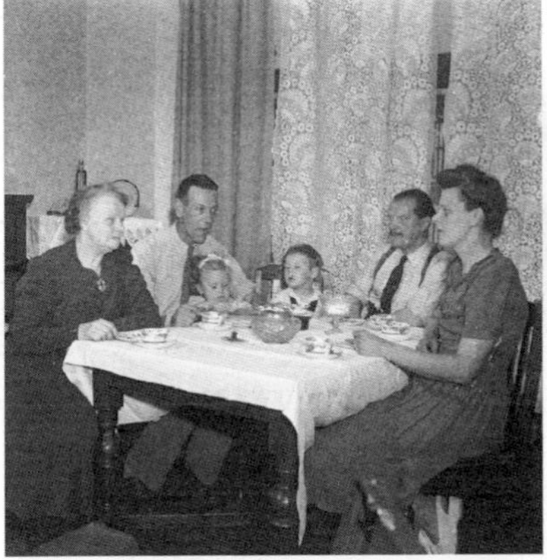

Do you think the role of the family has changed since the 1950s?

Discuss

Is the family an inevitable, unavoidable feature of society? In a small group, discuss possible alternatives to the family. What are the strengths and weaknesses of alternative ways of bringing up children, like the Kibbutz system in Israel or children's homes for children unable to live with their families, for example?

P1 The sick role

The concept of the 'sick role' was developed by functionalist sociologists. Parson's (1951) argued that individuals adopt a socially defined 'sick role' in modern society. Doctors play a key role in this through diagnosing illness and then defining an individual as officially 'sick'. Once a person is officially 'sick', they are free from any blame or guilt for being sick and are allowed to abandon their normal responsibilities and activities.

The sick role has both rights and obligations attached to it. For example, the sick person has the right to refrain from work and other normal social duties, but also the obligation to seek medical help and to return to full health as quickly as possible. This role is one way of dealing with ill health in society as it ensures the smooth functioning of society. The existence of the sick role ensures that the potential disruption disease and ill health could bring to society is kept to a minimum.

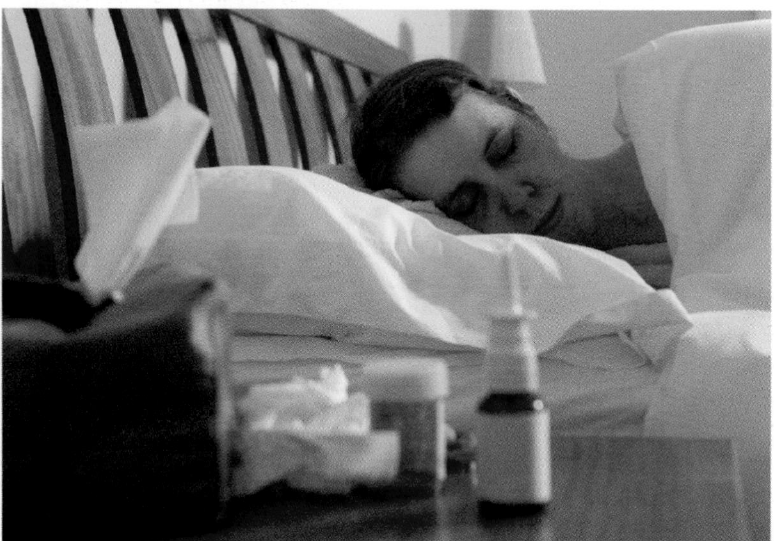

Weaknesses of functionalism

Functionalism was a popular and widely used sociological perspective in the middle of the twentieth century. Contemporary sociologists are now more critical of it because functionalism:

- ignores conflict and competition in society and paints an overly positive picture of the shared goals and values underpinning society
- focuses on the positive social functions of social institutions and roles and ignores any negative or harmful consequences; for example, adoption of the sick role by people with chronic problems and disability discourages full participation in society and may lead to dependency

Your assessment criteria:

P1 Explain the principal sociological perspectives

Reflect

Reflect on an occasion where you felt unwell and went to see your GP. Did you take on the 'sick role' when your doctor confirmed that you were 'sick'? How did your family and friends treat you differently when you were 'sick'? How did being defined as 'officially sick' affect your behaviour and relationships with others?

- is based on notions of value consensus and assumes that this underpins socialisation. However, in a diverse society many different, competing and at times antagonistic value systems coexist.

The Marxist perspective

Marxism is a political and sociological perspective based on the work of Karl Marx (1818–1883). Marx provided an account of the new class-based society that emerged after the industrial revolution. The Marxist perspective questions the functionalist idea that modern capitalist society is based on consensus (agreement) between the various social groups in society and harmony between social institutions. Instead, Marxists argue that society is really based on the unequal distribution of economic power and wealth.

Marxists believe that there are basically two social classes in capitalist societies, such as the UK. These consist of the **bourgeoisie** who own the 'means of production', and the **proletariat** who sell their labour to the owners of the means of production for wages. Marxists believe that the capitalist, bourgeois class exploit the proletariat and wield both economic and cultural power over them. This leads to a society that is characterised by antagonism and 'class conflict'.

Key terms

Bourgeoisie: *the class of wealthy people who own the means of production (factories, land etc.)*

Proletariat: *the class of poorer people who have to work for wages as they do not own the means of production*

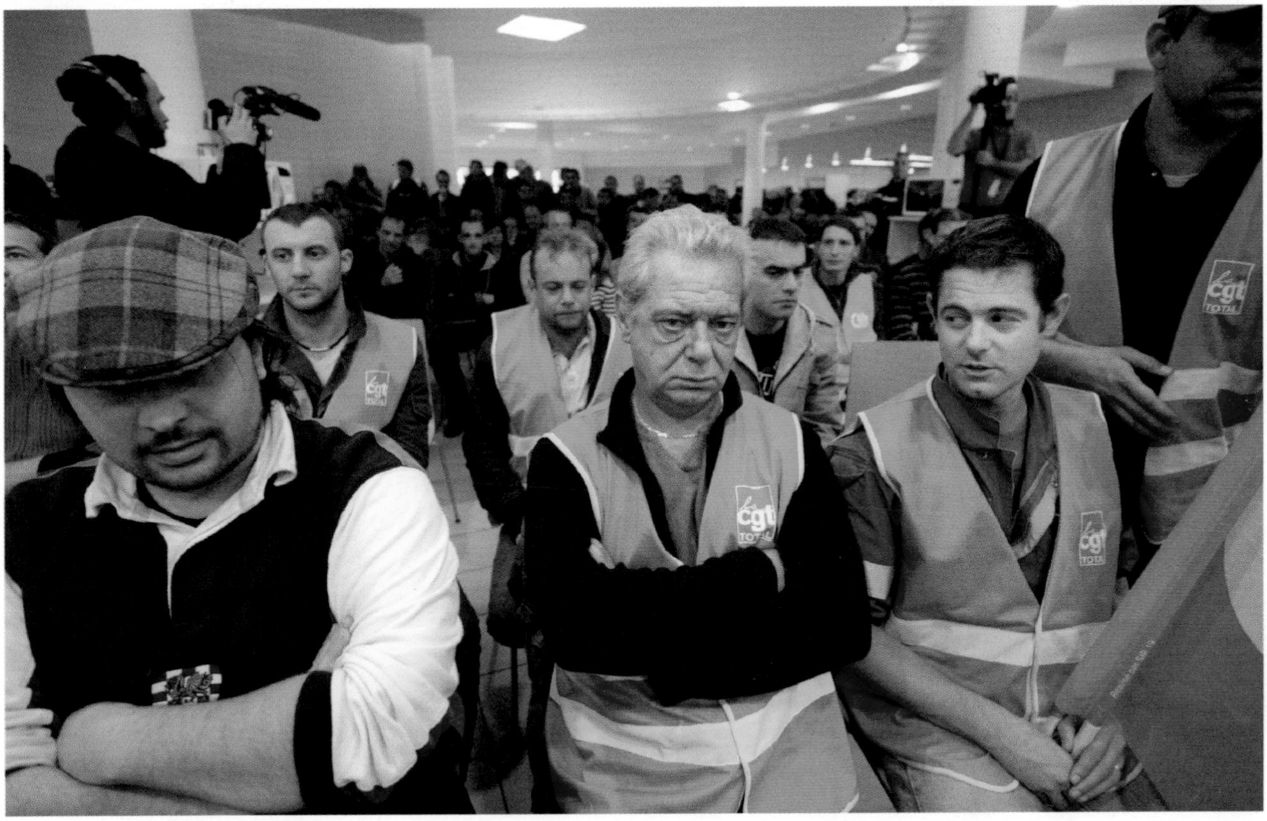

Are workplace strikes an example of class conflict?

P1 Ideology and oppression

Sociologists who use a Marxist perspective argue that the interests of the bourgeoisie are pursued at the expense of the proletariat, and vice versa. Marx himself argued that the bourgeoisie partly controlled society by developing and enforcing what he called a '**ruling ideology**'. This is a 'package of ideas' that protects and approves the interests of the bourgeoisie. For example, the belief that everyone can achieve success by working hard, that wealth is the best measure of success and that business owners and 'bosses' are morally entitled to keep profits for themselves are part of the ruling ideology in capitalist societies.

Marxist sociologists argue that by accepting a 'ruling ideology' the proletariat don't act in their own interests and are oppressed by a '**false consciousness**'. According to Marxism, revolution and a system of state controlled services would produce a better society that worked in the interests of everybody rather than a privileged, powerful bourgeois minority. For Marxists, society functions to keep the bourgeoisie in power and the proletariat in a subservient position. Society is organised to ensure that this relationship continues and that class conflict is minimised.

Weaknesses of the Marxist perspective

Marxism offered a powerful, radical alternative to the functionalist perspective and was widely used in sociology in the 1960s and 1970s. However, contemporary sociologists are likely to criticise the Marxist perspective because it:

- puts too much emphasis on social class and class conflict in particular
- it doesn't recognise how employers and employees in modern societies do have shared interests in the success of a business or organisation and that both 'sides' are often happy to co-operate
- focuses on the economy as the driving force of social behaviour and ignores other important influences such as gender, ethnicity and religion
- doesn't recognise that people are socially active, with some power and the ability to make choices and influence the direction of their own lives.

Your assessment criteria:

P1 Explain the principal sociological perspectives

Key terms

False consciousness: *a failure by members of the proletariat to recognise their real interests*

Ruling ideology: *the beliefs and values of the most powerful groups in society, which dominate ways of thinking in society*

Discuss

Why hasn't there been a revolution in the UK when society is so unequal?

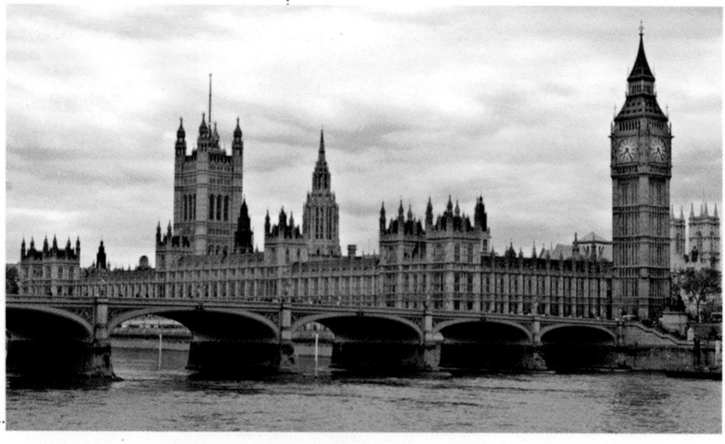

Do you think the interests of the the proletariat are represented in Parliament?

Case study

Lady Geraldine Ferguson-Carew employs Debbie Millar to clean the holiday cottages on her country estate. Debbie is paid the minimum wage for her work, but is very grateful for the opportunity to earn some money. There are few other employers in the rural area where she lives. Debbie and her employer are the same age but have very different social backgrounds. Lady Ferguson-Carew inherited her country estate from her father, a wealthy landowner and farmer. She has never had a job, other than running the estate. However, she believes that the hard work and good judgement of her ancestors has put her in the position she is in society today. She would like to pass on to her own children the country estate where she lives.

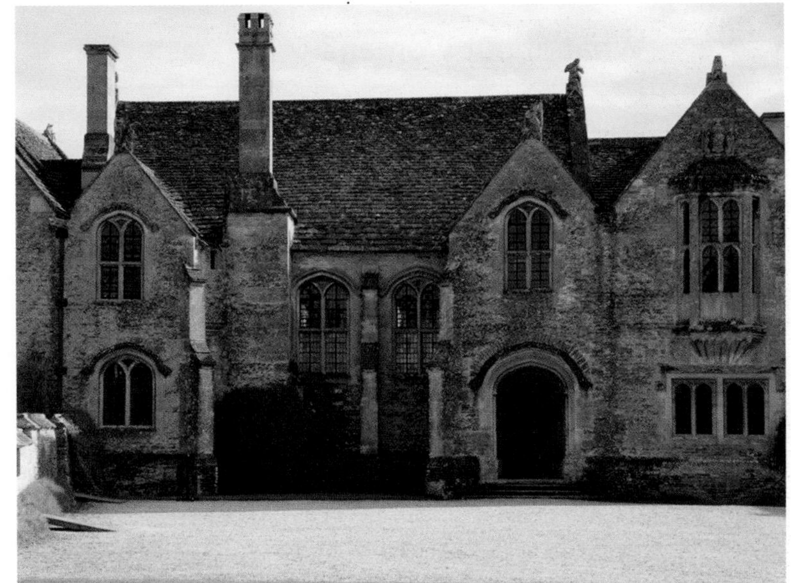

1. According to the Marxist perspective, who is a member of the bourgeoisie and who is a member of the proletariat in the case study?
2. How does Lady Geraldine Ferguson-Carew use a 'ruling ideology' to justify her position in society?
3. Why, according to the Marxist perspective, do the inequalities between people like Debbie Millar and Lady Geraldine Ferguson-Carew not result in more social conflict?

What do you know?

1. Identify two main features of the functionalist perspective on society.
2. Describe how functionalists explain the structure of society.
3. What is the 'sick role' and what function does it perform for society?
4. Identify two of the main features of the Marxist perspective on society.
5. Why, according to the Marxist perspective, is society characterised by conflict?
6. Explain why contemporary sociologists are critical of the Marxist perspective.

Feminist perspectives

Structural perspectives, such as functionalism and Marxism, view individuals as relatively powerless to influence their own destiny and life chances. Wider social forces are seen as more important in shaping society than individual social action. By contrast, the feminist and interactionist perspectives challenge this assumption. They see social action by individuals and groups who have shared interests (such as women), as central to the way in which people are responsible for making and remaking society.

Your assessment criteria:

P1 Explain the principal sociological perspectives

P1 What about women?

Feminism is a critical sociological perspective. It has played an important part in the way sociologists think about society since the 1960s. Feminists criticised both functionalism and Marxism for ignoring the specific experiences and concerns of women. The feminist perspective has been widely applied to areas such as the family, health and care, the education system and employment to highlight inequalities in the opportunities and experiences of men and women and to campaign for change. Marxist, radical and liberal feminism are the three main forms of feminism used in contemporary sociology.

Marxist feminism

Marxist feminists use the conflict model of Marxism to explain how women are exploited both in terms of social class and gender in a male dominated society. Women are oppressed and exploited, especially through unpaid domestic and child care work, by men. They are expected to meet the needs of men, looking after and supporting them, so that men can go out to work. Women are given the primary responsibility of caring for children and ensuring that the home is comfortable and clean. The 'culture of domesticity' and the housewife/mother role that is imposed on women are part of a false consciousness that restricts women's lives and limits their social, educational and employment opportunities. The Marxist feminist perspective offers a structural, conflict viewpoint of society (see the section on 'Functionalist and Marxist approaches') that prioritises the experiences of women.

Key terms

***Feminism:** a perspective that believes women are disadvantaged in society and should have equal rights with men*

Investigate

Are the old stereotypes of male 'breadwinners' and female 'housewives' dying out? What evidence is there to support the claims of Marxist feminists that women still lose out to men because of gender discrimination? Find and analyse data on housework, employment and educational attainment to assess the validity of the Marxist feminist perspective in contemporary society.

Radical feminism

Radical feminists view society in terms of a basic and profound conflict of interests between men and women. Society is seen as **patriarchal** and organised in a way that ensures men remain in a dominant position in relation to women. Radical feminists question many of the taken-for-granted female social roles (such as housewife/mother) and attitudes towards women, believing them to be a form of oppression. The answer to this for some radical feminists, is for women to avoid contact with men and to live separate lives. Some radical feminists did set up separatist women-only communities in the 1970s and 1980s which excluded men and which tried to avoid patriarchal forms of social organisation, such as 'family' structures. Radical feminism highlighted the way in which gender equality issues, including domestic violence and sexual assault, were a consequence of repressive male power. This was very influential in the creation of women's centres, rape crisis and domestic violence services and the idea that 'sisterhood' is a powerful way to challenge patriarchy.

Key terms

Patriarchal: *where power and authority are held by men*

Discuss

In a small group, discuss the pros and cons of a society which segregates men and women. What could be gained from reorganising society in this way? Would women's lives be improved or diminished in such as society?

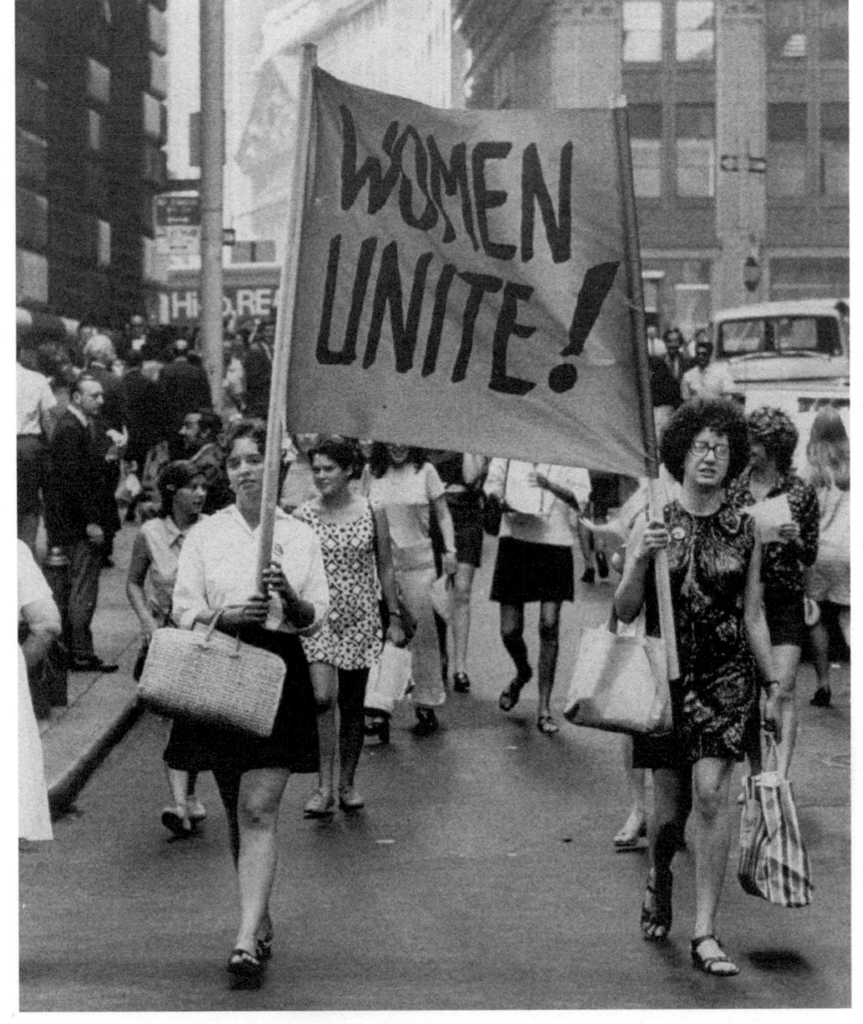

Reflect

Do you think that men and women have radically different interests and needs in relation to health and social care services? If so, what are they? You might like to think about the issue of single sex wards and being able to choose a doctor or other practitioner of the same gender.

P1 Liberal feminism

Liberal feminists adopt a reforming rather than a radical approach to women's experiences and opportunities within society. Liberal feminists are particularly concerned with achieving equality of opportunity in the society that we have rather than in overturning the current social system. The liberal feminist perspective has been used to identify and explore how sexual discrimination acts as a major barrier to women's equality, for example. The liberal feminist perspective questions the 'naturalness' of gender-specific roles (such as the domesticated housewife/mother and breadwinning husband/father) by pointing out that they are the result of social expectations and processes rather than biological differences between men and women. The liberal feminist perspective has also been used to challenge and change many examples of social disadvantage and gender discrimination, to develop laws on sex discrimination and equal pay and to challenge sexist ideas about women's roles, relationships and place in society.

Your assessment criteria:

P1 Explain the principal sociological perspectives

Reflect

Reflect on and compare the three approaches to feminism outlined in the text by creating and completing a table like the one below.

Issue	Marxist feminism	Radical feminism	Liberal feminism
1. What is the root cause of women's oppression in society?			
2. What should be done to change women's oppression in society?			
3. Is it possible to achieve gender equality in contemporary society?			

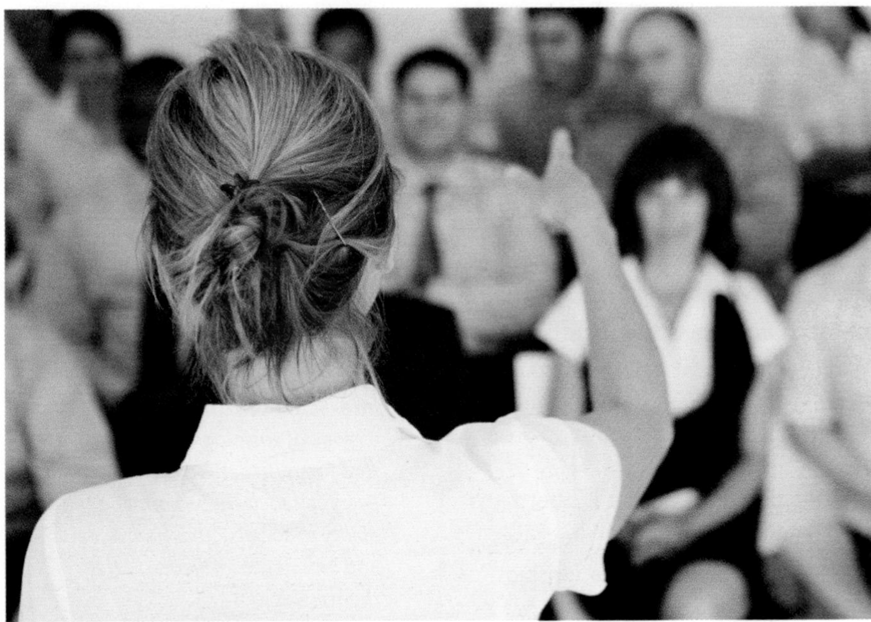

Has feminism helped to improve the position of women in the workplace?

Weaknesses and criticisms of feminism

Figure 7.6 identifies a number of specific criticisms of Marxist, radical and liberal feminism. In general, feminism has made a positive, constructive contribution to the sociological study of health and social care. It has drawn attention to the different needs and experiences of women as a group and the importance of gender as a social difference that makes a difference to people's lives.

Discuss

How do gender differences make a difference to women's lives and opportunities?

Figure 7.6 Criticisms of Marxist, radical and liberal feminism.

Feminist perspective	Weaknesses and criticisms
Marxist feminism	• Marxist feminists focus too much on class and ignore the powerful influence of other social factors such as ethnicity, age and disability on women's lives. • Some feminists reject the idea that gender inequalities are caused by capitalism (as opposed to patriarchy or unequal laws).
Radical feminism	• Radical feminists have tended to be white, middle-class women who haven't taken the experiences of black or working-class women into account. • Radical feminism's solution of separatism and their rejection of men as a whole is seen as extreme and off-putting because it undermines the interests and views of many women.
Liberal feminism	• Liberal feminists are criticised for accepting existing social inequalities (based on class and ethnicity) between women. • The liberal feminist goal of 'equality of opportunity' does not challenge the basic assumptions and way of organising society (e.g. roles in the family) that disadvantage women.

Interactionist perspectives

P1 What is interactionism?

Interactionism in sociology focuses on the role of social action, the ways in which individuals make choices and the meanings of social behaviour. This is a very different approach from the structuralist perspectives of functionalism and Marxism because it assumes that people, rather than big social forces, can make a difference to society and how we live our lives within it.

Sociologists who use interactionist perspectives believe that it's better to look at the **micro-social** behaviours of people and the social processes that occur in care settings (care practices, doctor–patient relationships, labelling processes) rather than at the **macro-social** structures and social trends that occur at a more distant, societal level. Interactionists look at society through a 'microscope', whereas structuralists look at society through a 'magnifying glass'.

Can you influence your own life chances?

The social action approach is based on the idea that people have sufficient power and influence to shape their own lives and destiny. For example, interactionists argue that people can create or construct their social experiences through the cultural meanings that they bring to different social situations. This sociological point is important for health and social care professionals because it suggests that an individual's problems or difficulties can best be understood by appreciating their cultural perspective and way of life. A health or social care professional who isn't culturally sensitive will assume that everyone views and experiences life in the same way. As a result, they may not be able to identify why a person has problems or the most culturally appropriate ways of supporting them.

Labelling theory

The interactionist perspective has been applied to the health and social care field in a number of ways. One of its uses has been in helping care practitioners understand what happens during face-to-face interactions. In particular, interactionism has shown how the **labelling** of behaviour is a social process that has implications for the way people are treated and identify themselves in health and social care settings. Labelling theory has been used to explain how the medical process of diagnosing health problems is, in fact, often a social process. For example, in the nineteenth century women who exhibited a range of symptoms, including crying and laughing for 'no reason', were diagnosed with the

Your assessment criteria:

P1 Explain the principal sociological perspectives

Key terms

Interactionism: *this term refers to a range of sociological perspectives that focus on detailed aspects of everyday social behaviour and the ability of social actors (individuals and groups) to influence society themselves*

Macro-social: *large-scale social structures*

Micro-social: *small-scale, detailed aspects of society or social behaviour*

Reflect

What do you do to try and take control of your life and influence your life chances? Can you think of any decisions or behavioural choices that you have made to shape your own health, wellbeing or opportunities in life?

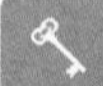

Key terms

Labelling: *applying stereotypical ideas to a person or group while ignoring individuality and differences*

Reflect

Why do you think people fear 'mental illness labels' and try to hide their own mental health problems as a result?

disease of 'hysteria'. Medical practitioners at the time believed 'hysteria' was caused by women trying to do activities, such as going out to work, that were beyond their natural abilities. The cure was rest and a return to domestic activity. However, there was no such disease. Labelling the symptoms as illness was in fact a way of controlling and oppressing women. Health and social care practitioners are now aware that using crude diagnostic labels such a 'hysteric', 'schizophrenic' or 'spastic' stereotypes a person in a negative way and can be discriminatory and unhelpful as a way of describing a person's care needs.

Weaknesses and criticisms of interactionism

Figure 7.7 identifies a number of specific criticisms of the interactionist perspective in sociology.

Reflect

Can you think of any medical 'labels' that may be seen as negative and unhelpful?

Figure 7.7 Criticisms of the interactionist perspective.

Issue	Criticisms
Focus	Interactionism focuses on detailed aspects of social life and ignores the bigger, structural picture. It doesn't see society as a social system.
Uses of research	Interactionist research tends to be small-scale and produces findings that are specific to the research setting. Findings can't be applied to society as a whole.
What makes society 'tick'	Interactionists don't take account of power in society, or consider how wider social forces or historical processes can influence social relationships and individuals' interactions.

What do you know?

1. Identify three forms of feminism.
2. Describe the main focus of liberal feminism and give an example of how this perspective can be applied in health and social care work.
3. Explain how feminist perspectives could help a health or social care professional understand the needs and experiences of people who use care services.
4. Identify two characteristics of the interactionist perspective that distinguish it from structuralist perspectives.
5. Describe an example relevant to health and social care of the use or influence of culture.
6. Explain what labelling theory involves and give a reason why health and social care professionals should understand it.

Collectivism, postmodernism and the New Right

The discipline of sociology is widely seen as being 'political' in the sense that it attracts people who are critical and wish to change society rather than just describe it. People with widely different viewpoints and ideas about how society *ought* to be organised have also contributed to sociological debate, particularly on health and social care and welfare issues.

Your assessment criteria:

P1 Explain the principal sociological perspectives

Collectivism focuses on state provision of services.

P1 Collectivism

The collectivist perspective to health and social care provision is also known as 'welfarism'. This sees the state, or the government, as having the main responsibility for providing care and welfare services in society. In particular, collectivism prioritises the needs of disadvantaged and vulnerable groups in society and develops services and forms of support to meet their particular needs. Disabled people, the unemployed and those on low incomes, children, older people, people with mental health problems and people who are sick are all examples of vulnerable groups who receive significant welfare support from government.

The collectivist perspective was expressed most clearly by the post-second world war labour government, which developed the 'welfare state' as a way of tackling major social problems in British society at the time. The collectivist ideas of this government led to the development of the National Health Service, primary and secondary schooling for all and a national system of social security benefits. As a consequence, the state's role in social welfare and care provision expanded significantly

Reflect

Do you have any strong views on how society could or ought to be changed for the better? Would you describe yourself as 'politically aware' in the way you think about these issues?

during this time. The collectivist approach to care and welfare saw the 'welfare state' grow until the late 1970s. Welfarism was gradually challenged because economic problems and a shift in political ideas caused a move away from collectivism during this period. The collectivist idea that the government should provide care and welfare services for all has weakened significantly and no longer informs government policy.

The New Right

The New Right perspective is more of a political philosophy than a sociological perspective. It is associated with branches of Conservative political thinking (especially **Thatcherism**) and the Republican Party in the USA. The New Right perspective has been most influential when used by politicians to suggest how society ought to be run rather than as a way of explaining social processes or of understanding social structure.

Users of the New Right perspective argue that governments should avoid regulating individuals' lives and should promote, or at least allow, individual freedom and liberty. New Right thinkers argue that the 'free market' will produce better solutions to social problems than government intervention. Individual responsibility and personal choice are seen as preferable to a state-controlled welfare system that is seen to be ineffective and the cause of 'welfare dependency'.

Discuss

How much responsibility should the government have for providing health, social care and welfare support? Is this the individual's responsibility or the responsibility of society collectively? Discuss this issue in a small group, identifying points of view and whether they support or reject the collectivist perspective.

Key terms

Thatcherism: *the policies promoted by Margaret Thatcher, the Conservative Prime Minister, during the 1980s*

Case study

Simon Chandler, aged 45, has mental health problems. He has received care and support from the NHS and voluntary sector organisations for his problems since he was 20 years old. Simon often felt frustrated with the services he received and has always said he would have a better quality of life if he was just given the money to buy care and support services himself. This has now happened! A new government initiative has developed a 'Personalisation Policy' for people with mental health problems. This involves giving service users direct control of a budget so that they can personalise their own care. Simon is very keen to take on this responsibility as he believes that he understands his own needs best.

1. How does the 'Personalisation Policy' express New Right ideas?
2. Can you think of any advantages or strengths of this way of funding care?
3. Can you think of any disadvantages or weaknesses of giving service users direct responsibility for buying services that meet their care needs?

P1 Deserving and undeserving?

The New Right perspective implicitly makes judgements about the 'types' of people there are in society. For example, it makes a distinction between those who are 'deserving' of welfare because they are in poverty or experiencing problems through no fault of their own, and 'undeserving' people who 'waste' their abilities and settle for a life on welfare rather than make a personal effort to better themselves. This way of viewing society assumes that:

- everybody can succeed if they want to and try hard enough
- society is 'naturally' structured to allow the 'best', the 'winners', to rise to the top and the 'worst', the less able and the 'losers' in life to sink to the bottom of the social hierarchy.

This way of viewing society is widely disputed and would be rejected by most sociologists. The main criticism of this perspective is that it accepts and legitimises social inequalities. Many sociologists would argue that the New Right approach fails to consider how cultural, political and economic barriers restrict the lives of marginalised, less powerful groups other than to say that people in these groups are somehow inferior and life's 'natural' losers.

Postmodernism

Postmodernism is a recent and quite controversial perspective in sociology. As its name suggests, this perspective is based on the idea that modern industrial society, in which social institutions, social roles and the beliefs people held were relatively clear and straightforward, is now in the past. Postmodern society is much less stable, more fragmented and fast-changing. It makes no sense to talk or think about 'The Family', for example, because family structure and people's roles and relationships within them are diverse. Similarly, in employment situations there is no longer a 'job for life' or a predictable career path available to most people. Working life – like social life in general – is seen as much less certain, more fragile and risky.

Postmodernists argue that society is not based on stable, relatively permanent social institutions that people can base their lives around. Instead, society is much more individualised and based on temporary associations between people and short-lived structures. People are no longer 'trapped' by their gender, ethnicity or social class – they are free to make their own decisions, to invent and reinvent a lifestyle that suits them and are less likely to see themselves as part of larger social groups with shared goals and interests, like 'the working class' or 'liberal feminists', for example.

Your assessment criteria:

P1 Explain the principal sociological perspectives

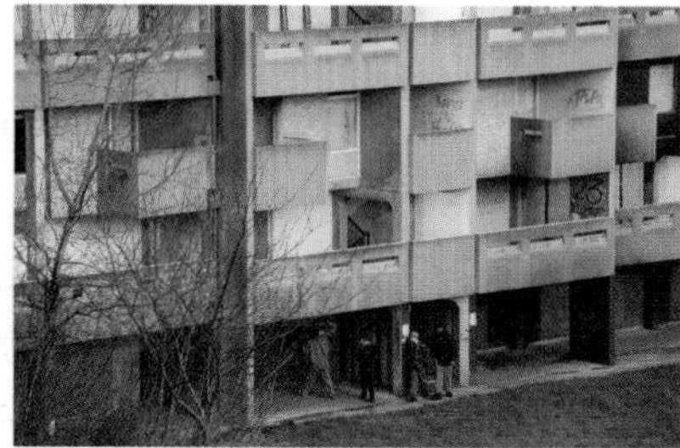

Does everybody get the same start in life?

Key terms

Postmodernism: *this sociological perspective stresses the uncertain, fragmented and fast-changing nature of modern society*

Reflect

Do you think postmodernists are right that society has become less stable, more fragmented and insecure than it was in the past? Or is there evidence that society remains a relatively stable and predictable backdrop to most people's lives?

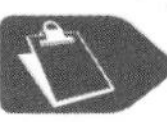

Case study

Kelly, aged 17, spends half of the week living with her mum and stepfather and the other half of the week with her dad and his partner Philip. Kelly describes all of these people as her parents and thinks of them as members of her family. Her sister Sophie only lives with her mum and stepfather and will only see her dad if he visits her at home. She doesn't like to talk about his relationship with Philip as she blames Philip for the break up of her family. Sophie says she 'doesn't believe in "The Family" any more'. Despite this, she feels secure living at home.

1. How can the family situation described in the scenario above be explained from a postmodern perspective?
2. What evidence is there in the scenario that contemporary society is no longer based on stable social institutions?
3. Is Sophie right not to believe in 'The Family'?

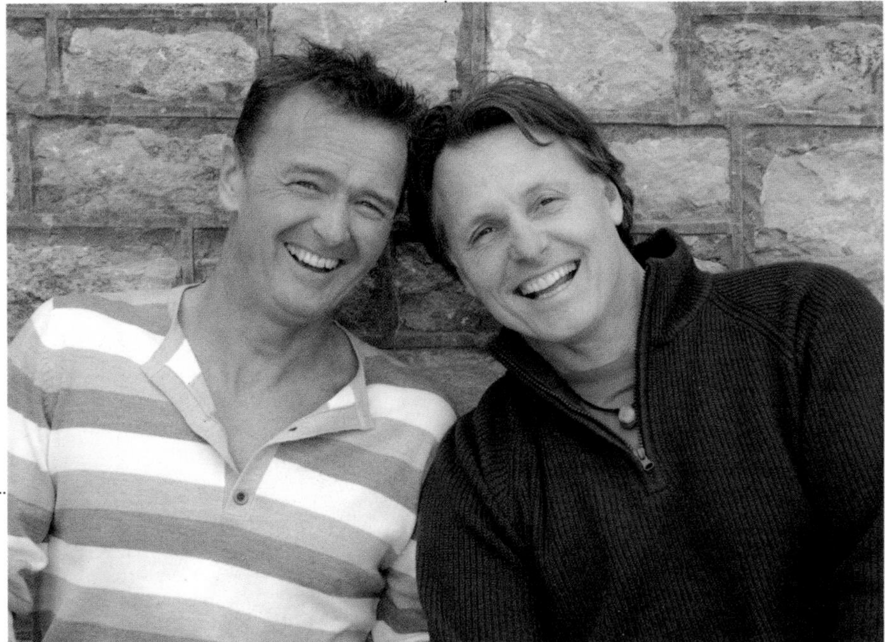

What do you know?

1. Describe the main focus of the collectivist perspective in health and social care.
2. Explain how the 'welfare state' expressed collectivist ideas.
3. Identify two features of the New Right perspective.
4. Explain how the New Right perspective approaches health and social care provision differently from the collectivist perspective.
5. Identify two of the claims made about society by the postmodern perspective.
6. Are postmodern ideas more compatible with those of structuralism or interactionism? Explain your views.

Concepts of health and ill health

It might seem a little odd to begin by wondering what 'health' is at this stage in your course. There seems to be general agreement in modern society that 'good health' is something that all people want to experience, and that people know what this involves. Sociologists argue that 'health' is quite a complicated concept, that there are a number of different ways of understanding it and that the way health is defined has implications for health policy and service provision. In sociological terms 'health' and 'illness' are contested concepts. This means that we cannot take the meaning of these words for granted.

Your assessment criteria:

P2 Explain different sociological approaches to health and ill health

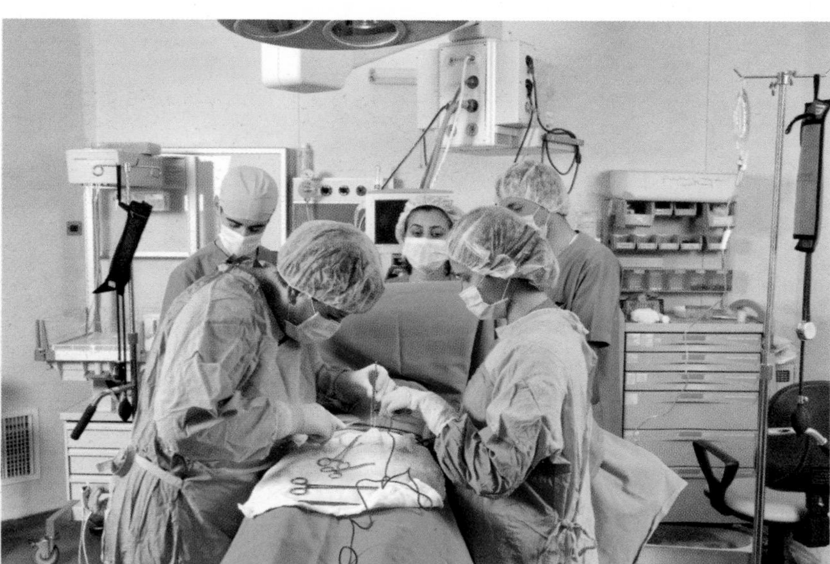

P2 What is 'health'?

If you wanted to find a definition of 'health', you might look in a dictionary or a specialist health and social care textbook. You would, no doubt, find a definition there. However, the surprising thing might be that you would find a variety of definitions of the same term, divided into 'positive', 'negative' and 'holistic' categories.

Positive definitions

The World Health Organisation (WHO) has defined health as being:

> 'a state of complete physical, mental and social wellbeing, not merely the absence of disease of infirmity' (WHO, 1946).

What the World Health Organisation is doing here is actually providing us with *two* definitions, and making it clear that it supports only the positive definition of health as ***a state of complete physical, mental and social wellbeing***. The key term here is 'wellbeing', which seems to suggest that the person feels good both mentally and physically, despite the existence of any 'objective' mental or physical infirmities.

A person with a disability who leads a full life and is content may be regarded as 'healthy'. The positive definition of 'health' is vague and unclear in 'medical' terms. It seems to suggest that 'health' has as much to do with general quality of life issues as it does with biology. Alternative health and complementary therapy practitioners tend to use this kind of definition as part of their practice more than traditional medical practitioners do.

Negative definitions

The second part of the quote from the WHO suggests that 'health' is the state of ***not*** having an illness, infirmity or disease. This is a more commonly used and accepted, though not necessarily a 'truer' or better way of defining 'health' in the UK. Using this definition, we would say that when a person feels unwell they are 'unhealthy', or lack 'health'. In other words, 'health' is defined by the absence of ill-health. Within this definition, a distinction is often made between **illness** and **disease**. Illness involves a person's own, or 'subjective', definition of their lack of health, of 'not feeling right' or 'feeling unwell'. However, disease is a biological state in which an individual's body is affected by some form of observable physical 'abnormality' or **pathology**. The simplest way to understand this is to view the body as a machine that may at times malfunction because, for some reason, one or more of the parts stops working. The damage to the machine part is 'disease'.

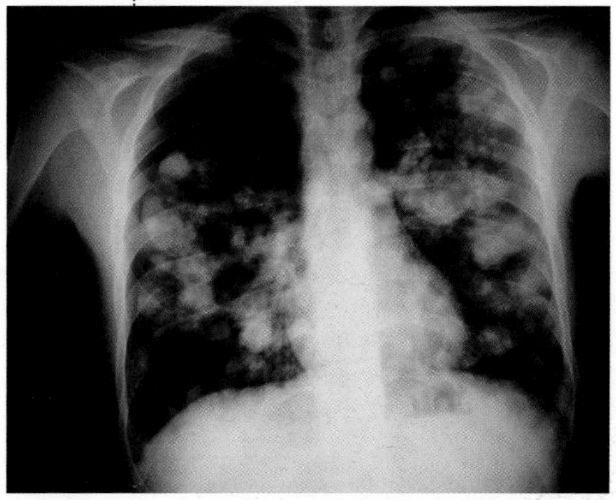

X-rays can reveal signs of disease.

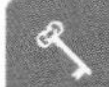

Key terms

Disease: *an abnormal state or disorder that can be observed and measured*

Illness: *a personally defined state of not being in good health*

Pathology: *the manifestations of a disease*

Currently, most health care practice and policy is based on this type of negative definition. Taking the machine metaphor we used earlier, it is the role of the doctor to identify physical faults and repair them. This is achieved through 'curative medicine', based on surgery and the use of pharmaceuticals (drugs) that alleviate biological disorder.

Discuss

Do you find the positive or negative definition of health most useful? Which type of definition do you tend to use when you think about your own health? Share your ideas with a group of classmates. Try to identify the similarities and differences between the ways each person thinks about health.

Your assessment criteria:

P2 Explain different sociological approaches to health and ill health

P2 Holistic definitions of health

The **holistic** approach to health suggests that we should take all aspects of a person's life into account when we're looking at their health. This approach is concerned with the 'whole person' and includes an individual's:

- physical (bodily) health and wellbeing
- intellectual (thinking and learning) wellbeing
- social (relationship) wellbeing
- emotional (feelings) wellbeing.

The term 'wellbeing' is linked to, but also different from, health. Wellbeing is used in Western societies to refer to the way people feel about themselves. If people feel 'good' (positive) about themselves and are happy with life they will have a high level of wellbeing, and vice versa. As individuals, we are the best judges of our personal sense of wellbeing.

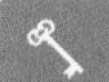

Key terms

Holistic: *taking into account all aspects of a person's life*

'Health' as a changing, subjective concept

The differences in defining 'health' that we have described above are very significant for the activities of health professionals and for health care provision in British society. However, it is now accepted that there is no absolute, fixed, 'objective' definition of what constitutes 'health'. The concept of health varies over time. What was considered an acceptable standard of physical 'health' 100 years ago would today be regarded as unacceptable and intolerable.

The biomedical model of health

The biomedical model is the dominant approach to health in contemporary Western societies and the one that most doctors use. Because the biomedical model is now so dominant it can be difficult to believe that it is a relatively recent way of thinking about and practising 'health' care, and that a range of credible alternatives also exist.

The biomedical model used by doctors assumes that:

- health is the absence of biological abnormality in the body
- doctors can use special 'scientific' methods and knowledge to observe the body, and to identify whether or not there are symptoms of any biological abnormality

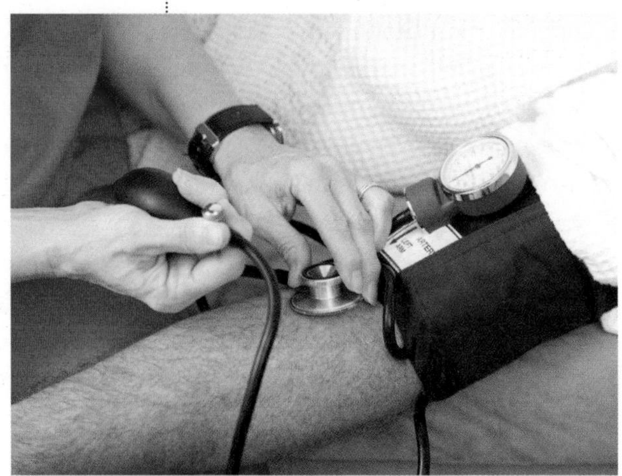

Taking a person's blood pressure can identify certain problems.

- the causes of ill health are located in the individual's malfunctioning biological system
- health can be restored by using surgery and drugs to correct the malfunctions that occur.

Acceptance of the biomedical model and its assumptions about health has resulted in particular types of health care services and health policies being developed in modern societies like the UK. The structure of the National Health Service is based primarily upon the activities of specialist doctors, seeking to cure the diseases that they have identified, for example. However, there is considerable doubt that this model actually reflects reality and, increasingly, the biomedical model used by the medical profession is being challenged.

Discuss

Why do you go to see a biomedical doctor when you are unwell? What do you expect to get from a biomedical approach?

The socio-medical model of health

Biomedical knowledge and medical practitioners have an important role to play in health care provision. Clearly, medicine does have a very important role to play in 'fighting' disease and 'saving lives', but there are plenty of arguments and sources of evidence to show that biomedicine is useful only for some of the 'health' problems that people face, rather than for everything. Sociologists have noted that the growth of interest in complementary therapies and public health has led to a shift towards 'social' models of 'health' and 'illness', and new, community-based approaches to the provision of services.

During the nineteenth century, the tradition of public health medicine developed alongside, but separate from, the biological/individual focus of the biomedical model. Both shared a negative definition of health as being the absence of illness. However, the public health model attempted, through preventive methods such as improving water supplies, and developing public housing programmes and health education campaigns, to prevent general ill health from occurring in society in the first place.

The public health approach adopts a socio-medical model of health. The real causes and origins of ill health are seen as being located in the environment rather than the individual. For example, poor housing and poverty are environmental factors that contribute to respiratory problems. The 'public health' solution is better housing, and programmes to tackle inequality and poverty. The medical model solution consists of antibiotics to treat the pathology, or malfunctioning, that is occurring in the individual's respiratory system.

Investigate

Use the internet and library sources to investigate the public health movement of the late nineteenth and early twentieth centuries. Find out how public health reformers achieved major improvements in mortality and morbidity rates by tackling poor social conditions and cleaning up the environment.

Models of health

P2 Disability and impairment

The concepts of disability and impairment illustrate the different approaches taken by the biomedical and socio-medical models of health. Impairment is a biomedical idea that focuses on weakness in or damage to some part of the individual's body or senses. An impairment may limit a person's ability to function independently or lead to them receiving support, assistance or adaptation aids to overcome it. By contrast, the term disability has become associated with the socio-medical model. A disability is seen as a problem that is created by society rather than something located within the individual. For example, it is the buildings and physical environment in society that dis-ables wheelchair users, rather than their physical impairment. In an accessible environment, a wheelchair user is not disabled at all. Disabilities, from a socio-medical perspective, are restrictions on access to ordinary social life caused by barriers that create disabling environments.

Your assessment criteria:

- **P2** Explain different sociological approaches to health and ill health
- **M1** Assess the biomedical and socio-medical models of health

Investigate

Carry out some observations around your school or college. Are there any parts of the building that are disabling to people who have physical or sensory impairments? Also try to identify ways in which your school or college has adapted the environment to make it more enabling for people with physical and sensory impairments.

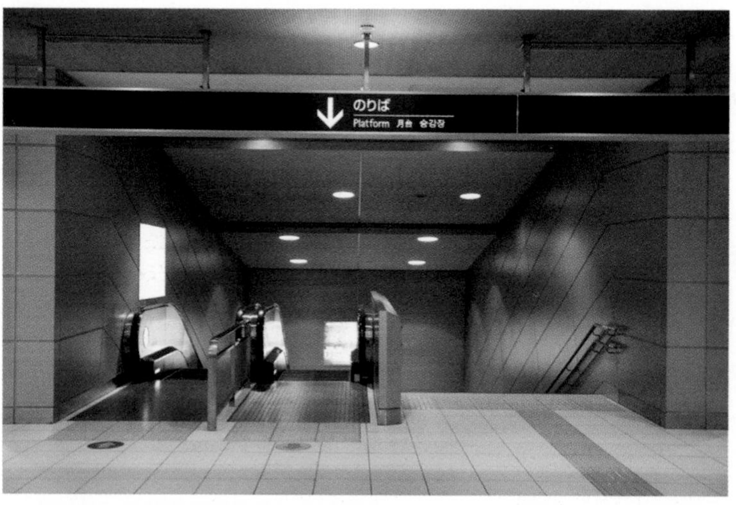

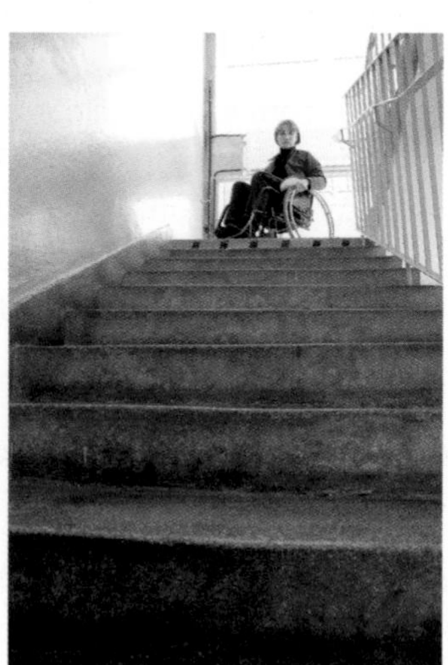

It could be argued that these environments disable wheelchair users.

M1 Assessing models of health

The biomedical and socio-medical models have a range of strengths and limitations. Examples are outlined opposite.

Model of health	Strengths	Limitations
Biomedical	• based on scientific knowledge and research • has provided many effective cures and treatments for disease and physical conditions	• focuses on the individual and pays insufficient attention to environmental and social factors associated with health problems
	• widely used and understood by health care practitioners in developed countries	• cannot explain illness or many mental health problems where there are no physical signs or symptoms to link to distress • treatments can be expensive and require training and expertise to deliver
Socio-medical	• focuses on population health and takes a broad range of factors into account in promoting this • offers a broader, more flexible and inclusive way of understanding health, illness and disability than the biomedical model • can explain why population level health improvements were achieved when social conditions (sanitation, clean water) improved in the late nineteenth century	• cannot be used to address an individual's health problems, especially where emergency care is needed • doesn't have a clear way of identifying or classifying health problems • changing the physical environment and health-related attitudes and behaviour are complex tasks, take time and rarely have an immediate impact on health experience

What do you know?

1. Identify three ways of defining 'health'.
2. Describe the negative definition of health and explain why medical practitioners tend to use this kind of definition.
3. Explain what the biomedical model of health involves.
4. How does the socio-medical model of health differ from the biomedical model?
5. How does the biomedical concept of impairment differ from the socio-medical concept of disability?
6. Assess the strengths and weaknesses of the biomedical and socio-medical approaches to health.

Discuss

Which of these two models do you find most persuasive? Which is best for understanding personal health? Which is best at explaining population health patterns?

Measurement of health

Patterns and trends in health and illness experience are usually expressed as statistics. Official government statistics on a wide range of health issues are compiled by the Office for National Statistics (www.ons.gov.uk).

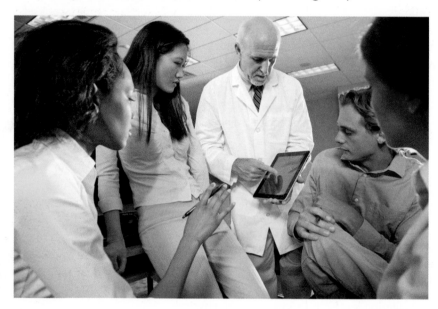

Your assessment criteria:

P3 Explain patterns and trends in health and illness among different social groupings

P3 Data sources

Data sources such as *Social Trends*, *Population Trends* and *Health Statistical Quarterly* are used to plan and commission care services. The data in these publications record patterns and trends over time in

- **mortality** (death) **rates**
- **morbidity** (illness) **rates**
- **disease incidence**
- **disease prevalence**

The data presented in official statistics may be analysed (or broken down) into patterns according to sex, age, social class, ethnicity or location. This enables health care planners to identify the service needs of particular groups within the population.

Other important sources of data on patterns and trends in health and illness experience include statistics compiled and published by non-governmental independent sector organisations and academic researchers in universities. Independent sector organisations such as charities, businesses and pressure groups may compile and publish data on specific health issues related to their particular interests. MIND, Cancer Research UK and the Help the Aged all provide specialist forms of support

Key terms

Disease incidence: *the number of new cases of a disease in a population during a specified time period*

Disease prevalence: *the total number of cases of a disease in a population during a specified time period*

Morbidity rate: *the number of people who have a particular illness in a year*

Mortality rate: *the number of deaths in a population in a year, usually expressed as death per thousand of the population*

for particular client groups and publish information on their websites and in regular reports. Academic researchers may also carry out detailed, specialist studies into the health and illness experiences of particular groups. They tend to publish their data in specialist academic journals.

Difficulties in measuring health

Statistical data on health and illness should provide an accurate summary of people's experiences. However, there are a number of reasons why this might not be the case. Some of these are related to:

- different ways of defining health (positive, negative, alternative)
- help-seeking behaviour – some people who are ill don't go to see a doctor, while others who are not really unwell do go!
- the diagnostic practices and experience of doctors – people with identical symptoms may be diagnosed with different conditions by different doctors or might be seen as malingering to get time off work or school, for example
- the real reasons for a person's death (for example, suicide, AIDS or drug overdose) may not be recorded on their death certificate, to avoid distress to relatives.

Data on patterns and trends in health and illness experience should also be treated cautiously because:

- the organisation compiling and publishing the data might have a particular reason or motive for presenting data in a way that will raise concern or generate support
- a publication, such as a newspaper or magazine, may present the data in a way that confirms the views or prejudices of its readers.

Because official statistics tend to present an incomplete picture of health and illness experiences in the population, sociologists describe them as being part of a **clinical iceberg**. That is, official statistics are only the visible part of health and illness experiences. The true or real patterns and trends are concealed beneath the surface.

Investigate

You know that governments compile and publish statistical data on mortality rates, morbidity rates, disease prevalence and disease incidence rates. But where does the raw data that make up these statistical trends come from? Investigate and produce a table identifying the sources of:

- *mortality data*
- *morbidity data*
- *disease incidence data*
- *disease prevalence data.*

Key terms

Clinical iceberg: *the idea that a lot of ill health and disease is concealed from the medical profession and is not reflected in health statistics*

Discuss

Why do you think a lot of illness and disease remains undiagnosed? Identify and discuss possible reasons for this.

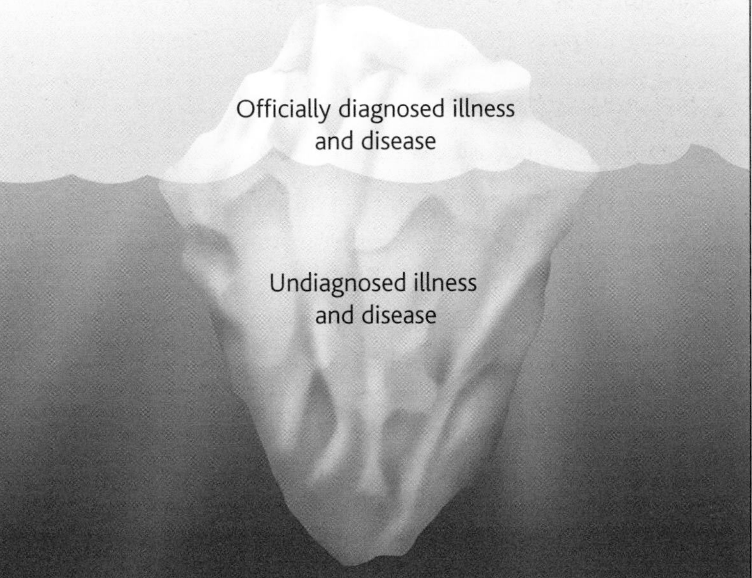

Figure 7.8 Clinical iceberg.

Morbidity and mortality rates

P3 Patterns and trends in morbidity and mortality

People generally assume that being 'healthy' depends partly on a person's genes and partly on their lifestyle. If we accept this and take genes and lifestyle out of the equation, it would be reasonable to say that everyone in society should have the same chance to experience 'good health'. However, this is not the case. Statistical data show that life expectancy and standards of health are closely linked to social factors, such as social class, ethnic origin, gender and geographical location.

Social class and mortality rates

Mortality rates describe the social distribution of death in society. In the early 1970s, the mortality rate among males of working age was twice as high for those in the lowest social class as for those in the highest. By the late 1990s, the figure was ***three*** times higher! Mortality rates fell by 40 per cent between 1970 and the late 1990s for social classes I and II, by 30 per cent for classes III and IV, but by only 10 per cent for class V (the lowest social class). These data show that the chances of people from the higher social classes dying early are falling faster than those of people from lower social classes. In other words, the difference in life expectancy is widening between the more affluent and the poorer groups in UK society. For men belonging to social classes I and II, life expectancy at birth increased by two years during the 1980s; yet for classes IV and V, the increase was only 1.4 years. Men could expect to live to 75 in the higher social classes, but only to 70 in the lower classes. Women could expect to live to 80 in the higher social classes, but to 77 in the lower classes.

If all males in England and Wales had the same death rates as those in the higher social classes, there would be 17, 200 fewer ('premature') deaths each year. Death rates are particularly higher for heart disease, suicide and accidents in adulthood, but infant mortality rates are also noticeably different. At present, five out of every 1000 infants from parents in the two higher social classes die at birth, but seven out of every 1000 infants from parents in the two lower social classes die at birth.

Your assessment criteria:

P3 Explain patterns and trends in health and illness among different social groupings

Investigate

Use the Office for National Statistics website (www.ons.gov.uk) to find evidence of links between social class and health experience. Try to summarise the data in your own words.

Discuss

Can you think of any reasons to explain why working-class people die sooner than middle-class people?

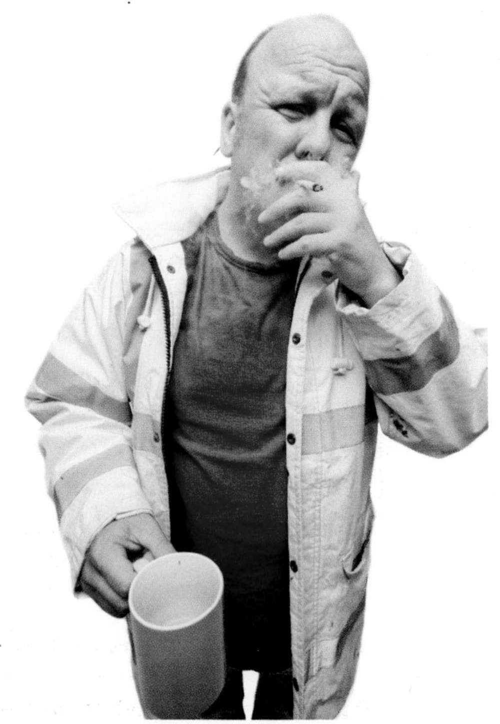

Social class and morbidity

Morbidity refers to levels of illness and disability in the population. Unlike death rates, there does not appear to be a decline in morbidity rates. At present, for those aged 45–64, 17 per cent of professional men reported a 'limited long-standing illness' (a chronic illness), compared with 48 per cent of unskilled males. For women of the same age, 25 per cent of professional and 45 per cent of unskilled women workers disclosed such a condition. A commonly used measure of poor health is obesity (linked, for example, to heart problems, one of the major killers in the UK): 25 per cent of women in class V were obese compared with 14 per cent in class I, while the relevant figures for men are 18 per cent compared with 11 per cent.

It's not just physical health that is linked to social class – so too is mental health. The table below shows the differences in mental health problems between social class groups for men and women. For women in particular, the chance of experiencing mental illness is much higher if they belong to one of the lower social classes. About 25 per cent of all women in classes IV and V suffered from mental disorder of some kind, compared with about 15 per cent of women from social classes I and II. What is also striking is the high proportion of *all* women suffering from some form of mental health problem.

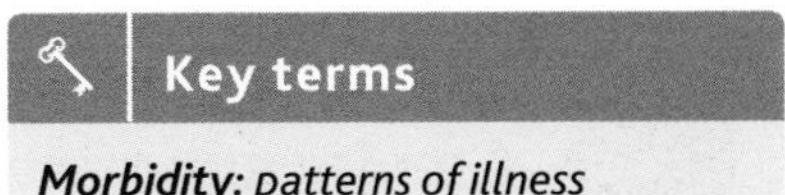

Key terms

Morbidity: *patterns of illness*

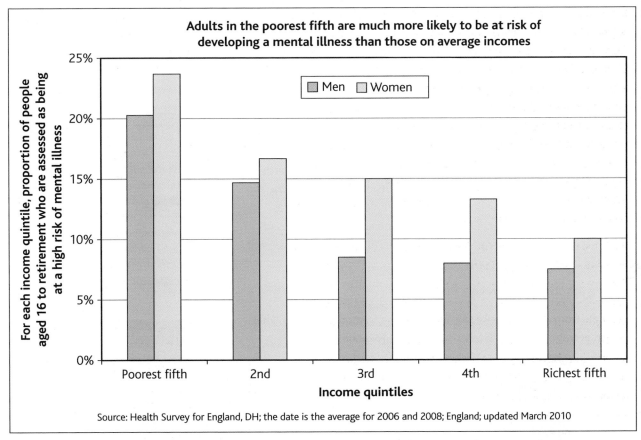

Reflect

Why do you think people in the lower social classes are more likely to be obese than people in the higher social classes? How would you explain this health pattern?

Adults in the poorest fifth are much more likely to be at risk of developing a mental illness than those on average incomes

Men
Women

For each income quintile, proportion of people aged 16 to retirement who are assessed as being at a high risk of mental illness

25%
20%
15%
10%
5%
0%

Poorest fifth
2nd
3rd
4th
Richest fifth

Income quintiles

Source: Health Survey for England, DH; the date is the average for 2006 and 2008; England; updated March 2010

Figure 7.9 The differences in mental health problems between social class groups for men and women.

Patterns and trends of health

P3 Gender and patterns of health and illness

Mortality rates for both sexes have been declining since the mid-nineteenth century. More recently, since 1971, death rates have decreased by 29 per cent for males and by 25 per cent for females, although women continue to have a longer life expectancy than men. Causes of death vary too, with males more likely to die from cancer and heart disease. The pattern of mortality varies too. The age-specific mortality rates for males are higher throughout life, but peak between 15 and 22, with the higher rates of death as a result of motor vehicle accidents. In childhood, boys are far more likely than are girls to die from accidents.

However, the differences are not so clear when it comes to morbidity. Overall, once age is taken into account, there is little difference in the proportions of males and females reporting limiting long-standing illnesses (women live longer and are therefore more likely to report ill health in their final years). During the child-bearing years of women's lives, they report significantly higher levels of illness. More than two-thirds of people with disabilities in Britain are women – although this is also likely to be partly due to the fact that women live longer than men and are therefore more likely to have disabilities.

Ethnicity and patterns of health and illness

Knowledge and understanding of the influence of ethnicity on health and illness is much less accurate and clear than it is for gender and social class. The main reason for this is that the statistics about ethnicity and health are usually based on information obtained on 'country of birth'. As a result, only those people actually born outside of the UK (in the Caribbean or the Indian subcontinent, for example) are identified as belonging to an ethnic minority. The health and illness experiences of British-born people of African-Caribbean or South Asian heritage are not included in the 'ethnic minority' statistics.

Bearing this statistical drawback in mind:

- people from African, Caribbean and Indian backgrounds have a higher than average chance of having a limited long-standing illness
- those from Bangladeshi and Pakistani backgrounds have the highest levels of long-term illness
- people of Chinese origin have the lowest levels of long-standing illness in the UK

Your assessment criteria:

P3 Explain patterns and trends in health and illness among different social groupings

Investigate

Construct a short questionnaire asking students from different ethnic backgrounds at your school or college about the number of times they've received hospital treatment and the reasons for this. Make sure that you ask each person to state their ethnicity so that you can analyse your findings according to ethnic group.

Investigate

Use the internet and library sources to find out ways of describing ethnicity, and links between ethnicity and health experience.

- children born to mothers from Caribbean and Pakistani places of birth have twice the average levels of infant mortality.

Mortality statistics don't show the same clear patterns as morbidity statistics. The table below illustrates differences in causes of death for people born in different countries, but resident at the time of death in the UK. Certain causes of death are closely linked to certain ethnic groups. For example:

- People from Scotland are the most likely to die from lung cancer, but they are far less likely to die from strokes than people from a West African background.
- People born in the Caribbean are much less likely to die from coronary heart disease than those from East Africa, but they are significantly more likely than them to have strokes.

Unlike the statistics we have looked at for gender or for social class, a much more complex pattern appears to exist here.

Discuss

How might a person's cultural background be linked to their health and illness experiences?

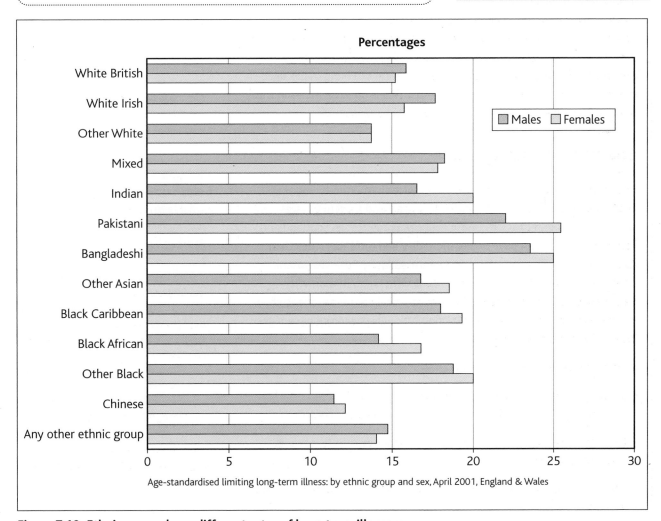

Reflect

Look at the data in Figure 7.10. What do they tell you about the links between ethnicity and morbidity?

Percentages

White British
White Irish
Other White
Mixed
Indian
Pakistani
Bangladeshi
Other Asian
Black Caribbean
Black African
Other Black
Chinese
Any other ethnic group

Males Females

0 5 10 15 20 25 30

Age-standardised limiting long-term illness: by ethnic group and sex, April 2001, England & Wales

Figure 7.10 Ethnic groups have different rates of long-term illnesses.

Age, locality and risk

P3 Age and patterns and trends of health and illness

Old age is commonly thought of as a life stage where people are more prone to physical illness and when they experience depression, grief and loss. There is some truth to this as older people are more likely to experience chronic health problems, life-limiting conditions and to experience the loss of partners, friends and other older relatives. However, this pattern does not mean that ill health is necessarily a consequence of ageing or that all older people are unwell or frail.

Risk behaviour

People who have lifestyles that involve high-risk activities like cigarette smoking, high alcohol consumption and unprotected sex are more likely to develop conditions that cause ill health and even premature death. Risk is one of the reasons for a difference between male and female patterns of mortality. In particular, the death rate of young males aged 17–24 is much higher than that of females. This is because males in this age group engage in more deliberately risky behaviour.

Locality and health

Statistics show there are noticeable differences in morbidity and mortality levels between the regions. Mortality and morbidity rates are highest in poorer regions of the country. For example, Scotland and north-east of England have higher morbidity and mortality rates than the south-east of England. Furthermore, research by Peter Townsend (1962) has demonstrated quite significant differences in morbidity between London boroughs. Ill health is more likely to be experienced by people who are poor. The poorer London boroughs therefore have higher morbidity rates.

Your assessment criteria:

P3 Explain patterns and trends in health and illness among different social groupings

Investigate

Interview a person who is much older than you (a relative or neighbour, perhaps), but the same gender, about the patterns and milestones of 'ill-health' they've experienced during their life. How do the older person's experiences compare with your own?

Reflect

Why do you think young men are more likely than young women to engage in behaviour that could be considered 'risky' for health and wellbeing?

Discuss

What kinds of behaviour do you think puts the health of 17–24-year-old men at risk?

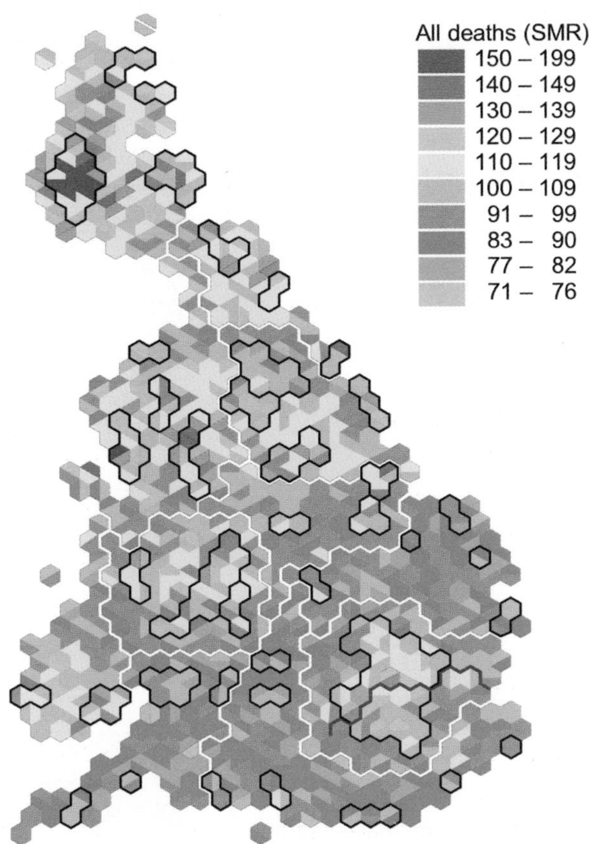

Map of all deaths in Britain (England, Scotland and Wales), from all causes, from 1981 to 2004 inclusive.

What do you know?

1. Identify three measures that are used to record levels of health and illness.
2. Describe two sources of health data.
3. Explain why measuring health is difficult.
4. What do statistics show about the links between social class and patterns of health and illness?
5. In what ways are patterns of health and illness gendered?
6. What do statistics show about the links between ethnicity and patterns of health and illness?

Sociological explanations of health and illness trends

The statistics outlined in the previous sections indicate that there are clear relationships between health and illness experience and social factors such as social class, ethnicity and gender, for example. But why should this be? How can the social patterning of health and illness experience be explained? Sociologists have identified a number of different ways of explaining the different patterns and trends in health and illness experience. These competing explanations are important because they have different implications for health policy and the provision of care services.

Your assessment criteria:

M2 Use different sociological perspectives to discuss patterns and trends of health and illness in two different social groups

M2 Artefact explanations

Artefact explanations challenge the truth of official statistics and research data on patterns of health and illness. They claim that the statistics misrepresent or fabricate reality and that the 'patterns and trends' shown by research are really a product of research processes rather than a reflection of any underlying reality.

The artefact approach challenges the statistics that link ill health to social class, for example. It suggests that the apparent 'growing health gap' between the higher and lower social classes is a statistical quirk rather than an accurate reflection of what is actually happening. The changing nature of employment in the UK over the past 30 years means that there are extremely few manual workers remaining. In other words, social class IV has shrunk to a very small proportion of the population while there have been very great increases in the middle and higher social classes.

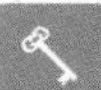 Key terms

Artefact: *something made by human beings*

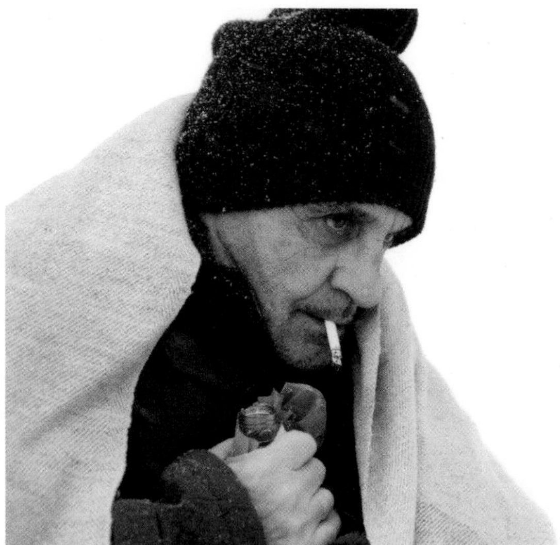

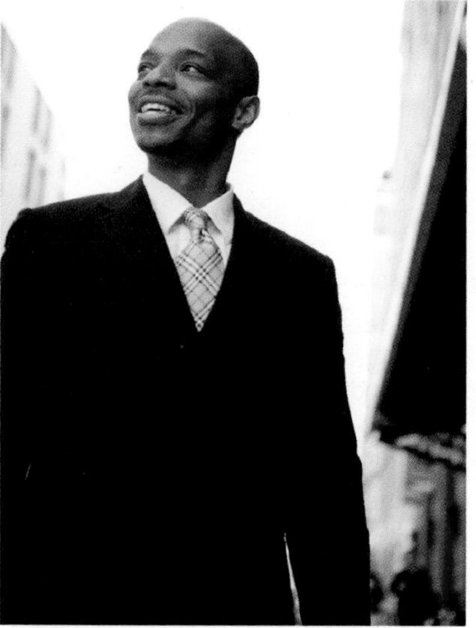

The artefact approach challenges the statistics that link ill health to social class.

According to people who offer an artefact explanation, this makes the 'growing health gap' between people in the higher and lower social classes meaningless. Although it is true that the gap in health may have increased between the lowest social class and the rest of society, the low numbers remaining in social class V mean that there is actually only a very small number of people whose health is not improving at the rate of the majority of society.

Natural and social selection

The natural and social selection explanation is based on evolutionary ideas. In basic terms, it explains patterns and trends in health and illness experience by claiming that those people who are fitter, more capable and who have better inherited health potential are less likely to find themselves in the lower social classes or suffering from long-term health problems. However, those in poor health are more likely to slip down the social scale, be unemployed or in lower-paid occupations and live in poorer social circumstances.

The evidence that exists partly supports this explanation, in that those with long-term illnesses and disabilities are likely to have poorly paid occupations, and are more likely to be reliant on welfare benefits. Poor health over a long period is also partly related to downward **social mobility**. We also know from statistical data that those in higher social classes have higher standards of health and less chance of mortality throughout their lives. Good health, however, is not a cause of *upward* social mobility so this can only be a partial explanation for the trends and patterns in health experience that exist.

Reflect

Have you ever completed a questionnaire or a form where you were unable to give the answers you wanted because of the way the questions were asked? How might this lead to inaccurate, artefact data?

Reflect

Make a list of factors (other than genes and natural ability) that could explain why people in higher social classes tend to experience lower illness and premature death rates than people in the lower social classes.

Key terms

Social mobility: *movement between social classes (up or down)*

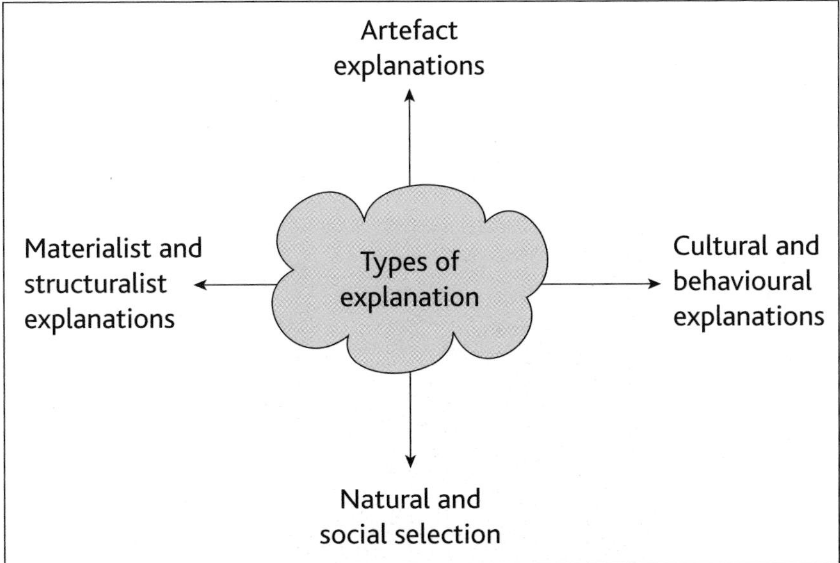

Figure 7.11 Ways of explaining health and illness experience.

M2 Cultural and behavioural explanations

Cultural and behavioural explanations of the patterns and trends in health and illness experience have until recently been a preferred explanation of governments. This type of explanation stresses that a person's lifestyle and the choices they make are the key to understanding their health and illness experience. There is evidence to support the claim that lifestyle choices and health behaviour, which may be linked to employment patterns, regional and class values, diet, alcohol consumption and level of exercise for example, are linked to health outcomes. Government health campaigns have therefore suggested that lifestyle changes can lead to higher standards of health and longer life expectancy.

The cultural version of this type of explanation suggests that cultural (or sub-cultural) beliefs, values and lifestyle practices can explain health and illness patterns within particular cultural groups within the population. The behavioural explanation suggests that the behaviours, choices or health-related practices of individuals and groups within the population provide the key to understanding patterns and trends. A more radical and critical version of this explanation suggests that advertising and the media place immense pressure on people to undertake potentially unhealthy patterns of eating, such as relying on convenience foods, and to suffer a lack of exercise (through car use).

Materialist and structuralist explanations

Materialist and structuralist explanations are based upon the argument that it is not personal choice that determines lifestyle, but *necessity* – based upon differences in income and/or power. For example, a study by Michael Marmot *et al.* (1991) found that the lower the grade of employees in the civil service, the greater the level of illness and higher the level of mortality. Indeed, civil servants in the lowest grades were three times more likely to die before pensionable age than those in the top grades. Marmot *et al.* (1991) argued that the most likely reason for this was the higher levels of stress found among the lower grades.

Materialist and structuralist explanations suggest that wider social forces, such as social class and ethnicity, and the material circumstances of people's lives are the key factors that affect health and illness experience. It is broad, long-standing social inequalities rather than personal choices or lifestyles that ultimately make a difference to people's health and illness experience.

Your assessment criteria:

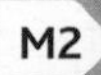

M2 Use different sociological perspectives to discuss patterns and trends of health and illness in two different social groups

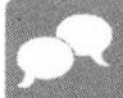

Discuss

How has your experience of health and illness been influenced by your lifestyle, behaviour or culture? Share your experiences in a small group and discuss the strengths and limitations of the cultural/behavioural approach as a way of explaining your experiences.

Reflect

How plausible are cultural and behavioural explanations? Do they place too much responsibility on individuals to live in a particular way? How might they be seen as 'victim-blaming'?

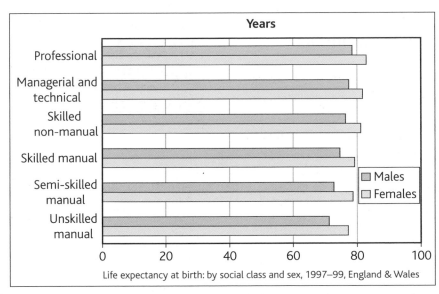

Figure 7.12 Life expectancy and social class.

Case study

Peter Townsend (1962), a pioneering sociologist, studied patterns and trends of health and illness experience in areas of the north-east of England and in London. He found that there was a close relationship between material deprivation (indicated by high levels of unemployment, low levels of car ownership and household overcrowding) and poor health, high levels of disability and low birth weight. Townsend argued that the living conditions and high levels of deprivation people experienced were not a lifestyle choice, but a state of life imposed on these people by the existence of extreme social inequality in certain parts of the UK. Ill health and early death are the outcomes, therefore, of poverty and inequality, and there is little that can be done to change behaviour while these conditions exist.

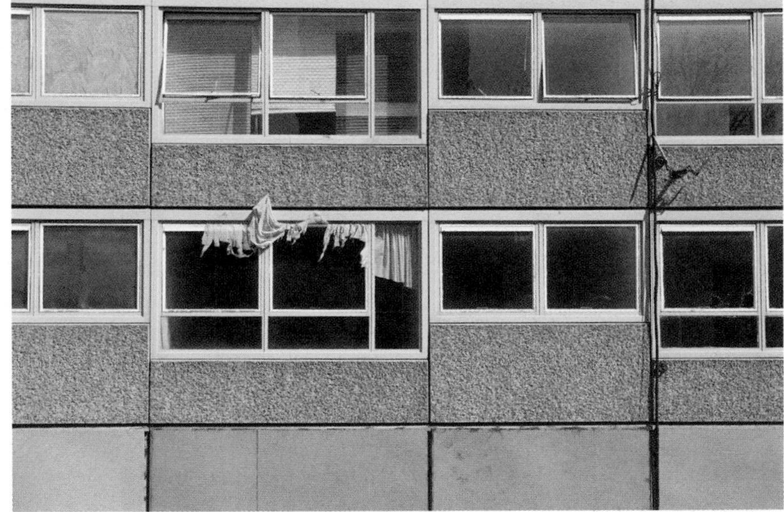

Townsend found links between material deprivation and poor health.

1. Which two explanations of health and illness patterns do Townsend's research conclusions reject?
2. What structural factors or material conditions does Townsend claim are linked to ill health and early death?
3. How, if at all, can health and social care services help to tackle the problems faced by people living in conditions of material deprivation?

D1 Evaluating sociological explanations

Your assessment criteria:

D1 Evaluate different sociological explanations for patterns and trends of health and illness in two different social groups

Figure 7.13 Examples of strengths and weaknesses

Type of explanation	Strengths	Weaknesses
Artefact	• Artefact explanations do expose technical problems in defining and measuring health.	• Repeated studies show that the links between social class and health are likely to be real.
Natural and social selection	• There is evidence that poor health leads to a decline in social class and occupational status. • It can partly explain the persistence of ill-health and high mortality in lower social class groups.	• This explanation doesn't explain how members of higher social classes who experience poor health maintain their social class position. • Why don't poor people in good health move up the social class scale?
Behavioural and cultural	• Health behaviours and lifestyle are linked to health outcomes. • This explanation also takes account of cultural differences. • It encourages individual responsibility for health and provides a focus for health policy.	• This can be seen as a victim-blaming explanation because it places too much responsibility for health outcomes on the individual. • This approach suggests that some behaviours and cultural practices are dysfunctional when they could also be seen as efforts to cope with adverse circumstances.
Materialist and structural	• It provides a way of explaining persistent population level health patterns and inequalities. • There is a lot of data supporting the claim that social factors (class, gender and ethnicity) do have an impact on health.	• It assumes that individuals are powerless to influence their health experience. • It relieves people of responsibility and blame for their lifestyles and the choices they make that are risky to health.

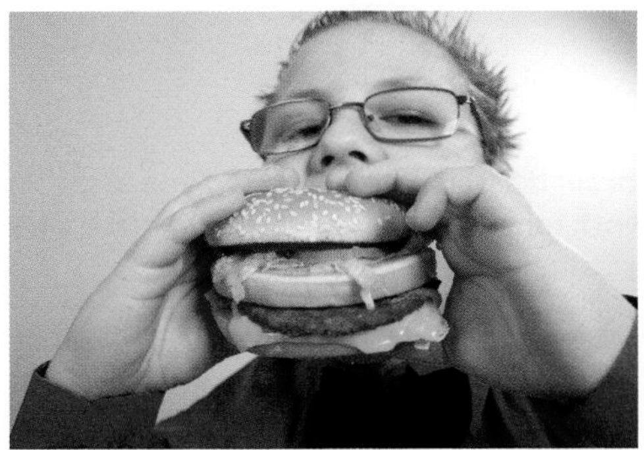
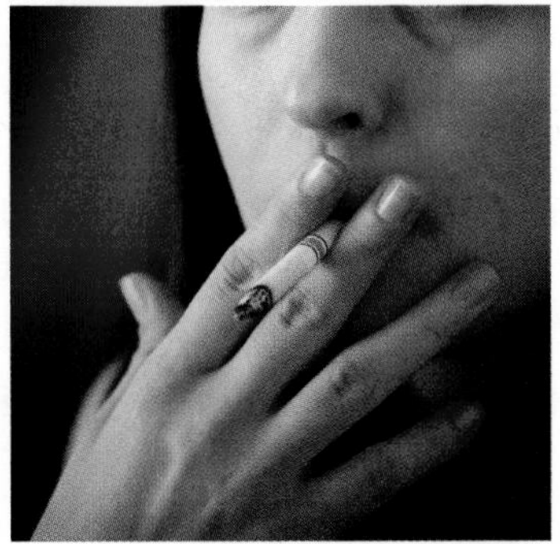
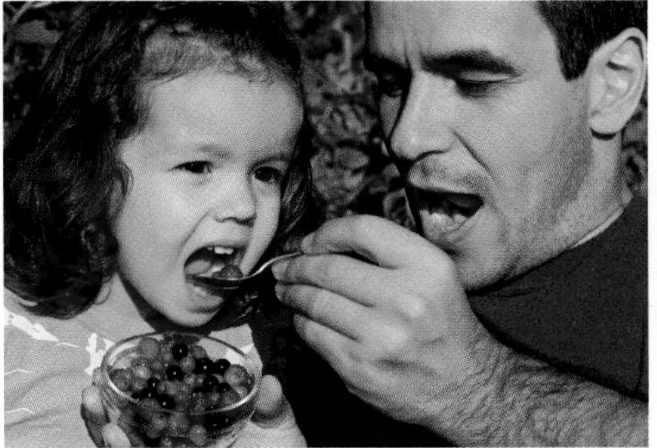
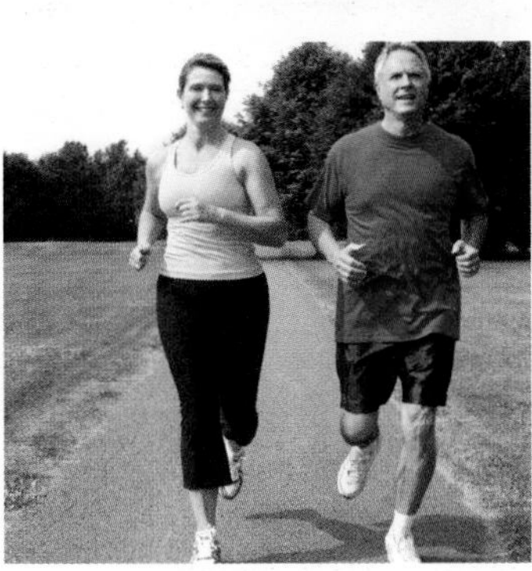

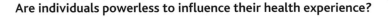

Are individuals powerless to influence their health experience?

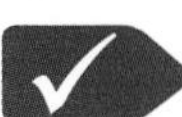

What do you know?

1. Identify three different approaches to explaining trends and patterns in health and illness experience.
2. What does the artefact explanation claim about the validity of health and illness data?
3. Explain the main claim of the natural and social selection explanation and its apparent weakness.
4. According to the cultural and behavioural explanation, what influence can individuals have over their experience of health and illness?
5. How does the materialist/structuralist explanation account for social differences in health and illness experience?
6. Which of the different explanations for health and illness patterns do you think provides the most plausible reason for the link between lower social classes and higher mortality rates?

Investigate

Using the internet or textbook resources, find out about the Acheson Inquiry (1998) into Health Inequalities. How did the Inquiry report account for the patterns of health inequality they discovered?

Assessment checklist

Your learning and level of understanding of this unit will be assessed through assignments given to you and marked by your teacher or tutor. Before you submit your assignment work for assessment you should make sure that you have produced sufficient evidence to achieve the grade you are aiming for.

To pass this unit you will need to present evidence for assessment which demonstrates that you can meet all of the pass criteria for the unit.

Assessment Criteria	Description	✓
P1	Explain the principal sociological perspectives	☐
P2	Explain different sociological approaches to health and ill health	☐
P3	Explain patterns and trends in health and illness among different social groupings	☐

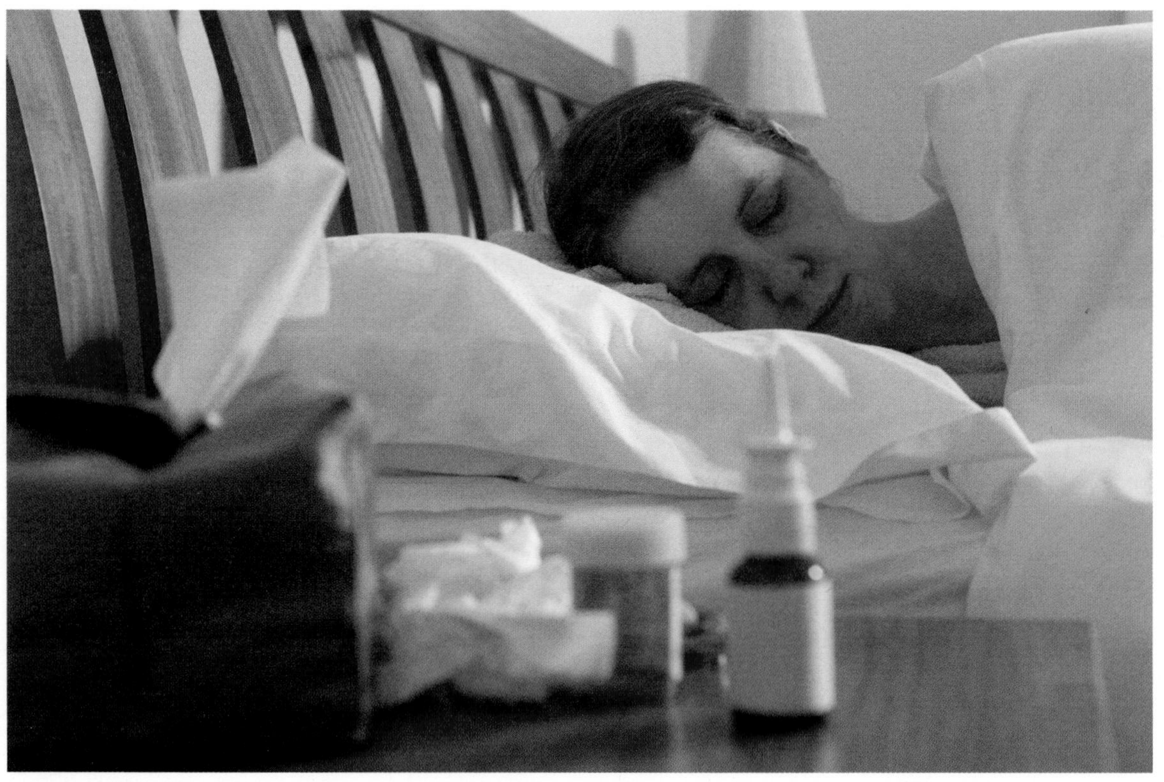

You can achieve a merit grade for the unit by presenting evidence that also meets all of the following merit criteria for the unit.

Assessment Criteria	Description	✓
M1	Assess the biomedical and socio-medical models of health	☐
M2	Use different sociological perspectives to discuss patterns and trends of health and illness in two different social groups	☐

You can achieve a distinction grade for the unit by presenting evidence that also meets all of the following distinction criteria for the unit.

Assessment Criteria	Description	✓
D1	Evaluate different sociological explanations for patterns and trends of health and illness in two different social groups	☐

References

Marmot M. Davey-Smith G. Stansfield S. Patel C. North F. and Head J. (1991) *Health Inequalities among British Civil Servants: The Whitehall Study II,* Lancet, 337

Murdock, G.P. (1949) *Social Structure,* New York, Macmillan

Parsons, T. (1951) *The Social System,* New York, The Free Press

The World Health Organisation (1946) *Constitution: Basic Documents,* Geneva, WHO

Townsend, P. (1962) *The Last Refuge,* Routledge and Kegan Paul, London

8 | Psychological perspectives in health and social care

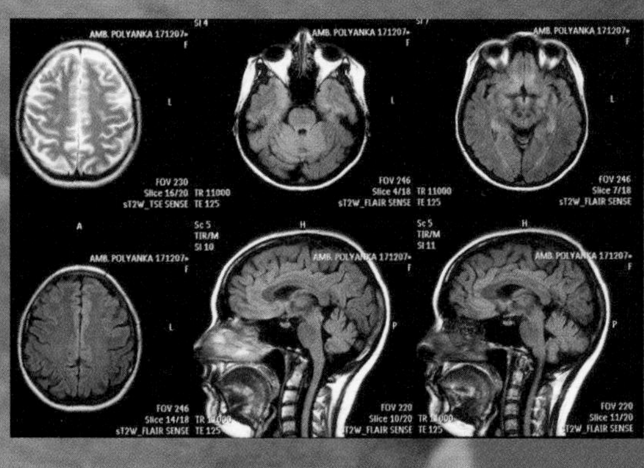

LO1 Understand psychological perspectives

- behaviourism
- social learning perspective
- psychodynamic perspective
- humanistic perspective
- cognitive/information-processing perspective
- biological perspective

LO2 Understand psychological approaches to health and social care

- behaviourism (understanding challenging behaviour, changing or shaping behaviour)
- social learning approach (promoting anti-discriminatory behaviour, using positive role models in health education)
- psychodynamic approach (understanding challenging behaviour, understanding and managing anxiety)
- humanistic approach (empathy, understanding, respecting other individuals, active listening, non-judgemental approach)
- cognitive approach (supporting individuals with learning difficulties, emotional problems, depression and post-traumatic stress disorder)
- biological approach (understanding developmental norms, understanding genetic predisposition, the effects of shift work)

The behaviourist perspective

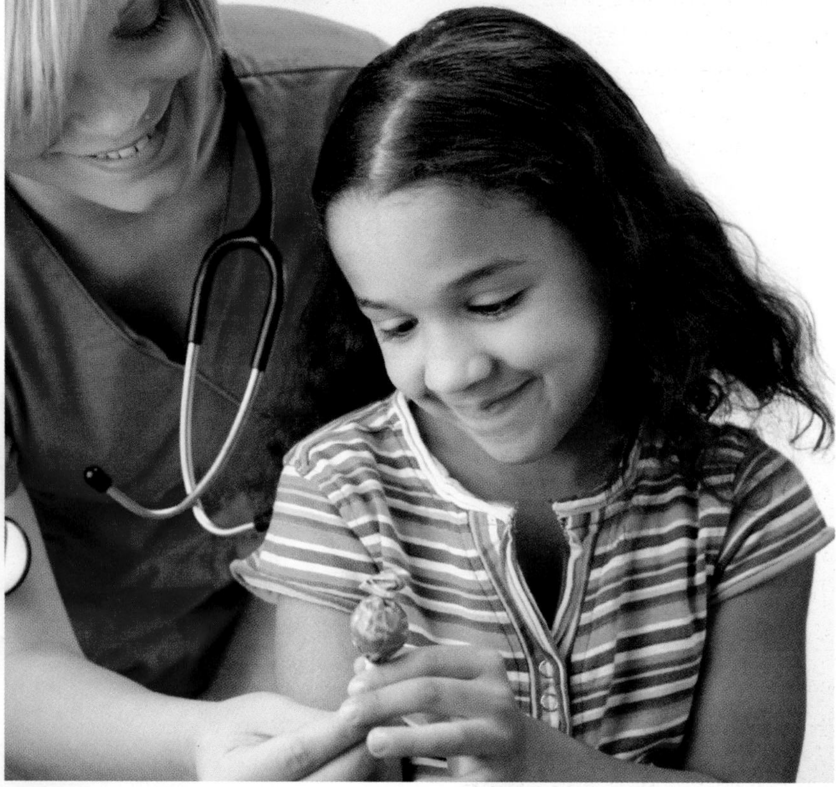

Behaviourists use rewards to reinforce desired behaviours.

Your assessment criteria:

P1 Explain the principal psychological perspectives

P1 Behaviourist approaches

Behaviourism was once the dominant perspective in psychology and was widely used in health and social care settings, but is now less influential than it once was. This approach in psychology focuses on behaviour that can be observed. It is sometimes also known as 'learning theory' because it focuses on the way that human beings learn and the impact this has on their behaviour and relationships. For example, behaviourists believe that people have to learn how to make and maintain relationships and that the way we cope with stress and pressure is also the result of what we have learnt from others.

Behaviourists claim that human behaviour is:

- learnt from experience
- likely to be repeated if **reinforcement** occurs.

Ivan Pavlov (1849–1936), a Russian physiologist, and B.F. Skinner (1904–90), an American psychologist, are the two theorists who are

Key terms

Behaviourism: *a psychological perspective that focuses on the process and impact of the ways we learn to behave*

Reinforcement: *the process by which a response is strengthened and thereby reinforced*

most closely associated with the behaviourist **perspective**. During experiments that were originally designed to investigate the process of digestion in dogs, Pavlov discovered that animal behaviours develop partly through **associative learning**. This relatively simple approach to promoting learning is now known as **classical conditioning** (see below). B.F. Skinner made a deliberate attempt to investigate animal learning using rats and pigeons to test his theory of instrumental learning. The learning process that he identified is now known as **operant conditioning** (see page 351).

Key terms

Associative learning: *learning that occurs as a result of classical conditioning*

Classical conditioning: *learning to make an association between two events*

Operant conditioning: *the use of consequences to influence the occurrence of particular behaviours*

Perspective: *a way of thinking about and looking at something*

Classical conditioning

The process and principles of classical conditioning can be illustrated by describing and explaining Pavlov's experiments.

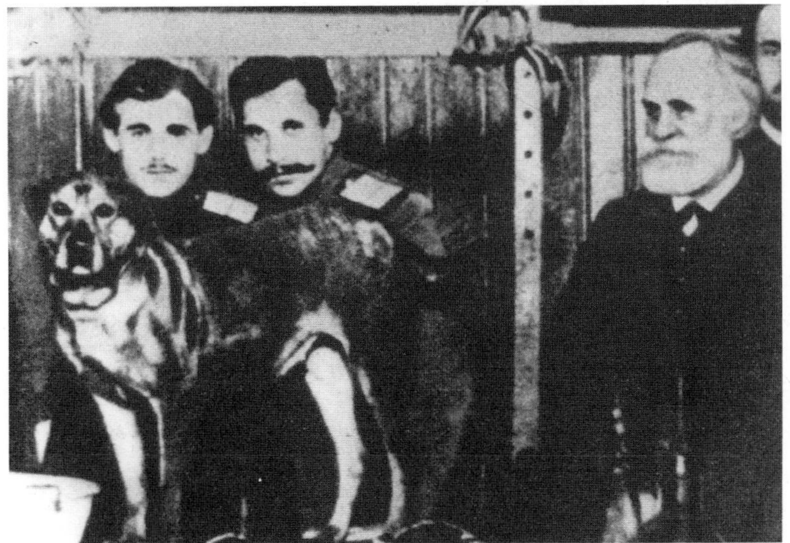

Ivan Pavlov (right) and one of the dogs from his experiments.

In Pavlov's experiments a dog was attached to a harness and to monitors that measured the rate at which it salivated. Pavlov thought he could learn more about digestion in dogs if he measured the amount of saliva they produced when food was presented to them. However, Pavlov noticed that the dogs used in his experiment didn't have to taste any food to begin salivating. They would salivate as soon as they realised food was being brought to them. For example, the dogs would begin salivating when they heard the footsteps of the approaching experimenter or laboratory assistant. This intrigued Pavlov because the belief at the time was that dogs and other animals salivated as a reflex response to food touching their tongues. Pavlov wondered instead whether the dogs were salivating because they had somehow learnt to associate food with the sound of the experimenter's steps; they were salivating in anticipation of the food. Pavlov worked out what was happening and, in the process, also identified the main principles of associative learning or classical conditioning.

Reflect

Can you think of anything that you have learnt through association? Think about sounds (e.g. songs), images (e.g. photographs) or smells (e.g. food cooking) that trigger off memories or particular thoughts when they occur.

P1 Understanding conditioning

Food automatically leads to salivation in dogs. This is known as an unconditioned response (UR). The food causing salivation is known as an unconditioned stimulus (US). Pavlov's experiment involved presenting a dog with food while he rang a bell. The aim was to see if the dog would learn to associate the bell with food. Repeated trials of this pairing (bell plus food) led the dog to associate the bell with food. In fact, after a short while the dog would salivate simply when the bell was rung (and no food was presented). Pavlov explained this by saying that the dog had developed or learnt a conditioned response (CR) of salivation in response to the conditioned stimulus (CS) of the bell. In simple terms, Pavlov's experiment demonstrates that animals learn their behaviours, in part, through conditioning processes. Human are animals too, so the principles of associative learning also apply to us! For example, road vehicle drivers have (usually) been conditioned to put their foot on the brake when they see a red traffic light.

Your assessment criteria:

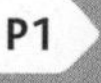

P1 Explain the principal psychological perspectives

Discuss

Can you think of any behaviours that humans learn through classical conditioning processes? Share examples with a small group of class colleagues and try to work out the UR, US, CR and CS in the situations you have identified.

Case study

Loud noises make babies cry because they are frightening. Cats don't usually cause babies to cry or feel frightened. Dominic, a 9-month-old boy, was used to seeing the cat from next door in the back garden of his family home. He hadn't shown any fear of cats until he witnessed a very loud cat fight between the neighbours' cat and an unknown cat, close to his pram. The fight and noise ended when Dominic's dad chased the cats away. Dominic now cries and seems frightened whenever he sees a cat.

1. Identify the unconditioned stimulus and the unconditioned response in this situation.
2. What is the conditioned response in this situation?
3. Explain how classical conditioning occurred in this situation.

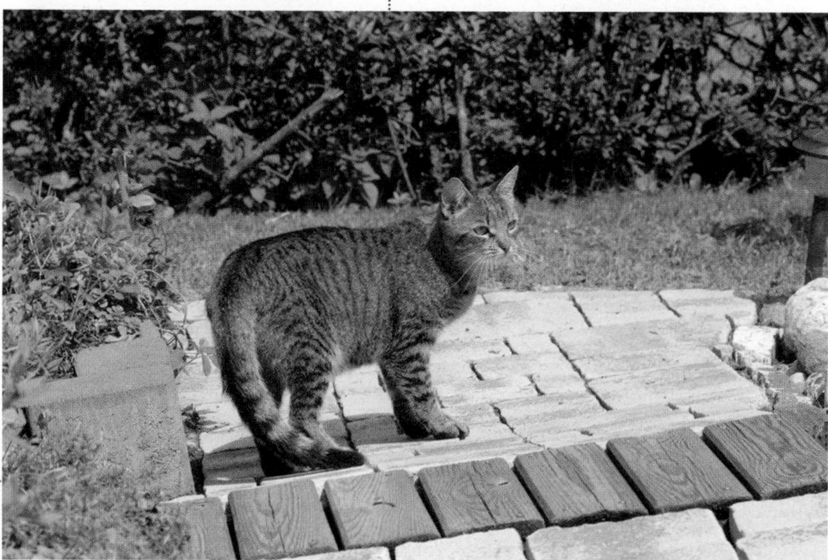

Operant conditioning

This aspect of behaviourism is associated with B.F. Skinner who used experiments with rats and pigeons to develop his **instrumental learning** theory. Skinner built a special box – now known as a 'Skinner box' – to facilitate the learning of new behaviours. The box contained a lever which, when pressed, released a food pellet or 'reward' to the rat in the box. After some trial and error, the rat learnt that lever-pressing had a consequence – it was rewarded with food. Skinner believed that the reward reinforced the rat's lever-pressing behaviour and made it more likely that this behaviour would be repeated in the future. It is because the rat requires a 'reward' that reinforces its behaviour that this is called instrumental learning.

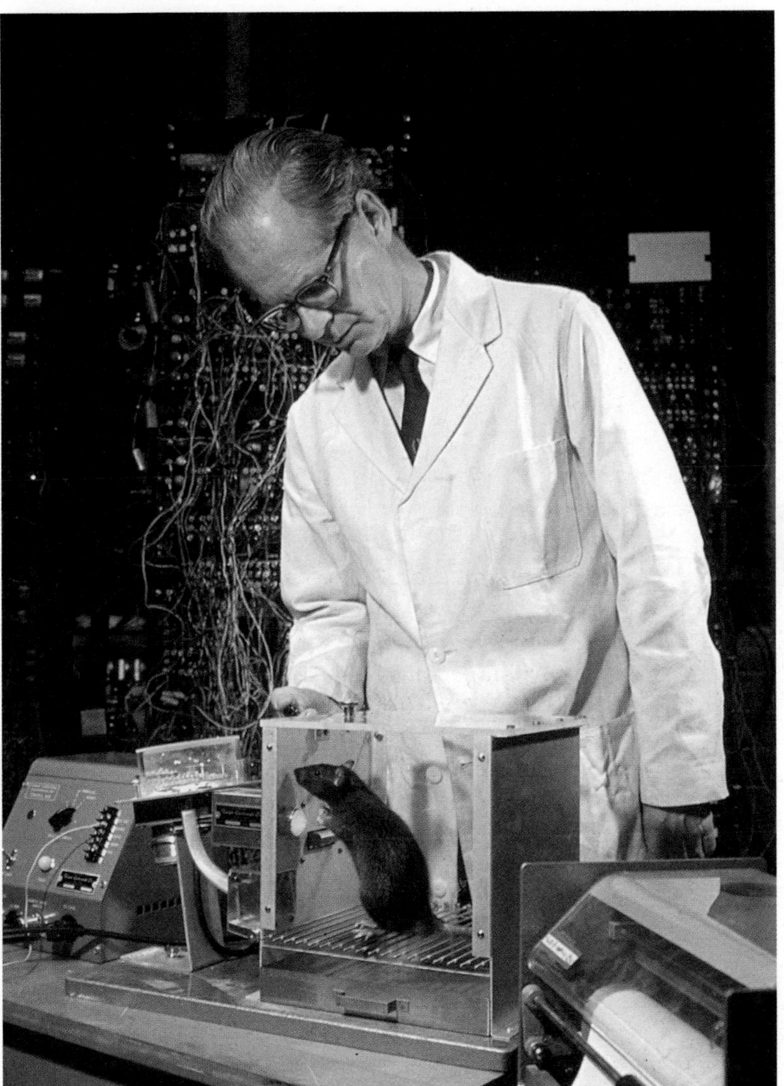

B.F. Skinner and his 'Skinner box'.

Key terms

Instrumental learning: *learning that occurs because it leads to a tangible reward, for example food or money*

Reflect

What are the similarities and differences between classical and operant conditioning? Try to identify one example of each.

Discuss

Can you think of any ways in which the behaviour of students like yourself is shaped by teachers using 'rewards'?

P1 Understanding reinforcement

Skinner's theory of operant conditioning is based on the idea that learning takes place through reinforcement. Skinner identified two types of reinforcement:

1. positive reinforcement where the consequences following a behaviour are experienced as desirable
2. negative reinforcement where carrying out a behaviour removes something unpleasant.

It is important to know that negative reinforcement and punishment are not the same. Negative reinforcement occurs when something unpleasant stops happening. This approach to reinforcement is rarely used in care work because care practitioners do not deliberately set up situations which are unpleasant. Punishment, by contrast, occurs when something unpleasant starts to happen. Behaviourists do not use punishment to change behaviour. They work, instead, through rewards.

Your assessment criteria:

P1 Explain the principal psychological perspectives

M1 Assess different psychological approaches to study

Reflect

Can you think of examples of punishments and negative reinforcements that are relevant to health and social care settings?

M1 Assessing the behaviourist approach

The strengths and weaknesses or limitations of the behaviourist approach to psychology are summarised in Figure 8.1 below.

Figure 8.1 An assessment of the behaviourist approach.

Strengths	Weaknesses or limitations
1. The behaviourist approach has been widely used in health care settings to successfully modify (e.g. phobias) and motivate (e.g. weight loss) behaviour change.	1. Behaviourism reduces human behaviour to a simple stimulus and response model. This fails to take into account inner mental processes or wider cultural and environmental influences on behaviour.
2. Behavioural assessment and treatment is relatively quick, inexpensive and solution-focused.	2. Some care practitioners and psychologists are critical of behaviourism for being manipulative and for failing to address the underlying causes of an individual's problems.
3. Changes in behaviour can be easily measured, monitored and observed.	3. Behavioural treatments work well in controlled environments, especially with animals. They have a more limited application to the real-world behaviour of human beings.

Case study

Jessica, aged 25, is agoraphobic and is afraid of going into crowded places. Kelly, a community psychiatric nurse, has assessed Jessica's behaviour. She and Jessica have now developed a behavioural plan to treat Jessica's agoraphobic behaviour.

- The first step is for Jessica to open her front door and simply stand on the step looking out. Kelly will reinforce this behaviour with encouragement and praise.
- Once Jessica can open the door and look out for 5 minutes without experiencing panic feelings, she will move on to walking down the path to the gate. Kelly will again provide encouragement and praise verbally.
- The next step is for Jessica to walk with Kelly to a café she really likes at the end of her street.
- The goal of the treatment plan is for Jessica to be able to catch a bus to her busy local supermarket and do some shopping there.

1. What kind of conditioning approach is being used to treat Jessica's agoraphobia?
2. How is Kelly reinforcing changes in Jessica's behaviour in this example?
3. Why is Jessica's consent to this treatment plan essential for it to succeed?

What do you know?

1. Identify three of the main characteristics of the behaviourist perspective in psychology.
2. Describe the process of classical conditioning, using the terms *unconditioned stimulus* and *conditioned response* somewhere in your answer.
3. Describe two forms of reinforcement used in operant conditioning.
4. Explain the difference between punishment and negative reinforcement.
5. Outline two criticisms of the behaviourist approach.

The social learning perspective

The social learning perspective and the humanistic perspective (see page 360) both focus on the psychological aspects of human relationships and on the influence other people have on our psychological development and experiences.

Your assessment criteria:

P1 Explain the principal psychological perspectives

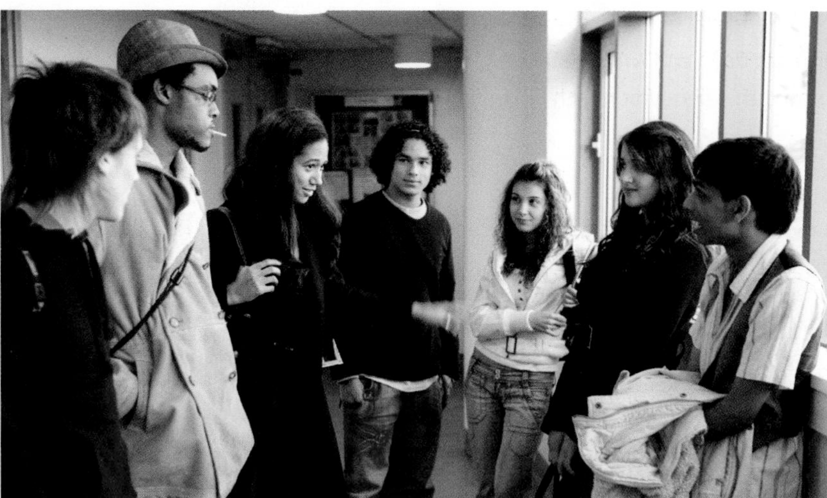

Social learning theory focuses on the influence people have on each other's learning and behaviour.

P1 The work of Albert Bandura

Albert Bandura, born in 1925, is the psychologist responsible for developing some of the main principles of the **social learning perspective**. He recognised that behaviourism could only explain how people learn directly through experience. People, and other animals, also learn *indirectly* by observing and imitating the behaviour of others. As a result, this perspective focuses on the effects that other people, such as parents, teachers, friends, peer group members, celebrities, sports performers and pop stars, for example, can have on an individual's development and behaviour. In particular, social learning theory argues that some behaviours are acquired or learnt through **imitation** of admired people or **role models**.

Bandura (1965) argued that we learn through a process of imitating role models, but also that we only imitate those behaviours we see as being in our interests. Social learning theorists like Bandura say that for behaviour to be imitated it must be rewarded or reinforced in some way. This can occur through '**vicarious** reinforcement' where an individual experiences reinforcement indirectly by seeing their role model being reinforced. For example, when children see their favourite footballer get away with some foul play, score a goal and then get lots of congratulations and cheers from team mates and

Key terms

Imitation: *copying a model or example*

Role models: *people who inspire others to imitate or be like them because of their desirable characteristics*

Social learning perspective: *a psychological perspective that focuses on the influence and impact that relationships and interactions with other people have on human development and behaviour*

Vicarious: *something that is felt indirectly by imagining what another person is feeling or experiencing*

supporters, they may decide to copy this aspect of their admired role model's behaviour the next time they play football themselves.

The social learning theory approach also suggests that learning and the development of behaviour sometimes occur with the need for direct reinforcement. Admired people (role models) are able to influence an individual's behaviour and identity if the individual is motivated to be more like their role model. People are motivated to be more like their role models if they admire or desire the personal attributes or qualities associated with them.

P1 The effects of groups on behaviour

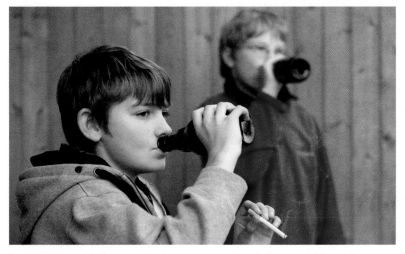

'Peer pressure' plays an important part in adolescents' learning and behaviour.

The basic claim of social learning theory is that the presence of other people has a big influence on our behaviour. At some point, you have probably had the experience of feeling that others are putting pressure on you to change your mind or to behave in a particular way. Psychologists interested in 'majority influence', also known as 'group pressure', have studied how individuals' attitudes, beliefs and behaviours tend to conform to those of the majority.

Deutsch and Gerard (1955) claim that people conform to **normative** influences (based on the desire to be liked and accepted) and informational influences (based on the desire to be right). A person might change the way they dress, speak or style their hair because of normative influences, for example. By contrast, a student nurse who closely observes qualified nurses to find out how to behave on the ward or in team meetings is using informational influence to change his or her behaviour.

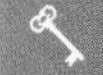

Key terms

Normative: *something that is regarded as normal, expected or standard*

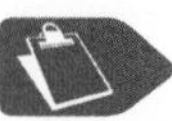

Case study

Danny is a mental health nurse. He has spent the past 3 years working in an in-patient unit with people who are receiving treatment for diagnosed mental health problems. Danny has just got a new job, working in the community team. This will involve going to the homes of people who are experiencing problems or who have been referred by a GP, to assess their mental health. Danny isn't sure how to approach his new work role. Should he be very open with people that he is assessing their mental state, that others believe they might have a mental illness and that they might need treatment? How should he behave when he arrives at a person's house? Should he dress differently? Danny has asked himself lots of questions like this. He has come to the conclusion that:

- his work-related speech and behaviour will need to change
- he should observe the other community nurses closely to work out the acceptable ways of behaving in community situations.

1. Who are the sources of 'normative influence' in this scenario?
2. Describe how Danny's behaviour may be affected by normative influences when he begins his new job.
3. Explain how the concept of 'informational influence' can be used to explain the way Danny adapts to his new work role.

Your assessment criteria:

P1 Explain the principal psychological perspectives

P1 Investigating group pressure

Solomon Asch (1956) carried out what is now a classic psychology study into the effects of groups on behaviour. Asch was interested in finding out how people would behave when they were exposed to group pressure in a situation where members of a group all selected an obviously wrong answer to a specific question. Asch asked seven male students to look at two cards. The 'test' card showed one vertical line. The other card showed three vertical lines of different lengths. In turn, the seven participants were asked which of the three lines was the same length as the 'test' line. Out of the seven participants in each 'trial' only one was a genuine or naive participant. The other six were always accomplices of the experimenter. They were pretending to be genuine participants but, in fact, deliberately gave the wrong answer to the question in 12 of the 18 tests. The genuine participant was always the last but one to answer the question in each trial.

Investigate

Carry out a small-scale investigation in your school or college to test Asch's claims about majority influence or group pressure. Alternatively, ask several of your friends or class colleagues whether 'peer pressure' (majority influence) has ever caused them to behave in a particular way. Does their experience support Asch's claims about majority influence?

So, what happened? The genuine participants conformed to incorrect answers 32 per cent of the time despite the fact that the correct answer was always obvious. In interview afterwards, some of the genuine participants claimed that the obviously wrong answer was correct while others said they didn't want to be the only person choosing the correct answer in case they were ridiculed or excluded by the group. However, most of the genuine participants who conformed by choosing wrong answers doubted their own judgement and thought that they must be wrong if everyone else had choosen a different line. Asch (1956) argued the results showed that majority influence, or group pressure, does affect the way that people behave. His results provide evidence that an individual can be influenced by a group.

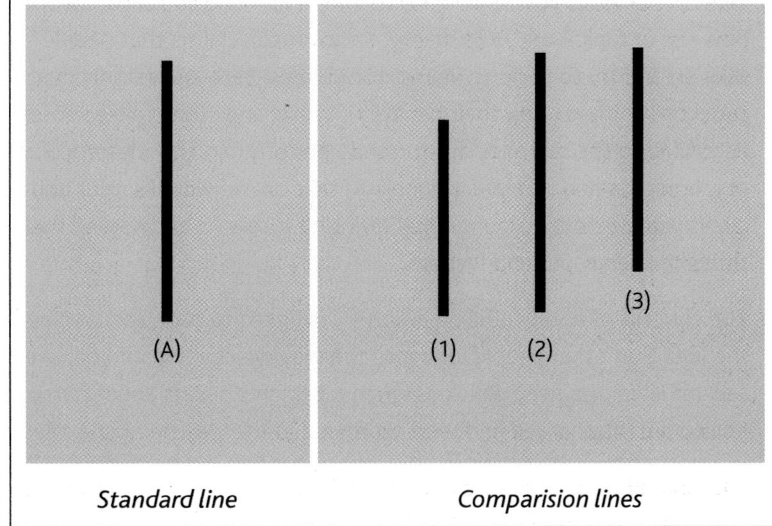

Figure 8.2 Asch's standard and comparison lines.

Effects of culture and society on behaviour

In addition to being part of different groups in society (family, friendship and peer groups, for example), we all contribute to and are affected by culture and the wider society in which we live. Culture consists (partly) of the shared values, norms, language, customs and practices of a group. The UK is a multicultural society in which a variety of cultural influences co-exist. Social learning theory suggests that we need to understand how culture can influence behaviour to understand the people we work with. It is important not to assume that the behaviour of the **indigenous** white majority population of the UK is the norm and that deviation from this by other ethnic groups is 'abnormal' in some way. Cultural influences do, for example, affect the use of eye-contact, touch and proximity during interpersonal interaction. Social learning theory draws attention to the way that different cultural and societal factors affect, and can be used to understand, human development and behaviour.

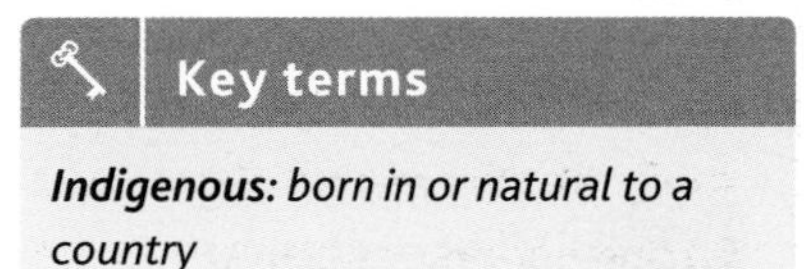

Indigenous: *born in or natural to a country*

P1 Role theory and self-fulfilling prophecy

The social learning theory perspective has produced a range of useful concepts or ideas that psychologists and health and social care workers now use in their work. Role theory, for example, claims that people take on and try to perform valued social roles. Because an individual takes on multiple roles, their behaviour will change (and make sense) according to the role they are currently performing. This idea encourages psychologists and care practitioners to take an individual's roles and circumstances into account when trying to assess or understand their thoughts, behaviour and feelings.

The concept of a self-fulfilling prophecy is linked to both social roles and the idea that other people influence the way we develop and behave. A self-fulfilling prophecy develops when a person's beliefs about him or herself are internalised and then expressed in the way he or she relates to others. For example, if a person develops a belief that they are not very capable, don't deserve respect or are somehow less important than others, the way they interact may reflect this (being submissive, withdrawn and accepting of personal criticism). The response of others – perhaps dominating, taking advantage of or overlooking the person's needs – then reinforces these beliefs. That is, the beliefs become a self-fulfilling prophecy. The phrase 'people get what they expect' captures the essence of this concept. People with high self-esteem, who expect to be treated favourably because they believe they deserve to be, tend to generate this behaviour from others, and vice versa for people with low self-esteem. In both cases the ways in which people present themselves and play their social roles trigger particular types of responses from others.

Your assessment criteria:

P1 Explain the principal psychological perspectives

M1 Assess different psychological approaches to study

Reflect

Are you persuaded by the self-fulfilling prophecy claim that people 'get what they expect' in life? Are there any limitations to or weaknesses in this claim?

Case study

Jonjo, aged 22, has been homeless for the last 5 years. He is dependent on alcohol and smokes cannabis whenever he can. Jonjo left home at the age of 16 when his parents threw him out. The last straw, as far as his parents were concerned, was his conviction for possessing cannabis. Jonjo says that he was 'harassed' by the Police, by his parents and by his GP who all treated him as a 'drug addict' when he began smoking cannabis at school. He says that being prosecuted and labelled made him start to think there was something 'wrong' with him. As a result he began to spend more time with friends who also smoked cannabis. This escalated to the point where Jonjo would spend most of the day trying to get cannabis, regularly getting into trouble with the Police for petty crime. Jonjo says he learnt to think of himself as a 'pot head' – which is what one police officer called him.

1. How did the ideas other people had about Jonjo's behaviour affect his self-concept?
2. What factors caused Jonjo's drug-taking behaviour to escalate?
3. Explain how the Jonjo's situation can be explained by the concept of a self-fulfilling prophecy.

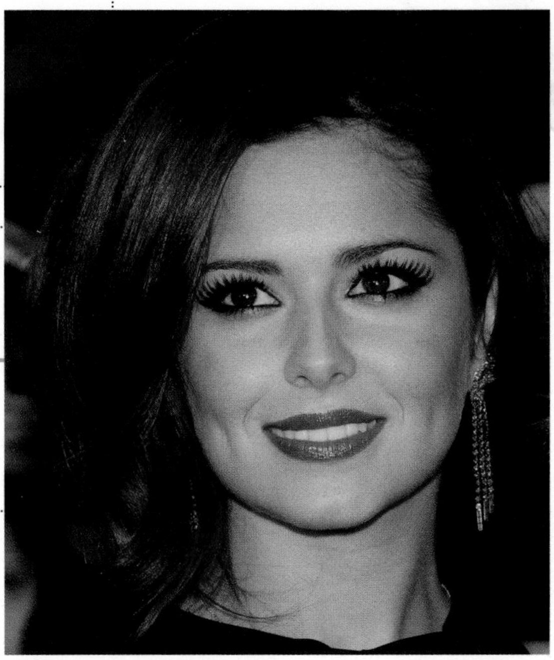

Social learning theory asserts that people learn behaviours, attitudes and values from role models such as Cheryl Cole.

M1 Assessing the social learning theory approach

The strengths and weaknesses or limitations of the social learning theory approach to psychology are summarised in Figure 8.3 below.

Figure 8.3 An assessment of the social learning theory approach.

Strengths	Weaknesses or limitations
1. Recognises that influences on human behaviour are broader and more complex than simple stimulus-response factors.	1. Ignores the role of biology and thinking (cognition) in human learning and behaviour.
2. Shows how other people (role models) play a key part in the way people learn behaviour, as well as attitudes and values.	2. Doesn't recognise the roles of the unconscious and early experiences in understanding an individual's behaviour.
3. Sees the person as making some active choices (through observation and imitation) in what they learn and how they behave.	3. Ignores the human experience of emotions and the powerful ways they can affect learning, behaviour and development.

The humanistic perspective

There are parallels between the humanistic perspective and the social learning perspective (see page 354) as both focus on the influence of other people on our development. The humanistic perspective became popular in psychology and began to influence health and social care practitioners from the mid-20th century onwards. Abraham Maslow (1908–70) and Carl Rogers (1902–87), both America psychologists, are now seen as the pioneers of this perspective. The humanistic perspective adopts a **holistic** approach to human experience. It is concerned with uniquely human issues and experiences such as the self, **self-actualisation** and individuality.

Your assessment criteria:

- **P1** Explain the principal psychological perspectives
- **M1** Assess different psychological approaches to study

Key terms

Holistic: *relating to the study of the whole person rather than focusing on a specific aspect or part of them*

Self-actualisation: *achieving your potential*

P1 Human needs and motivation

Abraham Maslow (1943) was interested in motivation and the way this affects human behaviour. He wanted to show that humans do not react blindly to situations or stimuli as behaviourism implies. He believed that a person's behaviour and development is needs-driven. You are probably already aware of Maslow's idea that human behaviour is linked to a 'hierarchy of needs'.

Maslow's humanistic approach to development and behaviour is based on the belief that human beings have a number of different types of need and that these needs must be met or satisfied in a particular sequence before the person can develop further. Specifically, a person's basic physiological needs must be met first, before they can satisfy their safety and security needs. Their behaviour will then be motivated by a desire to satisfy their love and emotional needs. When these are satisfied, the person will be motivated to meet their self-esteem needs. At this point, the individual is in a position to focus on achieving their full potential or self-actualisation needs.

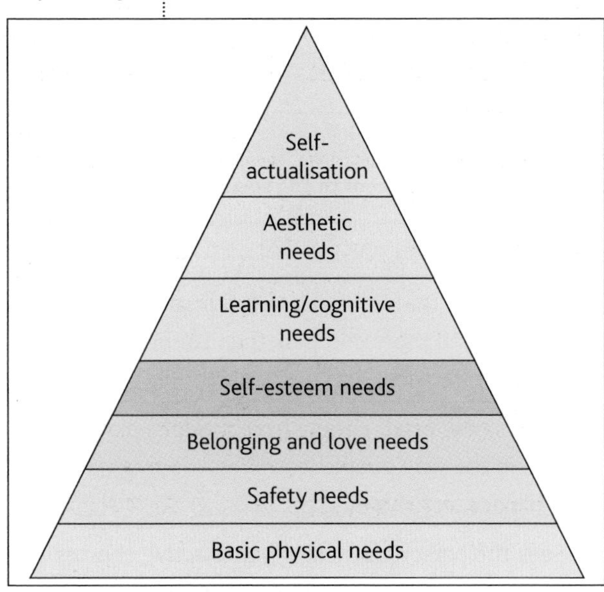

Figure 8.4 Maslow's hierarchy of needs.

Maslow's contribution to the humanistic perspective focuses on the way in which human behaviour and development is motivated by distinctly human qualities and needs.

Understanding and using the self

Carl Rogers (1961) was interested in the development of the self. He focused on the capacity that people have for self-direction and for understanding their own development needs. Rogers noted that an individual's self-concept is strongly influenced by the judgements they make about themselves and by what they believe others think about them. For example, a negative self-concept can develop if a person **internalises** critical comments that others make about them ('you're hopeless') and then think and act as if this is true. Rogers was also concerned with the importance of self-esteem and the role of the 'ideal self' in the way that we make judgements about ourselves. Humanistic psychologists such as Rogers (1961) claim that a mismatch between the ideal self and actual self can lead to psychological and emotional problems.

Key terms

Internalise: *incorporate into yourself attitudes and values that have been learnt*

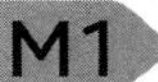

M1 Assessing the humanistic approach

The strengths and weaknesses or limitations of the humanistic approach to psychology are summarised in Figure 8.5 below.

Figure 8.5 An assessment of the humanist approach.

Strengths	Weaknesses or limitations
1. Recognises that the complexity of human emotions and relationships affects the way people develop and behave.	1. Based on relatively vague, unscientific concepts that can't be tested easily.
2. Provides useful concepts for developing supportive and ethical human relationships.	2. Encourages people to focus on self-fulfilment and perfecting themselves – can be seen as narcissistic.
3. Sees people as capable of resolving their own problems in an individual way.	3. Focuses on the individual rather than on the influence of others or their broader social or cultural surroundings.

What do you know?

1. How, according to social learning theory, are some human behaviours learnt or acquired?
2. Describe how a role model can influence a person's development and behaviour.
3. Explain how 'majority influence' (group pressure) can affect a person's judgement and behaviour.
4. What is a self-fulfilling prophecy?
5. Summarise Maslow's explanation of human development.
6. According to Carl Rogers, how does self-esteem develop?

The psychodynamic perspective

This perspective focuses on the deep psychological aspects of human relationships. It is strongly associated with the work of Sigmund Freud (1920) and the treatment of 'abnormal' behaviour.

Your assessment criteria:

P1 Explain the principal psychological perspectives

P1 Freud's influence on the development of psychoanalysis

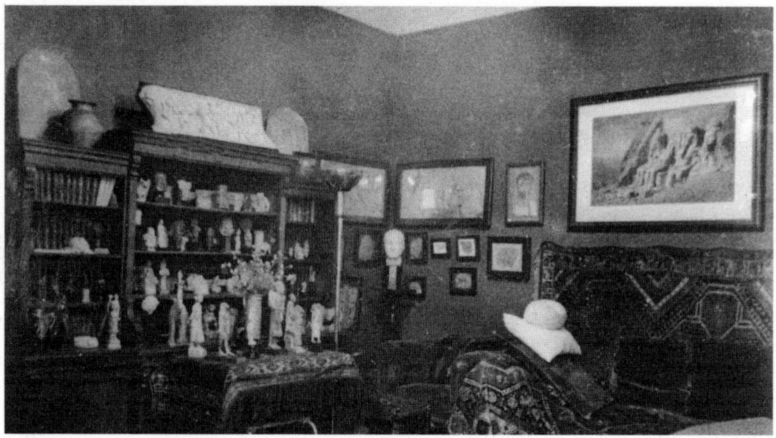

Freud's couch and consulting room.

Sigmund Freud (1856–1939) used his experiences as a therapist with mentally disordered people to develop his psychoanalytic ideas. He was particularly interested in the connections between abnormal behaviour and unconscious underlying psychological processes. The psychodynamic perspective in psychology now covers more than Freud's original psychoanalytic ideas. Other theorists and practitioners developed and extended Freud's work throughout the 20th century. Erik Erikson (1902–94) was one of these people. Inspired by Freud's work, Erikson produced a theory of psychosocial development (see page 366) that has influenced the work of many psychologists, educators and health and social care practitioners.

The unconscious mind

Freud argued that human behaviour and thinking can be motivated by unconscious processes. Freud claimed that the human personality or psyche consists of three interrelated structures – the id, ego and superego. According to Freud, the id and superego are always in conflict. The id, or unconscious part of the personality, is focused on getting what it wants. It consists of sexual, aggressive and loving instincts and wants immediate gratification. The superego is the last part of the personality to develop as a result of socialisation. It is driven by morals and a sense of right and wrong – it is the person's conscience. The ego tries to balance the demands of the id and superego. It is the conscious, rational part of the personality.

The psychodynamic perspective suggests that unconscious forces and conflicts cause psychological disturbances. Such disturbances are driven by memories, feelings and past experiences that are locked away in the unconscious but 'leak out' in dreams, slips of the tongue ('Freudian slips') and displacement behaviour. Early childhood experiences are seen as particularly important in creating unresolved psychological conflicts that become locked into the unconscious.

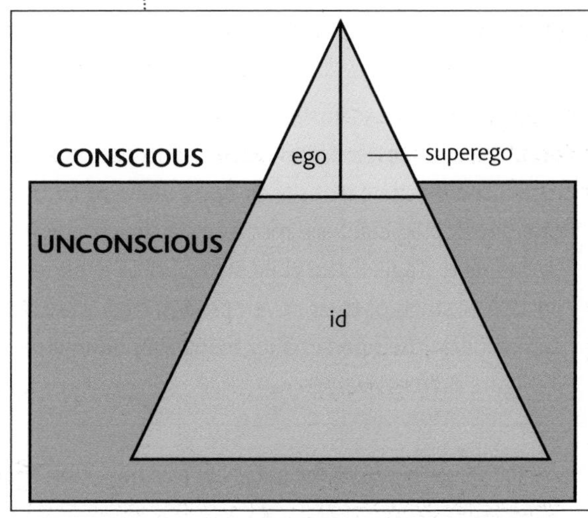

Figure 8.6 The conscious and unconscious parts of the mind.

Importance of early experiences

From a psychodynamic perspective, a person's early childhood experiences play a crucial part in their later psychological and emotional development. Traumatic and confusing events are **repressed** or pushed into the unconscious because they are too painful or because the child cannot deal with them. However, the distressing feelings associated with these events don't disappear. They 'leak out' in dreams, irrational behaviour and in psychological distress.

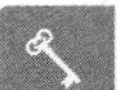

Key terms

Repressed: *involuntary psychological exclusion of desires and impulses (wishes, fantasies or feelings) from consciousness and holding or subduing them in the unconscious*

Case study

Daniel Joseph, aged 29, was recently offered a new job with better pay in a different part of the country. This would involve leaving his home area and living away from his friends and family. After receiving the job offer he developed symptoms of physical illness, particularly pains near to his heart. Daniel described his symptoms as 'heartache' and felt unable to take the new job. Once he'd written a letter saying that he could not accept the job, his symptoms disappeared. Daniel's doctor told him that there was no obvious physical cause for his chest pain and that he was physically healthy.

1. What kind of mental conflict was Daniel experiencing?
2. Which aspect of Daniel's mental conflict do you think he was aware (or conscious) of?
3. How can the concept of the unconscious mind help you to explain Daniel's health concerns?

Discuss

What is a 'Freudian slip'? Have you ever made one or been present when this has happened to somebody else? How does psychodynamic theory explain the 'Freudian slip'?

P1 Early psychosexual development

Freud believed that human beings go through several stages of psychosexual development. During this process a child's libido (energy) is focused on the part of their body relevant to that stage. If the needs of a developing child are met at a particular stage, they can move on to the next stage. If the child struggles or experiences conflict at a particular stage of their development, they may become 'fixated'. This can result in their personality being shaped in a particular way, as shown in Figure 8.7 below.

Your assessment criteria:

P1 Explain the principal psychological perspectives

Figure 8.7 A summary of the stages of psychosexual development.

Stage of development	Focus	Reasons for and effects of 'fixation'
Oral (0–18 months)	Mouth (sucking, licking, biting)	• Child weaned too early – may develop pessimistic, sarcastic personality. • Child weaned too late - may develop gullible, naively trusting personality.
Anal (1–3 years)	Toilet training	• Child pressurised to begin toilet training, or caught in a battle of wills about it, may retain faeces to deny parental control and satisfaction – may lead to obstinate, miserly or obsessive personality. • Lack of toilet training boundaries – may lead to messy, creative and disorganised personality.
Phallic (3–6 years)	Sex and gender	• Child may be filled with anxiety and guilt about unconscious rivalry with same sex parent for affection of opposite-sex parent. • Boys experience 'castration anxiety'; girls experience 'penis envy'. • If not resolved, child may become homosexual or lesbian which Freud believed 'abnormal'.
Latency stage (6 years to puberty)	Social pursuits, e.g. friendships, sport, academic achievement	• Not strictly a psychosexual development stage. • Focus is on social development.
Genital stage (puberty to maturity)	Sexual relationships	• More easily negotiated if no previous fixations. • If earlier conflicts resolved, will have the ability to form warm, loving heterosexual relationships.

Ego defence mechanisms

Freud believed that the ego uses 'defence mechanisms' to protect itself and balance the demands of the id and superego. Within the psychodynamic perspective, ego defence mechanisms are seen as a way of protecting the ego from distress and are used to cope with everyday life. Defence mechanisms allow us to unconsciously block out experiences that overwhelm us (see Figure 8.8 below).

Ego defence mechanisms are seen as natural and normal but can cause psychological problems if they are used too often.

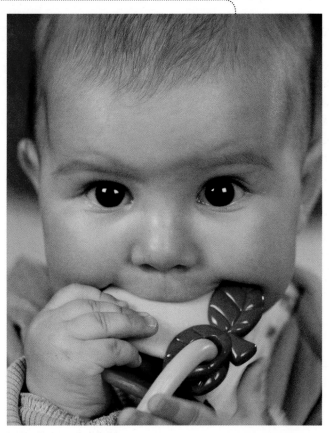

Which Freudian stage of development is this child in?

Figure 8.8 Examples of ego defence mechanisms.

Defence mechanism	Effect	Example
Repression	Forgetting an event or experience.	Having no recollection of a serious car crash.
Regression	Reverting to an earlier stage of development.	Bedwetting when a sibling is born or school begins.
Denial	Pushing events or emotion out of consciousness.	Refusal to accept a substance misuse problem.
Projection	Personal faults or negative feelings are attributed to someone else.	Accusing a colleague of being thoughtless when feeling this way oneself.
Displacement	Redirecting desire or other strong emotions onto another person.	Shouting at your partner instead of your best friend.

P1 Erik Erikson's psychosexual theory

Erik Erikson (1968) developed a theory of psychosexual development based on the ideas of Freud. He believed people experience several stages of psychosexual development over their lifetime and that social relationships play a significant part in this. Erikson rejected Freud's emphasis on unconscious forces and individual gratification. Instead he argued that an individual's development is motivated by a human need to be accepted by society and to live a meaningful life. Erikson developed his theory around the idea that people face and have to tackle a series of psychosocial crises in life. Each has a different social focus, as shown in Figure 8.9 below.

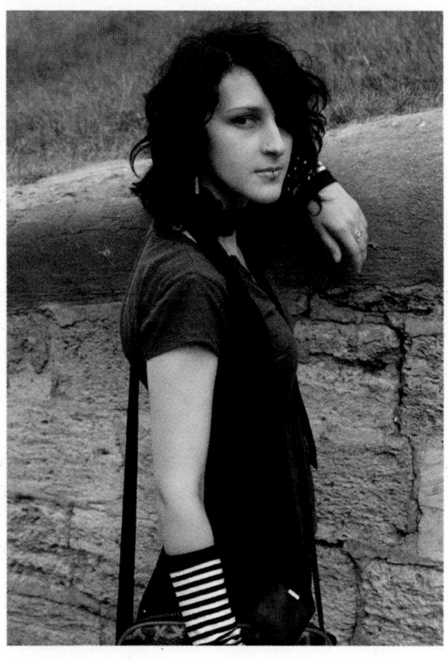

Identity formation is a key developmental issue during adolescence.

Your assessment criteria:

P1 Explain the principal psychological perspectives

M1 Assess different psychological approaches to study

Figure 8.9 Erikson's stages of psychosexual development.

Development stage	Key focus	Positive outcomes	Negative outcomes
Stage 1 (0–1 years)	Parenting	Dependable, responsive and caring parenting leads to *trust*.	Lack of warmth, affection and consistency leads to *mistrust*.
Stage 2 (1–3 years)	Becoming more independent	Being supported in independence leads to *autonomy*.	Being criticised and over-controlled leads to *self-doubt* about competence.
Stage 3 (3–6 years)	Engaging with the wider world	Being encouraged to try out new skills leads to *initiative*.	Being restricted leads to a sense of *guilt* and lack of confidence.
Stage 4 (6–12 years)	Understanding how things are made and work	Ability to succeed leads to *industry*.	Being pushed too hard on tasks leads to *inferiority*.
Stage 5 (12–18 years)	Identity development	Experimentation leads to a *secure identity*.	Inability to experiment leads to *role confusion* and negative identity.

M1 Assessing the psychodynamic approach

The strengths and weaknesses or limitations of the psychodynamic approach to psychology are summarised in Figure 8.10 below.

Figure 8.10 An assessment of the psychodynamic approach.

Strengths	Weaknesses or limitations
1. Effective for treating mild, anxiety-based problems but less suitable for treating more serious and enduring mental health problems.	1. Based on a theory and concepts that are difficult for many people to grasp, and which some distrust or find hard to believe.
2. Recognises the influence of the unconscious and the individual's 'inner' mental and emotional life on behaviour, emotion and development.	2. Places the therapist in a very powerful position – they are seen as having the 'expertise' to analyse and treat the individual. This may lead to abuse of power or may feel disempowering for those receiving treatment.
3. Aims to find and resolve the root causes of an individual's problems.	3. Can be very time-consuming, taking a long time to resolve an individual's problems or reduce their distress.

What do you know?

1. Identify two pioneers of the psychodynamic perspective in psychology.
2. Describe the parts played by the id, ego and superego in the human personality.
3. Explain the role of the unconscious in human behaviour.
4. Identify the stage of childhood psychosexual development that is linked to toilet training.
5. Describe the effects of two ego defence mechanisms on behaviour, giving an example of each.
6. Explain what Erikson meant by the term 'psychosexual crisis'.

The cognitive/information-processing perspective

Both the cognitive/information-processing perspective and the biological perspective (see page 372) take a scientific approach to human psychology, identifying links between the brain (or human body), behaviour, thinking and emotions.

Your assessment criteria:

P1 Explain the principal psychological perspectives

P1 The brain is like a computer

The cognitive/information-processing perspective compares the human mental processes taking place in the brain to software running on a computer. This perspective rose to prominence in the late 1950s when it started to challenge the narrow focus that behaviourism had on observable behaviour. Cognitive psychologists believed that internal mental processes should also be studied alongside behaviour. Psychologists and care practitioners using this perspective now typically study or work with people experiencing perceptual, memory, language and intellectual development or thinking problems; that is aspects of **cognition**, or the way the brain works.

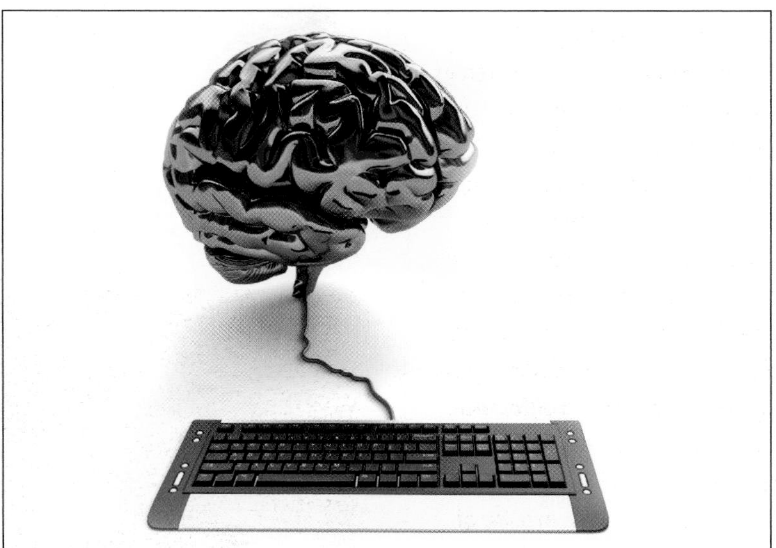

Figure 8.11 The brain as a computer.

Jean Piaget (1896–1980)

Jean Piaget was a Swiss psychologist who pioneered the cognitive approach in his work on children's thinking and learning. Piaget believed that children's thinking and intelligence developed over time as a result of biological **maturation**. He developed a stage-based theory of

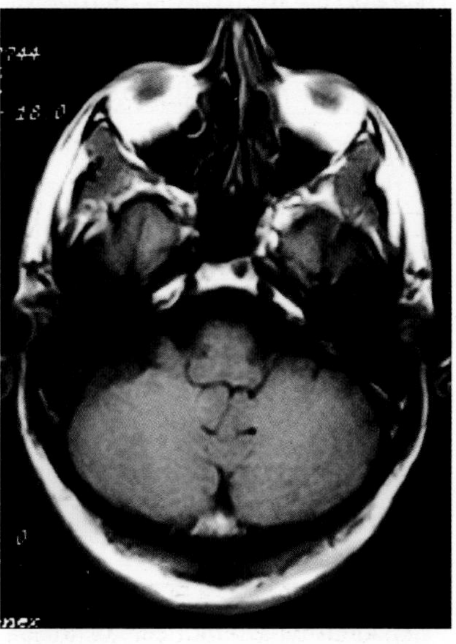

Key terms

Cognition: *mental activity*

Maturation: *the process of becoming fully developed or grown up (mature)*

cognitive development in which each stage built on a previous one, as shown in Figure 8.12 below.

Piaget's theory claims that cognitive development occurs when the child's brain has matured so that it is 'ready' for development. He argued that new information and experiences are gradually **assimilated** into the child's existing thinking. When this happens, the new experiences are **accommodated** by modifying existing thinking.

Key terms

Accommodated *existing thinking is modified to take account of new learning*

Assimilated: *taken in or incorporated*

Conservation: *the ability to think logically*

Figure 8.12 Piaget's stages of cognitive development.

Stage	Stage name	Age (years)	Focus of development
Stage 1	Sensorimotor	0–2	The world is experienced via motor activity and the senses.
Stage 2	Pre-operational	2–7	Language develops with memory. The child is egocentric and unable to think logically.
Stage 3	Concrete operational	7–11	The child can understand **conservation** but can't solve problems mentally.
Stage 4	Formal operational	11+	The child can use abstract thoughts and is able to represent problems.

Case study

Jean Piaget used a number of different experiments to investigate how children think about the world. He used conservation tests with children in the pre-operational and concrete operational stages of development. One of these tests involved using three glasses and a specific volume of water. Two of the glasses were identical in shape and size – small and wide. The third glass was much taller and thinner. Piaget would begin by showing the children the three glasses. In the first stage of the experiment, the two small wide glasses contained equal amounts of water. The taller, thin glass was empty. Stage two involved pouring water from one of the small wide glasses into the taller, thin glass. When the children were asked which glass contained the most water, they should have said there was no difference. However, children in the pre-operational stage would typically say the taller, thin glass contained most water. This is because their stage of intellectual development did not allow them to work out that, in spite of the change in shape of the vessel, the volume of water remained the same.

1. How old are children in the pre-operational stage of intellectual development?
2. Why do you think that the children typically said there was more water in the taller, thinner glass?
3. Which intellectual concept had the pre-operational children not yet developed?

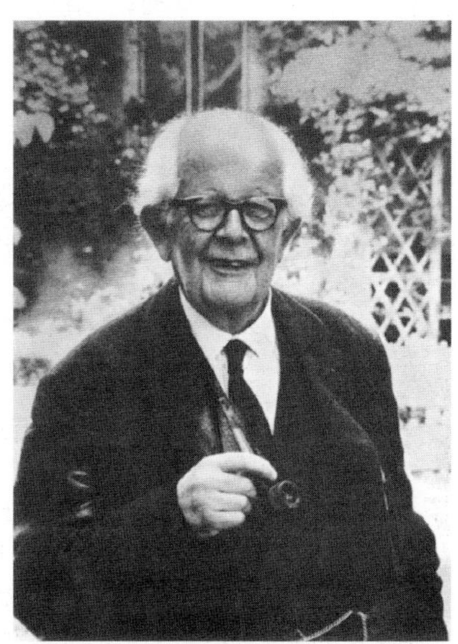

Jean Piaget (1896–1980).

P1 George Kelly (1905–66)

George Kelly used a cognitive approach to develop personal construct theory. He saw the individual as a 'scientist' making predictions about the future, testing them and revising or acting on them according to 'evidence'. Personal construct theory claims that people have to develop constructs to interpret and make sense of the environment in which they live. Because our environments are continually changing, we have to process lots of information and integrate it into the way we think about the world. We do this by developing and using new constructs in an adaptive way. Kelly argued that people construct and reconstruct a future for themselves, even 'reinventing' themselves, by changing their habitual ways of thinking about themselves and their environment.

Your assessment criteria:

P1 Explain the principal psychological perspectives

M1 Assess different psychological approaches to study

Case study

Yasmin, aged 28, recently lost her mother to breast cancer. Yasmin had always thought of her mother as a major source of support and strength in her life. During her mother's illness, Yasmin gradually got used to the idea that her mum was dying, but was still grief stricken when she finally died. Three months later, Yasmin has now decided that she can also be strong and supportive for her own daughter and that she will be able to live a happy, fulfilling life without the support of her mum.

1. Describe how Yasmin's experience of loss unsettled the way she viewed herself and the world.
2. Which of Yasmin's personal constructs has changed over the last 3 months?
3. How does a cognitive approach to psychology help to make sense of Yasmin's recent behaviour and development?

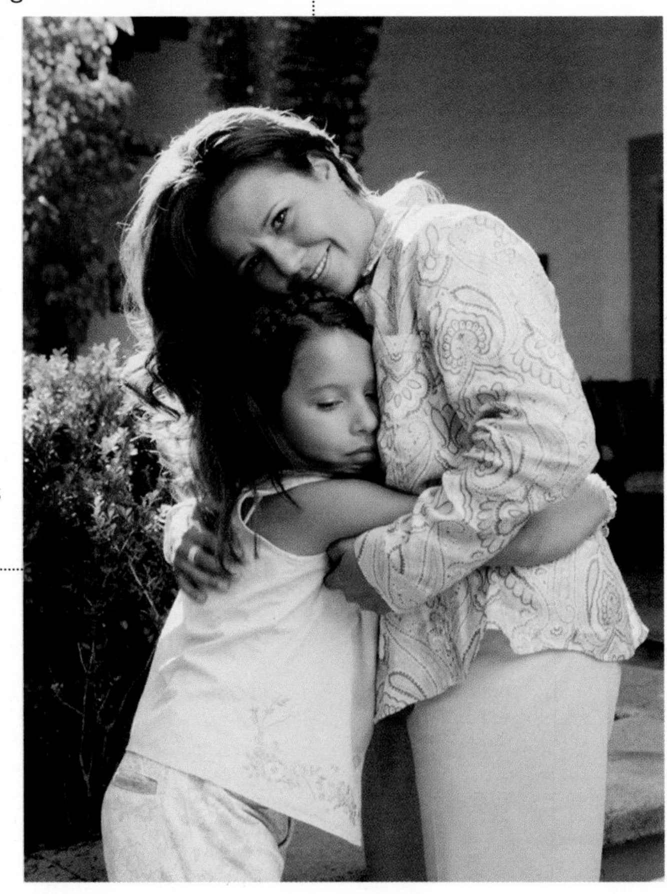

M1 Assessing the cognitive/information-processing approach

The strengths and weaknesses or limitations of the cognitive/information-processing approach to psychology are summarised in Figure 8.13 below.

Reflect

Can you think of any events or experiences in your life that have caused you to change the way you think about or present your 'self' to others? Does Kelly's personal construct theory help you to understand why and how this occurred?

Figure 8.13 An assessment of the cognitive/information-processing approach to psychology.

Strengths	Weaknesses or limitations
1. Research studies show that cognitive therapies (see Figure 8.14) are very effective for people suffering from mental disorders.	1. The cognitive approach seems to suggest that people can simply think their way out of problems and be self-sufficient. This fails to recognise the social, cultural and biological complexity of many health and social care problems.
2. The cognitive approach deals directly with the thoughts or emotions that are causing a person distress.	2. The cognitive approach doesn't seek out or address the origins of irrational thinking or emotional problems. It simply addresses the symptoms.
3. The approach recognises that a person's mental abilities develop and change over time.	3. People aren't totally controlled or purely influenced by brain activity – human behaviour and experience are the result of complex interactions between a variety of nature and nurture factors.

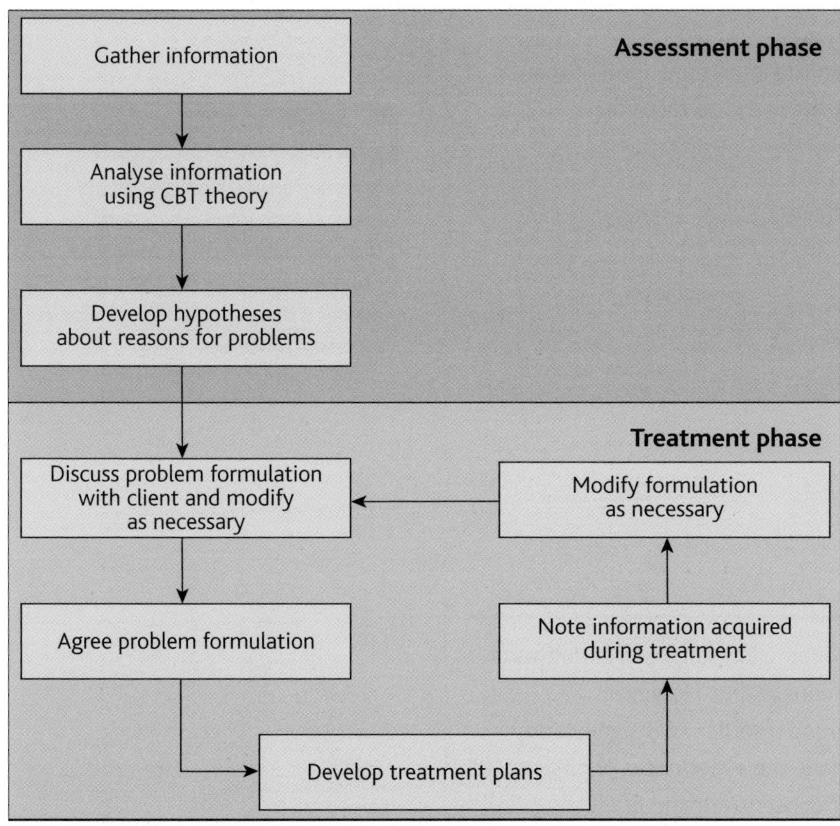

Figure 8.14. The Cognitive Behavioral Therapy (CBT) process.

The biological perspective

There are parallels between the cognitive/information processing perspective (see page 368) and the biological perspective as both take a scientific approach to human psychology.

Your assessment criteria:

P1 Explain the principal psychological perspectives

P1 Human biology and behaviour

The biological perspective in psychology applies the principles of biology to physiological, **genetic** and developmental aspects of human behaviour. The physiological strand of this approach focuses on nerves, neurotransmitters, brain circuits and basic biological processes, particularly maturation. A second strand of the biological perspective, known as evolutionary psychology, claims that many behaviours are deeply rooted in processes of **natural selection**, having been bred into the human population over time. Those behavioural characteristics that are **adaptive** are passed on to the next generation through selective breeding. Those that aren't adaptive are not selected and disappear. As a result, users of this approach claim that, to understand a particular type or example of human behaviour, we need to identify what natural selection designed it to do.

Biological psychologists are interested in the interconnection of mental and physiological processes. As a result they tend to focus on:

- sensation and perception
- motivated behaviour (hunger, thirst, sex)
- learning and memory
- emotion
- sleep and biological rhythms
- reasoning and decision-making.

Key terms

Adaptive: *behaviour that enables a person to adjust to another person or situation*

Genetic: *resulting from biological inheritance or heredity*

Natural selection: *reproduction of characteristics that increase an organism's chances of survival*

Discuss

In a small group, identify a list of physical or psychological conditions that you think have a biological basis. Consider what evidence there is that connects these conditions to biological factors or processes.

Case study

Jean Bains, aged 55, has suffered from depression since early adulthood. Most of the time her mood is low but manageable. However, approximately every 6 or 7 years her mood disorder gets significantly worse. Her energy levels drop significantly, she experiences poor sleep, finds it very hard to motivate herself or concentrate and gradually neglects herself. When this happens, Jean's psychiatrist changes her medication and refers her for a course of electro-convulsive therapy (ECT) at the local psychiatric unit. Jean seems to really benefit from this – her mood lifts quite quickly, she becomes much more motivated and is capable of looking after herself again.

1. Which aspects of Jean's depression have a biological component?
2. How might a biological psychologist explain the origins of Jean's depression?
3. Can you think of any think of any limitations or criticisms of the kinds of treatment Jean receives to deal with her depression?

Gessell's theory of maturation

Arnold Gessell (1880–1961) outlined a theory of development based on the claim that development occurs as a result of maturational processes. In effect, human development occurs in response to a sequence of biologically-based changes in the human body – especially the brain. The individual is seen as maturing through several different but linked stages of growth and development in which a predictable, biologically-based 'programme' of maturation unfolds. For example, foetal development during pregnancy follows a fixed, predictable set of stages until the foetus is ready to be born. From birth, a genetic 'programme' causes the baby to develop into a child, and the child into an adolescent. Maturational processes then lead on to the developmental changes that occur in adulthood and, finally, a progression into old age.

Gessell claimed that this process of change and development follows a relatively predictable pattern because it is 'hard wired' into the human genome. From this perspective, maturational processes drive human physical, psychological and emotional development, with the environment providing only background support rather than playing a leading role. This contrasts with humanistic and learning theory where nurture effects are seen as having a paramount influence on the individual's development.

Investigate

Find out how a human embryo develops and changes into a foetus, and what happens during each trimester of a woman's pregnancy. Produce a summary of the main maturational changes that occur at each stage.

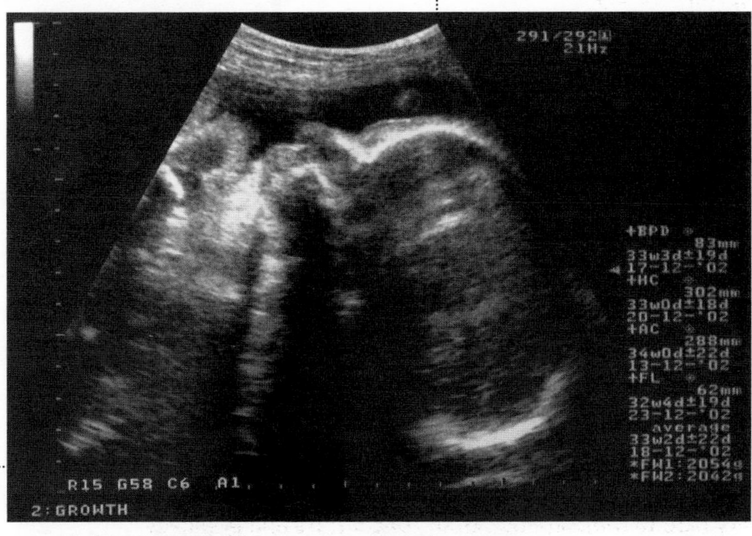

Foetal development is a maturational process.

Your assessment criteria:

P1 Explain the principal psychological perspectives

M1 Assess different psychological approaches to study

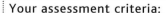

P1 Physical and physiological influences on behaviour

Biological psychologists study the ways that different parts of the brain, such as the right and left hemispheres, operate and affect human functioning. Movement, language and emotion are all influenced by particular parts of the brain, for example. When an area of the brain is damaged, or temporarily impaired by illness, drugs or other substances, a person's behaviour and mental abilities can be affected. Characteristic behaviours (tremors, impulsiveness or disinhibition, for example) can occur or the person can lose some functional ability (such as speech, memory or judgement).

Biological psychologists are also very interested in physiological processes, particularly the influence of neurotransmitters, on behaviour and mental state. Serotonin and dopamine are two neurotransmitters that are thought to have a strong influence on a person's mental state (see Figure 8.15).

Figure 8.15 Linking neurotransmitters to mental state.

Neurotransmitter	Psychological effects
Low serotonin levels	Increased risk of depression, suicide, impulsive aggression and alcoholism.
High serotonin levels	Fearfulness, obsessive behaviour, shyness and lack of self-confidence.
High dopamine levels	Increased risk of schizophrenia and experience of hallucinations.

Similarly, the release of hormones from a person's endocrine glands can have a powerful effect on their behaviour and how they feel. Melatonin, released from the pineal glands, acts on the brain stem to synchronise an individual's patterns of sleep and activity. Usually, the pineal gland responds to the external environment by releasing more melatonin as daylight fades, promoting sleep. Melatonin production is reduced as daylight returns. Similarly, you are probably aware of the link between testosterone and a person's level of aggression. The release of testosterone into the blood is linked to an increase in aggressiveness.

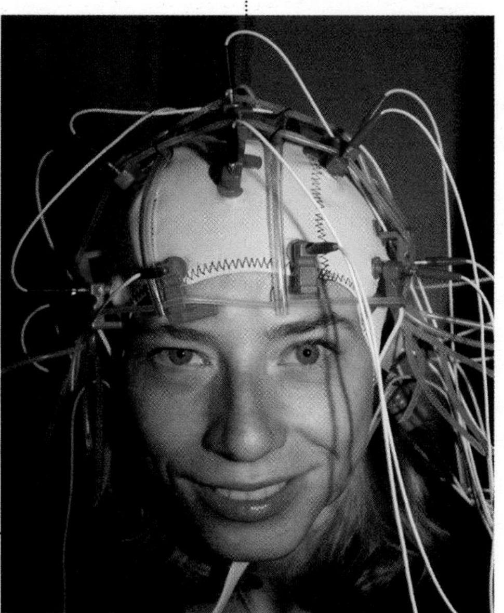

Neuropsychologists investigate brain function in a scientific way.

M1 Assessing the biological approach

The strengths and weaknesses or limitations of the biological approach to psychology are summarised in Figure 8.16 below.

Figure 8.16 An assessment of the biological approach to psychology.

Strengths	Weaknesses or limitations
1. Biological processes can be observed (e.g. brain scans) and measured (e.g. serotonin levels), enabling causes of psychological problems to be identified.	1. Complex human behaviours can't always be reduced to physical causes. Other environmental factors and inner mental processes may play a part too.
2. The claims and theories of biological psychology apply to all human beings, making them very useful to practitioners working with diverse populations.	2. This approach doesn't explain why individuals from different ethnic and cultural backgrounds may have different patterns of behaviour. As human beings with the same physiology, according to the biological approach, we should all behave in a very similar way.
3. Treatments that correct physiological problems and imbalances can be developed and used in a precise, evidence-based way.	3. Biological explanations of psychological problems tend to lead to biological treatments. These are not always successful and may have side-effects (medication) or cause physical damage (psycho-surgery).

What do you know?

1. Identify two psychologists who developed and used a cognitive/information-processing approach to psychology.
2. Describe the main features of Piaget's theory of children's intellectual development.
3. What are the main strengths and weaknesses of the cognitive perspective in psychology?
4. What do biological psychologists investigate?
5. Using your own words, summarise Arnold Gessell's theory of maturation.
6. Using two examples, explain the links between human physiology (the biological approach) and an individual's behaviour or mental state.

Investigate

Investigate the use of physical treatments that tend to be associated with the biological approach to psychological distress. These include:

- *medication*
- *electro-convulsive therapy*
- *psychosurgery*
- *physical exercise.*

Produce a summary explaining what each treatment involves, highlighting the connection between an individual's physiological processes and their behaviour or psychological experiences.

Behaviourism in care practice

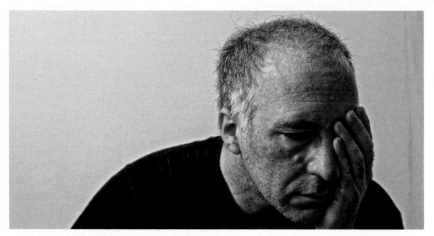

Behavioural techniques are used to treat a variety of psychological problems.

Your assessment criteria:

P2 Explain different psychological approaches to health practice

P2 Using behavioural techniques in health and social care

At the beginning of this unit (see page 348), we saw how the behavioural perspective focuses on the way people learn behaviours. The two behavioural approaches to learning – classical conditioning and operant conditioning – can be applied as part of treatment and therapy approaches in health and social care settings. Psychologists and care practitioners use behavioural techniques to change **maladaptive** and **challenging behaviours**, and to stimulate and shape new forms of behaviour.

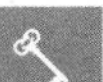

Key terms

Challenging behaviour: *behaviour that goes beyond expected social boundaries and that is seen as risky or threatening by others*

Maladaptive: *something that is unconstructive or disruptive*

Changing maladaptive and challenging health behaviour

Psychologists and health care practitioners are sometimes asked to work with people whose problems are the result of maladaptive behaviours. This means that their ways of coping with particular situations or stresses in life are damaging to themselves or others. Heavy drinking or drug-taking in response to stress and avoidance of travelling by aeroplane for fear of dying are examples of maladaptive behaviours. The concepts of association and reinforcement can be used to trace the origins of these kinds of behavioural and emotional problems and can help care practitioners understand an individual's behaviour.

Aversion therapy

Aversion therapy is a form of classical conditioning that uses **negative reinforcement** to change maladaptive behaviour. It has been used as a treatment for alcoholism, for example, where the patient is given a drug (Antabuse) that is perfectly safe and which has no side-effects – until the person drinks alcohol. When alcohol is consumed, the person feels very unwell and may be violently sick. Over time, the person learns to associate these unpleasant feelings and experiences with alcohol and stops drinking to avoid them. The same technique is used when a child's nails are painted with a bitter-tasting solution to deter nail biting.

Treatment of phobias

Phobias (see Figure 8.17) are often treated using a technique called **systematic desensitisation**. This involves reducing and ultimately removing the power of a maladaptive association by gradually exposing the person to the thing they find frightening. To do this, the care practitioner and the phobic person first create a 'hierarchy of fear'. The treatment stage involves gradually exposing the person to varying degrees of fear, while also helping them to relax and cope with each exposure. The goal is for the person to face the situation or object that they are phobic about without worrying. Systematic desensitisation has been used effectively to help people overcome all kinds of phobias, from agoraphobia (fear of open spaces) to fear of spiders, that cause distress and disrupt people's lives.

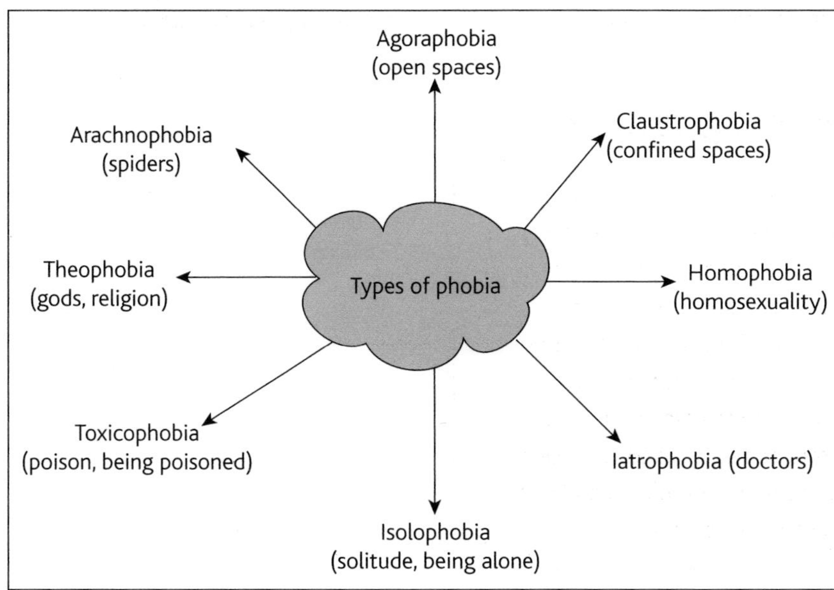

Figure 8.17 Types of phobia.

Investigate

People overeat and gain weight for a variety of reasons. Losing weight is also a notoriously difficult thing to do. Part of the reason for this is that people find changing their behaviour patterns very difficult.

1. *Note down possible reasons why some people develop a habit of overeating.*
2. *Could overeating be described as either a challenging or a maladaptive behaviour?*
3. *What behavioural approaches could be used to encourage overweight people to stop overeating?*

Key terms

Negative reinforcement: *the removal of a discouraging or negative stimulus associated with a behaviour*

Systematic desensitisation: *a behavioural technique that exposes an individual to a threatening stimulus in relaxed conditions until the anxiety response disappears*

Investigate

Investigate one of the following phobias, identifying the source of an individual's fear and the likely impact on their behaviour and lifestyle:

- *agoraphobia*
- *social phobia*
- *homophobia.*

P3 Changing and shaping social behaviour

The principles of operant conditioning can be used to stimulate or shape behaviours using behaviour modification techniques. These use reinforcement (and to a lesser extent punishment) to change and shape an individual's behaviour. Typically, this involves establishing a system of 'token' rewards to reinforce desired behaviours. For example, parents and child care practitioners sometimes use 'reward' stickers to encourage young children to learn to use a potty or toilet instead of wearing a nappy.

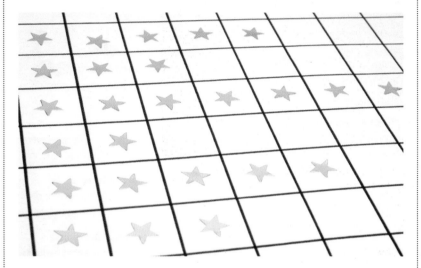

Token economy systems were a common feature of mental health and learning disability services until the 1980s. They were generally used to motivate and reinforce the development of self-care skills (getting dressed, having a wash, taking part in activities) in unmotivated people who had lived in large institutions like mental hospitals for many years. In modern care settings, care practitioners are more likely to use **social reinforcement** in the form of verbal praise ('Well done, that's really great!') to encourage desirable health behaviours and to build up the self-esteem and self-confidence of people who use the service.

Your assessment criteria:

P2 Explain different psychological approaches to health practice

P3 Explain different psychological approaches to social care practice

D1 Evaluate two psychological approaches to health and social care service provision

Key terms

Social reinforcement: *forms of verbal praise and encouragement*

Discuss

Think of as many different positive words or phrases as you can that could be used as social reinforcement for people with low self-esteem or low self-confidence. Make a list and discuss your examples with those of class colleagues.

P2 Changing challenging behaviours

Challenging behaviour is any form of behaviour that is out of keeping with the expected standards or patterns of behaviour in a culture or society. In effect, it is behaviour that 'challenges' normal expectations and standards. It may be the intensity, frequency or duration of the behaviour that is unusual and which puts the person or other people at risk. Challenging behaviour is usually associated with adults who have learning disabilities, mental health problems or dementia and with children experiencing 'tantrums'. Self-harm, violence, inappropriate sexual behaviour, selective incontinence and vandalism are all common types of challenging behaviour. Behavioural analysis and treatment of challenging behaviour tries to identify the causes, triggers and consequences of the behaviour. Operant conditioning principles are then used to help the person develop new, more socially acceptable ways of behaving.

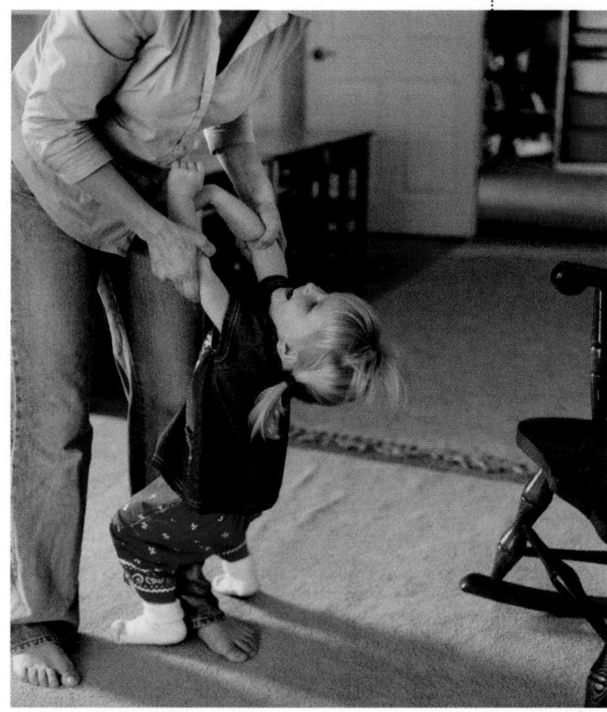

The behavior of young children can be very challenging at times.

D1 Evaluating behaviourism

Figure 8.18 An evaluation of behaviourism.

Strengths	Weaknesses/limitations
1. Behaviourism is a scientific and testable way of understanding and treating psychological problems.	1. Views human behaviour as being like a ping pong ball, continually being batted between stimulus factors and automatic responses.
2. Has many practical uses and can help people to modify or change their behaviour relatively quickly.	2. Ignores the influence of human consciousness, emotions and thinking abilities on human psychological development and experience.
3. Provides a way of understanding individual differences in behaviour because it focuses on an individual's particular circumstances and ways of responding.	3. Restricts its focus to observable behaviours only, ignoring a range of other factors (the unconscious, genetics, cognition, biological processes) that can influence psychological experiences.

Reflect

On balance, are you persuaded that behaviourism has a useful part to play in health and social care settings? What, for you, are its main strength and its main limitation?

The psychodynamic approach in care practice

The psychodynamic perspective has been widely used as a way of providing psychotherapy for people with behavioural, mental health and emotional problems. Various forms of individual and group psychodynamic therapy are used in primary and secondary health care settings in the UK. A basic principle of the psychodynamic perspective is that unconscious forces influence an individual's behaviour and thinking, and can cause distress. Care practitioners using a psychodynamic approach need to be skilled at understanding how disturbed thinking or behaviour may be a symptom of deeper, unconscious troubles.

Your assessment criteria:

P3 Explain different psychological approaches to social care practice

M2 Compare two psychological approaches to health and social care service provision

D1 Evaluate two psychological approaches to health and social care service provision

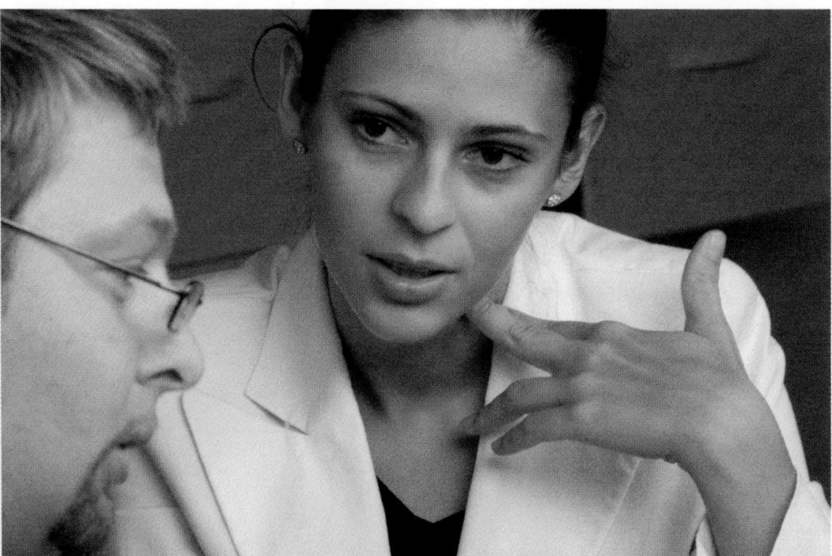

Psychodynamic practice focuses on inner mental processes.

Reflect

Why might it be helpful to ask an adult who is self-harming about the things that happened to them in childhood or adolescence? What is the psychodynamic rationale for this?

P3 Understanding challenging behaviour

The psychodynamic perspective can help care practitioners to understand the 'hidden' causes of challenging behaviour that can't otherwise be explained. For example, a child's bedwetting or an adult's self-harming behaviour may be linked to their early experiences, problems with psychosexual or psychosocial development or may be understood as ego defence mechanisms. In this way, behaviour that is apparently inexplicable, bizarre or 'bad' makes sense, can be discussed and addressed more constructively.

Understanding and managing anxiety

People often use defence mechanisms to try to control their anxieties without being aware that they are doing so. Their anxieties may then manifest themselves in physical symptoms and illnesses. This can be very difficult to deal with, both personally and for health care staff – the person has some physical symptoms but there is no obvious physical or medical cause. In circumstances like these, particularly where the symptoms have been long lasting, a psychodynamic approach can be helpful in revealing the psychological root causes of the person's problems and can also provide a way of addressing them.

Reflect

What kinds of behaviours indicate that a person is experiencing anxiety? Are you aware of having any anxiety-related behaviours (nail-biting, pacing about, hair-chewing)?

M2 Comparing behaviourism and the psychodynamic perspective

Figure 8.19 A comparison of behaviourism and the psychodynamic perspective.

Behaviourism	Psychodynamic perspective
1. Focuses on observable behaviours only. This means behaviourists deal with a person's current problems not things from their past.	1. Focuses on 'inner' mental processes that are inaccessible and can't easily be controlled by the individual.
2. Offers a relatively quick and cheap way of treating the behavioural symptoms of psychological problems.	2. Usually involves establishing a long-lasting relationship to get to the root causes of a person's problems. This is time-consuming and expensive.
3. Sees behaviour as the key aspect of human psychology and doesn't deal with issues in a hypothetical or subjective way – not interested in 'inner processes'.	3. Sees the human mind as a 'deep, dark dungeon' filled with an individual's demons and nightmares – this is very negative.
4. Based on relatively simple, effective principles.	4. Based on relatively complex theory that is difficult to test or evaluate for effectiveness.
5. Reductionist and deterministic. It reduces human psychology to a stimulus-response level and assumes that behaviour is determined by learnt responses.	5. Also reductionist and deterministic. It reduces human psychology to unconscious processes and unobservable mental structures that are seen to control or determine mental processes and emotional experiences.

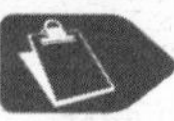

Case study

Gregor Russell is a specialist mental health nurse who uses a psychodynamic approach with people who are referred to the mental health unit where he works. This is a typical day in Gregor's life:

8.30am	Arrive for multidisciplinary team meeting. Discuss new referrals and clients' progress.
9.00am	Check referral reports for new clients, noting problems and therapy received so far.
10.00 am	Meet new client for initial assessment. Discuss difficulties and the way psychodynamic therapy works.
11.00–1.00pm	See clients already engaged in therapy for one-to-one sessions.
2.00pm	Receive and discuss telephone referral with social worker. Agree to assess client's suitability for psychodynamic therapy.
3.00pm	Facilitate group session for clients with significant anger and personality issues.
4.00pm	Meet colleague for supervision session.
5.00pm	Catch up with email, post and admin.

1. Identify two concepts that are likely to play an important part in Gregor's approach to psychological problems.
2. Briefly explain how psychodynamic therapists like Gregor work with clients.

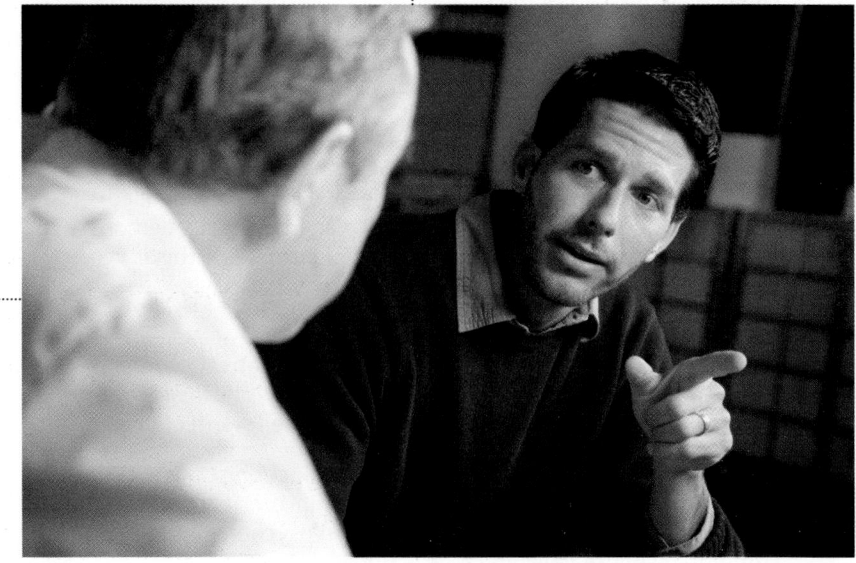

D1 Evaluating the psychodynamic approach to health and social care provision

Figure 8.20 An evaluation of the psychodynamic approach.

What does it offer?	What are its limitations?
1. Psychodynamic therapies are effective with certain types of people (articulate, introspective) and certain types of disorders (anxiety-based, linked to attachments and early experiences).	1. Psychodynamic therapies tend to focus on past experiences rather than the current difficulties a person faces.
2. These therapies seek out the root causes of people's problems and try to resolve them.	2. Digging deeply into a person's problems and past experiences can produce more distress (making the person feel worse) before a solution is found and symptoms are relieved.
3. The psychodynamic approach can be used with individuals or groups.	3. Costly and time-consuming, requiring a specially trained therapist.

Reflect

On balance, are you persuaded that psychodynamic theory has a useful part to play in health and social care settings? What, for you, are its main strength and its main limitation?

What do you know?

1. Identify two ways of using the behavioural perspective in health and social care practice.
2. What behavioural principle is aversion therapy based on?
3. Describe the process of systematic desensitisation.
4. How can operant conditioning principles be used to promote and shape an individual's self-care skills?
5. What is social reinforcement and how can it be used in health and social care settings?
6. Explain how behavioural principles can be used to help an individual experiencing post-traumatic stress disorder?

Social learning theory in care practice

Concepts and principles from the social learning perspective, along with those from the humanist perspective (see page 360), are widely used as part of care relationships and helping interventions.

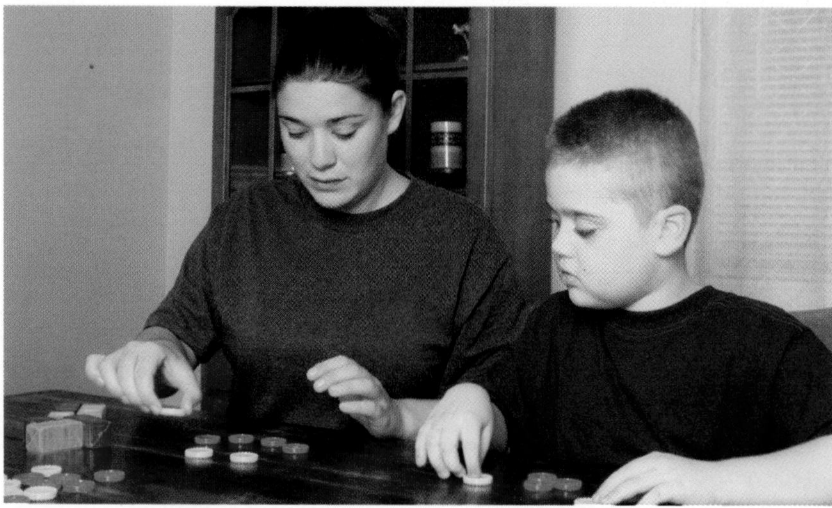

Imitation is a key concept in social learning theory.

Your assessment criteria:

P2 Explain different psychological approaches to health practice

P3 Explain different psychological approaches to social care practice

P2 Applying social learning theory

Social learning theory focuses on the influence that other people, particularly **role models**, can have on an individual's development and behaviour. The idea of modelling and learning through **imitation** has been used to promote anti-discriminatory behaviour and to persuade people to improve their health-related behaviours. Being anti-discriminatory and promoting health and wellbeing are key features of the care practitioner's role for many people working in the health and social care sectors.

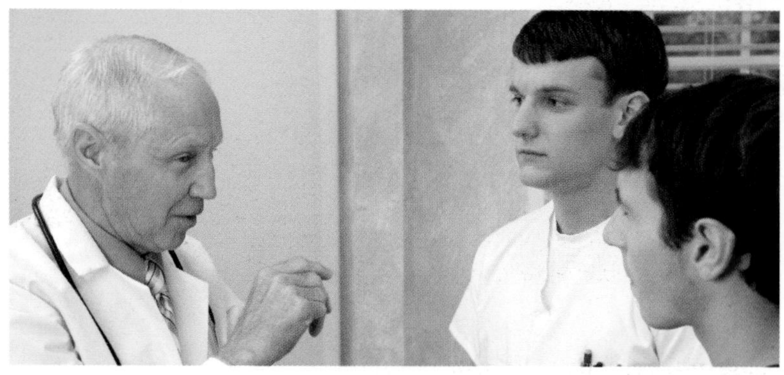

Experienced practitioners are important role models for less experienced trainees in health and social care settings.

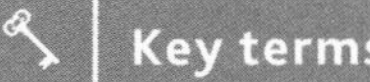

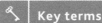

Key terms

Imitation: *copying*

Role models: *People who inspire others to imitate or be like them because of their desirable characteristics*

P3 Promoting anti-discriminatory behaviour and practices

A role model is somebody who is admired and whose behaviour and values are seen as desirable. Care practitioners tend to be committed to promoting equality and challenging discrimination in their everyday work. Expressing anti-discrimination values in the way that they relate to and interact with people and modelling behaviours that promote equality and fairness may encourage others (colleagues and people who use services) to imitate this kind of behaviour. In this way, the social learning perspective informs the approach care practitioners take in care relationships.

Case study

Analise is an educational psychologist in an integrated children's services team. She uses social learning theory in her practice. This is an example of her daily activity:

9.15am	Arrive at primary school to discuss problematic behaviour of Child A with headteacher and classroom teacher.
10.00am	Observe Child A in class and during break time.
12.00pm	Talk to class teacher and teaching assistant over lunch about their approach towards and feelings about Child A. Explain how to model and reinforce acceptable classroom behaviour.
1.00pm	Talk with Child A, mother and classroom teacher about behaviour issue. Agree some 'goals for the week' to work on when at school.
2.00–3.30pm	Meeting at SureStart centre to discuss referrals and review needs of current service users.
4.00pm	Meet with local group of Special Educational Needs Coordinators (SENCOs) to discuss inclusion and anti-discrimination strategies.
5.00pm	Write up notes and deal with admin.

1. Identify two social learning theory concepts that are likely to play an important part in Analise's approach to children's developmental and psychological problems.
2. Briefly explain how a psychologist like Analise might use the concept of role modelling in her work with Child A.

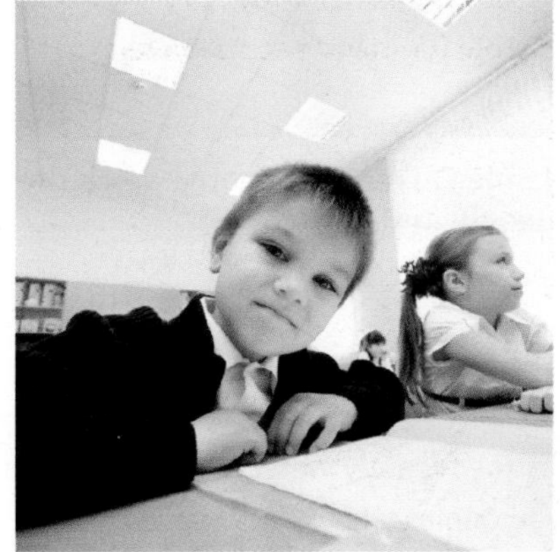

P2 Using positive role models in health education

As you learnt earlier in this unit (see page 385), role models can use the influence they have over people who aspire to be like them to shape the health behaviours of the wider public. The concepts of role modelling, vicarious reinforcement and imitation have been widely used by health education campaigners to raise awareness of a range of health issues, including diet, exercise and breast cancer for example, in ways that encourage people to change their behaviours. Diet, weight loss and healthy eating issues have been promoted by a range of celebrity chefs, such as Jamie Oliver, Hugh Fearnley-Whittingstall and Gordon Ramsey, over the past 5 years. Similarly, television and radio chat shows, and events such as the London Marathon frequently feature celebrities who are promoting health-related causes while also encouraging fans to change their health behaviour. The use of role models like celebrities and sports performers in health education programmes is a deliberate attempt to draw on social learning principles.

Your assessment criteria:

P2 Explain different psychological approaches to health practice

D1 Evaluate two psychological approaches to health and social care service provision

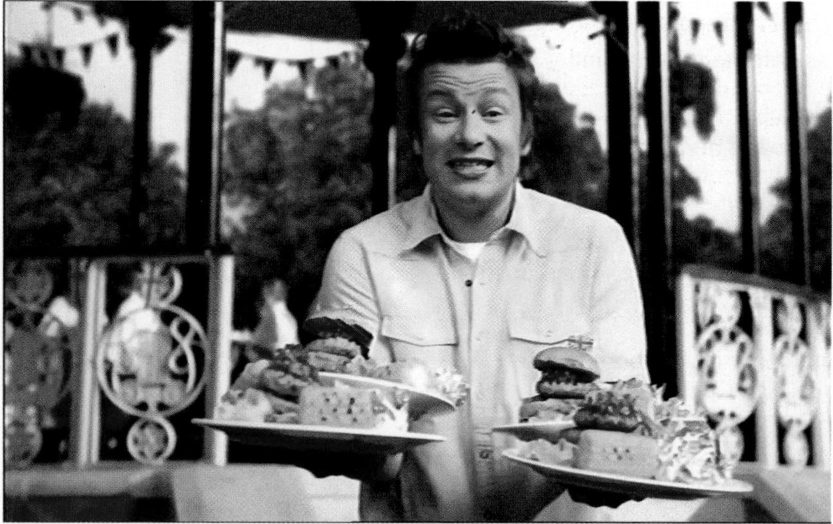

Jamie Oliver has become a healthy-eating role model for many people in the UK.

Reflect

Has your health behaviour ever been influenced by a celebrity (or a non-celebrity) role model? Think about how role models have influenced your thinking and behaviour about food, physical appearance or exercise, for example.

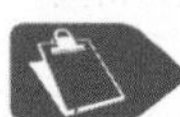

Case study

Joe recently watched a documentary about the impact of infertility on couples who wish to have children. He was moved by the story told by a pop star he admires who had been trying to start a family for the last 10 years. The celebrity was very open about the impact of infertility on his marriage and also on his self-esteem. When Joe saw an advertisement for a 10-mile fun run in aid of a fertility charity and noticed that the pop star would be running too, he decided to take part himself. Joe's physical fitness improved considerably as a result of the 3 months of training he undertook to prepare for the run. At the end of the run, Joe also had a strong sense of emotional wellbeing and satisfaction, and felt he had achieved something important.

1. Which social learning theory principles help to explain Joe's behaviour and feelings in this scenario?
2. How has a role model helped to deliver health education messages in this situation?
3. What psychological impact did the use of a role model have?

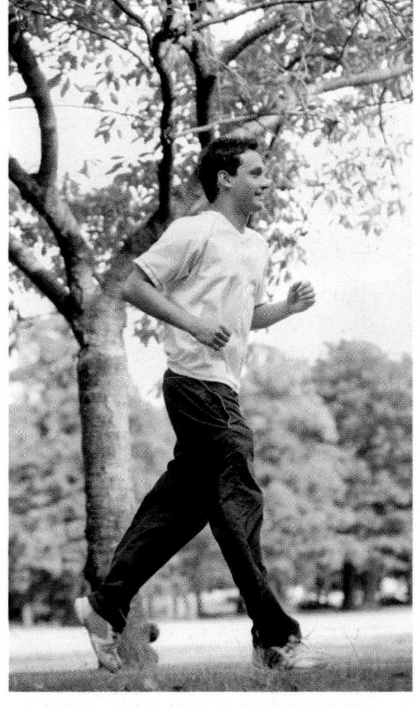

D1 Evaluating social learning theory

Figure 8.21 An evaluation of social learning theory.

What does it offer?	What are its limitations?
1. Combines behaviourist with cognitive principles. This provides a powerful, practical way of promoting learning and behaviour change.	1. Does not take into account different levels of ability or an individual's stage of intellectual development – it assumes everyone is capable of learning through observation.
2. The principles of social learning theory are simple, widely used and are seen as effective in educational settings and in care settings where teaching living skills is a feature of care practice.	2. Does not take into account the fact that people learn through experimenting and innovating, as well as by observing and imitating others – it underplays creativity.
3. Outcomes can be easily observed and are measurable.	3. Doesn't explain how to motivate people to learn through imitation – it just suggests that this is what happens and that all people can be motivated in the right circumstances.

Reflect

On balance, are you persuaded that social learning theory has a useful part to play in health and social care settings? What, for you, are its main strength and its main limitation?

Humanism in care practice

P3 P4 Applying the humanistic perspective

Humanism informs many approaches to counselling and therapy (see Figure 8.22) and also features in care relationships.

Carl Rogers' person-centred approach to counselling (see page 360) is now widely used and very influential in the health and social care sector. The concept of unconditional positive regard is central to this and is seen as a way of boosting an individual's self-esteem. Unconditional positive regard involves accepting and validating an individual's experiences, feelings, beliefs and judgements unconditionally and in a non-judgemental way. The aim of this is to help the person to develop a positive self-image and greater self-acceptance.

Empathy and understanding

Empathy involves listening and trying to understand another person's situation or feelings. This is often quite difficult to do and is distinct from **sympathy**. The listener needs to put aside any preconceptions they have in order to recognise how the person is struggling to deal with specific problems. They need to 'tune in' to the person's feelings and use their own emotions intelligently to experience empathy. The humanistic concept of empathy is now widely accepted as an important part of care relationships and health and social care practice generally. Health and social care practitioners generally recognise empathy as important and try to use it in their care practice.

Respecting individuals and being non-judgemental

There is wide acceptance in the health and social care sectors that an individual's needs, identity and preferences should always be respected. It is good practice not to criticise or make personal judgements about people who are receiving care, for example. Humanistic psychologists argue that we need to try to identify with other individuals – which can be difficult because of social differences – in order to avoid discriminatory practice and to provide services that meet each individual's needs

Your assessment criteria:

P2 Explain different psychological approaches to health practice

P3 Explain different psychological approaches to social care practice

Key terms

Empathy: *trying to understand another person's situation or feelings*

Humanism: *a psychological approach that emphasises the personal worth of each individual*

Sympathy: *sharing the feelings of others*

Reflect

Can you think of a situation in which you have been able to empathise, rather than sympathise, with another person?

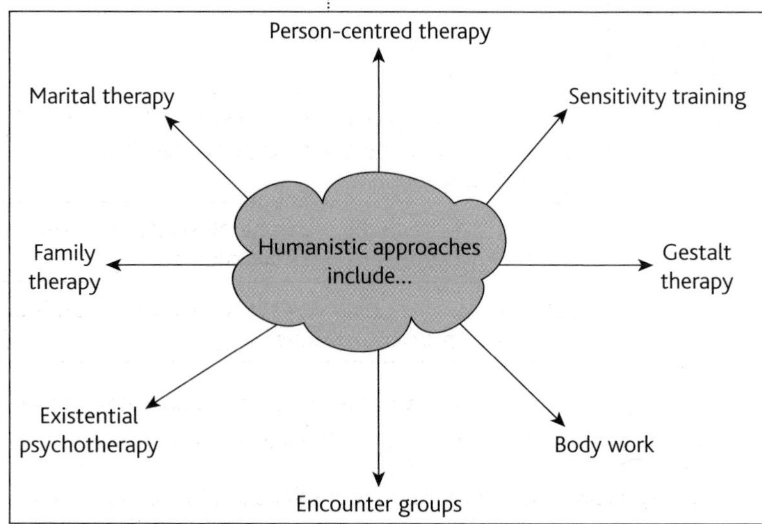

Figure 8.22 Humanistic approaches to counselling and therapy.

and preferences. In this way, the humanistic principle of valuing the personal worth of each individual is being put into practice.

Active listening

Active listening (see page 20) is an important means of putting the humanistic concepts of empathy, unconditional positive regard and respect for individuals into practice. Active listening involves actively focusing on and noticing what a person communicates, both verbally and non-verbally. This enables the listener to focus on the words a person is speaking, as well the emotions behind them. The humanistic perspective provides good theoretical reasons for using active listening in a wide range of care settings and contexts.

Reflect

Reflect on ways in which care workers, teachers or others in positions of authority have shown respect towards you? What did they do, what impact did this have on you and why was it important to be respected?

Case study

Trevor Jones is a counsellor working in a primary health care centre. This is a day in Trevor's working life:

8.00am	Attend referral meeting with GPs, community nurses and social workers. Discuss new referrals.
9.00am	See first client for continuing counselling (sixth out of 12 sessions). Discuss progress, feelings and strategies for coping with low mood.
10.00am	Write up notes and catch up on admin and telephone calls.
11.00am	See second client for review session. Agree very little progress made to reduce substance misuse. Discuss motivation and option of in-patient treatment.
12.30–1pm	Admin, post, emails and report-writing.
2.00pm	Facilitate 'Moving on' group for recently bereaved people. Discuss and listen to experiences, fears and coping strategies.
3.00pm	See third individual client for initial assessment and discussion of suitability for counselling.
4.00pm	Visit local homelessness project to give talk to staff on the role and process of counselling.

1. Identify two concepts that are likely to play an important part in Trevor's approach to a client's psychological problems.
2. Briefly explain how humanistic counsellors like Trevor work with clients.

M2 Comparing social learning theory and the humanistic perspective

Figure 8.23 A comparison of social learning theory and the humanist perspective.

Social learning theory	Humanistic perspective
1. Focuses on the observation of others' behaviour and imitation as key ways of developing behaviour.	1. Focuses on the importance of human relationships and the human capacity for self-understanding and personal development.
2. Focuses on environmental and cognitive factors and suggests that behaviour is influenced by others, rather than being the responsibility of the individual.	2. Not reductionist or deterministic. It recognises that human psychology and behaviour is complex and influenced by many factors.
3. Helpful for understanding how the context or circumstances of a person's life can affect their behaviour and development.	3. Humanistic concepts are widely used in health and social care settings, particularly in the way care practitioners develop and use care relationships.

Your assessment criteria:

M2 Compare two psychological approaches to health and social care service provision

D1 Evaluate two psychological approaches to health and social care service provision

Reflect

Do you think that social learning theory and the humanistic perspective are complementary or contrasting psychological approaches?

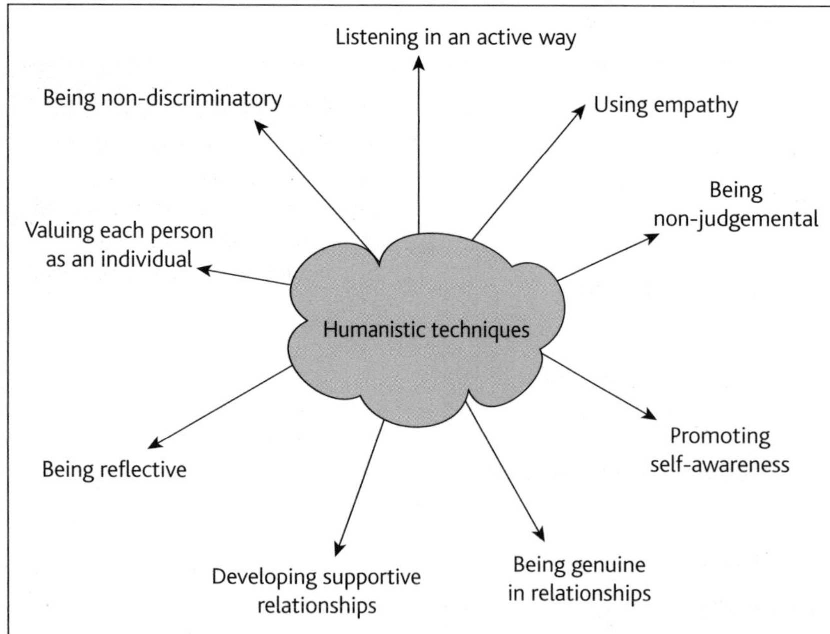

Figure 8.24 Humanist psychology has had a significant influence on the way care workers practise.

D1 Evaluating the humanistic perspective

Figure 8.25 An evaluation of the humanistic perspective.

Strengths	Weaknesses or limitations
1. The humanistic perspective encourages psychologists to accept that there is more to human behaviour and psychological experience than observable behaviour.	1. The humanistic focus on the individual and self-fulfilment can be seen as selfish and narcissistic.
2. Humanism is based on a positive view of human nature that emphasises individual responsibility.	2. Critics see the humanistic perspective as assuming an overly optimistic view of the world. It doesn't recognise that some people are unable to achieve self-fulfilment because they face significant social disadvantages, for example.
3. The ideas and concepts of the humanistic perspective are flexible and can be applied widely in health and social care settings.	3. The ideas and theories of the humanistic perspective can't be tested. They are seen as vague and unverifiable by those who want scientific evidence of effectiveness.
4. The humanistic perspective is based on values that are inclusive and supportive of all human beings.	4. The humanistic perspective suggests that everyone is capable of achieving self-actualisation and self-fulfilment. This may only be true of very talented and socially advantaged people.
5. The humanistic perspective is very client-centred and has enabled a large counselling industry to grow and develop.	5. Humanistic psychology ignores the unconscious – it recognises only those thoughts and behaviours that people are aware of.

What do you know?

1. Identify one way in which the principles of social learning theory can be used in health or social care practice.
2. What part can positive role models play in promoting health and wellbeing?
3. Outline two strengths and two contrasting weaknesses of social learning theory.
4. Identify three humanistic concepts that are used in health and social care work.
5. Describe how the focus of the humanistic perspective compares to that of the social learning theory perspective in psychology.
6. Outline two strengths and two contrasting weaknesses of the humanistic psychological perspective.

Reflect

On balance, are you persuaded that the humanistic perspective has a useful part to play in health and social care settings? What, for you, are its main strength and its main limitation?

The cognitive approach to care practice

Both the cognitive perspective and the biological perspective (see page 396) take a 'scientific' approach to psychological problems and care practice, and focus on links between the human body (or brain) and psychological experience or processes.

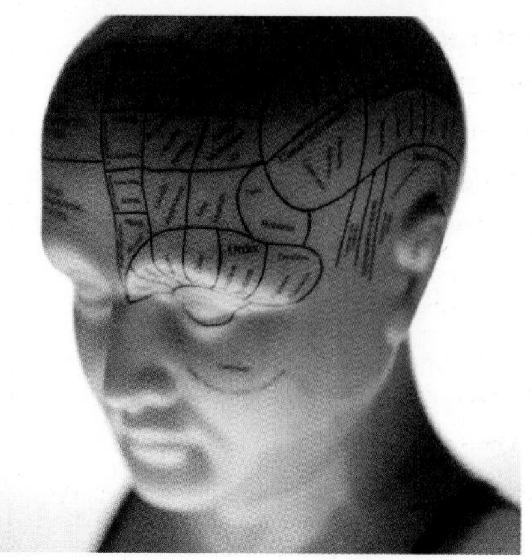

Cognitive psychologists take a scientific approach to psychological problems.

Your assessment criteria:

P2 Explain different psychological approaches to health practice

P3 Explain different psychological approaches to social care practice

P2/P3 Applying the cognitive approach to health and social care practice

Many contemporary psychologists would describe themselves as cognitive psychologists. The cognitive approach – and the view that mental events are characterised by an information-flow that has to be processed – is also very popular in health and social care settings. Specialist counsellors and therapists using forms of cognitive therapy, as well as doctors, nurses and other health care practitioners and social care workers who incorporate cognitive techniques into their relationship-building and intervention strategies, all draw on the idea of a cognitive triad (see Figure 8.26). This sees links between thinking, emotion and behaviour, but also recognises that the brain's ability to process information is central.

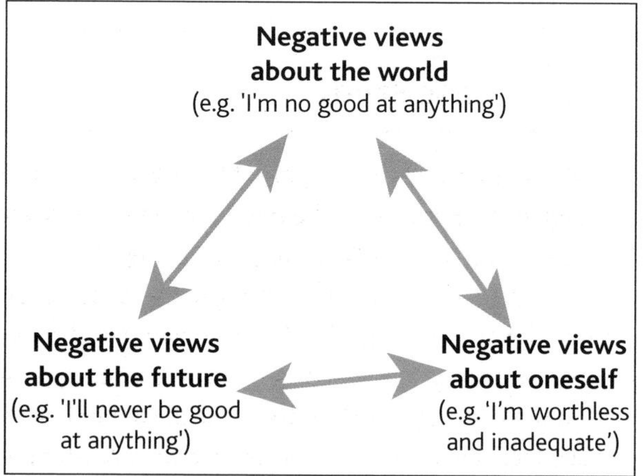

Figure 8.26 Aaron Beck's cognitive triad.

Supporting people with learning disabilities

The cognitive perspective has been used in care work with a variety of different service user groups. For example, cognitive approaches can be used to help people who 'misread' or misinterpret situations. This can happen to people with learning disabilities who may become confused and overwhelmed by the demands and complexities of everyday life. Cognitive approaches can be used to identify thinking errors and to develop new ways of learning and coping.

Supporting individuals with depression

Cognitive therapies are widely used to support people with emotional problems (especially anxiety and depression). They focus on helping people to identify, challenge and change negative or irrational patterns of thinking and are an effective way of reducing mental distress. The goal is to improve self-esteem and to contain the individual's behaviour.

Cognitive behaviour therapy (CBT) was developed by Aaron Beck to treat depression. Beck identified a 'cognitive triad' (see Figure 8.26) based on a negative self-appraisal that leads to negative beliefs about the world and the future – which the individual sees themselves as powerless to overcome. The aim of CBT is to challenge negative thoughts and to enable each person to develop an alternative, positive view of the world. A 'thought diary' may be used to collect or catch 'negative automatic thoughts' and to identify patterns of negative thinking. The care practitioner and client can then work out ways of challenging these patterns. A key strategy is to consider the evidence for the negative thoughts and what the alternatives might be. Once they have learnt some new coping strategies, CBT enables the individual to identify and deal with their own thinking errors.

Discuss

Are there circumstances in which the goal of changing a person's pattern of thinking about themselves or the world generally might be inappropriate, unacceptable or even unethical?

Case study

Sally gave birth to her daughter Meeka 6 weeks ago. Sally stayed in hospital for 4 days after the birth of Meeka to recover from her caesarean operation. Sally felt relaxed and well during this time but was very happy to go home. Since returning home, Sally has started to experience overwhelming feelings that Meeka might die. She has been very tearful and depressed, has had little or no appetite and is now extremely reluctant to let Meeka out of her sight. Sally feels she is the only person able to look after Meeka properly. She has developed a strict routine for Meeka (feeding, changing, sleeping) and is unable to vary this. Sally believes that if Meeka doesn't wake up and feed at the right times, she might not have enough energy and will die.

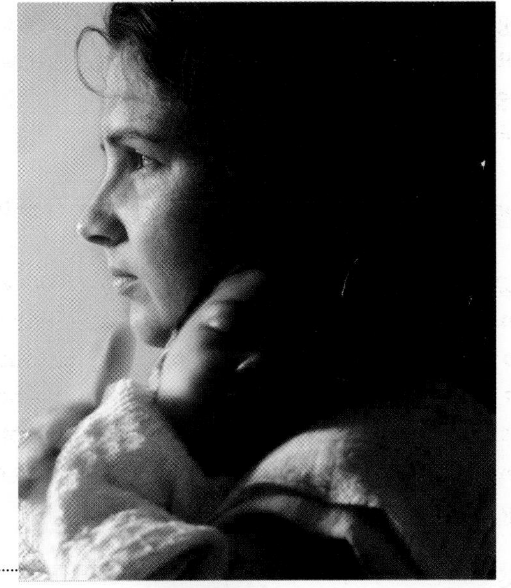

1. Which aspects of Sally's thinking seem to be negative and irrational?
2. How might a cognitive approach help to explain Sally's current problems?
3. Suggest how a care practitioner could use cognitive therapy to help Sally with her current problems.

P2 Supporting individuals with PTSD

Post-traumatic stress disorder (PTSD) is a mental health problem experienced by people who have been exposed to traumatic and frightening events, for example soldiers, victims of crime and people who have suffered serious abuse. Typically, an individual suffering from PTSD may become emotionally distressed and very frightened when a stimulus reminds them of a traumatic event, causing them to re-experience associated feelings. For example, a car backfiring may bring back memories and feelings associated with gun fire, or an unexplained noise downstairs may cause the person to re-experience a burglary. As a result, people with PTSD are often very anxious, have poor sleep and poor concentration, and may be **hyper-vigilant** because they believe the event could recur. This may lead to the person using avoidance strategies, becoming withdrawn and estranged from others, and developing maladaptive feelings and behaviours as ways of coping.

Mental health workers who support and treat people suffering from PTSD try to help them to make new associations (about the event and its consequences) and to reframe their thoughts in a way that leaves the traumatic event in the past. The goal is to ensure that the person doesn't feel the events are recurring in the present. Classical and operant conditioning techniques are combined in this kind of behavioural treatment. Treatment aims to remove the association between fear-inducing stimuli and the past event, while also minimising and controlling the physiological effects of fear, panic and anxiety through systematic desensitisation (see also page 377).

Your assessment criteria:

P2 Explain different psychological approaches to health practice

D1 Evaluate two psychological approaches to health and social care service provision

Key terms

Hyper-vigilant: *extremely watchful and alert to danger*

Investigate

Find out about the work of Combat Stress (www.combatstress.org.uk) and the way in which the organisation offers psychological support and treatment for ex-services personnel suffering from PTSD and other psychological conditions.

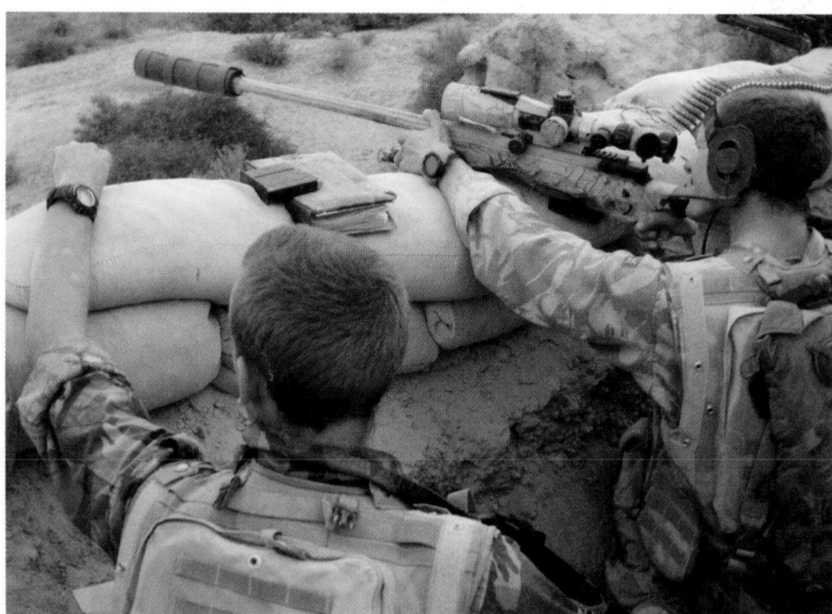

PTSD is associated with experiences of extreme personal threat.

D1 Evaluating the cognitive approach to health and social care provision

Figure 8.27 An evaluation of the cognitive approach to health and social care provision.

What does it offer?	What are its limitations?
1. A scientific, evidence-based approach to psychology.	1. It is criticised for treating a person's symptoms rather than the causes of their problems.
2. It can be applied quite widely in the health and social care field.	2. It is reductionist and deterministic, suggesting that complex human psychological processes and experiences can be explained largely in terms of brain functioning.
3. A relatively quick, low cost and effective way of helping people to deal with personal distress and cognitive problems.	3. The cognitive approach ignores the influence of human emotions, consciousness and free will on behaviour and psychological experiences.

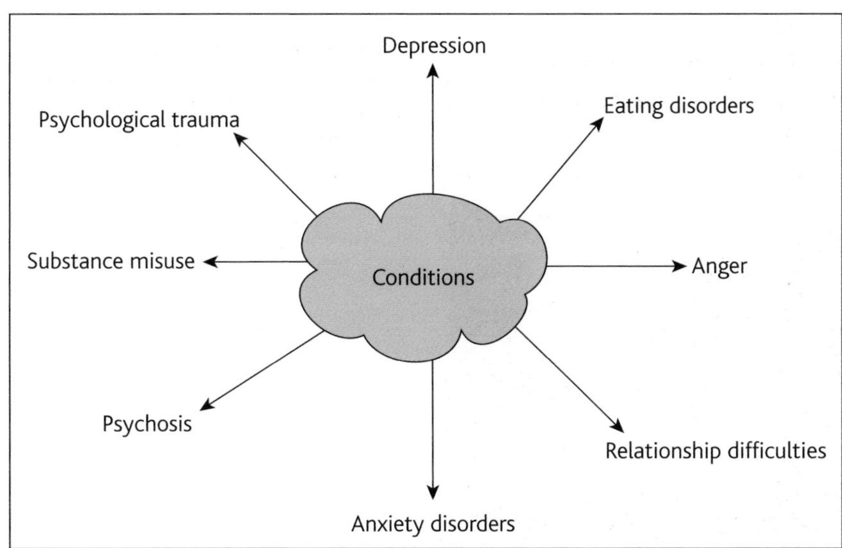

Figure 8.28 Conditions that can be treated using a cognitive approach.

The biological approach to care practice

P2 Using a biological perspective in health and social care practice

The biological perspective has a long history in psychology. Many of the pioneers of psychology were interested in physiological issues and stumbled upon the connections between the body and mind almost by accident. The biological perspective now enables us, via tools like **MRI** and **PET** scans, to explore the human brain and nervous system in detail. Researchers can investigate the effects of brain damage, drugs, and disease on psychological functioning in ways that were simply not possible in the past. As a result, the biological perspective has been used to help care practitioners understand a range of disorders that have significant psychological symptoms. These include:

- Parkinson's disease
- Huntington's disease
- Alzheimer's disease
- clinical depression
- schizophrenia
- autism
- anxiety
- substance misuse.

Your assessment criteria:

P2 Explain different psychological approaches to health practice

P3 Explain different psychological approaches to social care practice

Key terms

MRI: *Magnetic Resonance Imaging scan*

PET: *Positron Emission Tomography scan*

Investigate

Investigate the psychological symptoms that are associated with one or more of the conditions listed on the left.

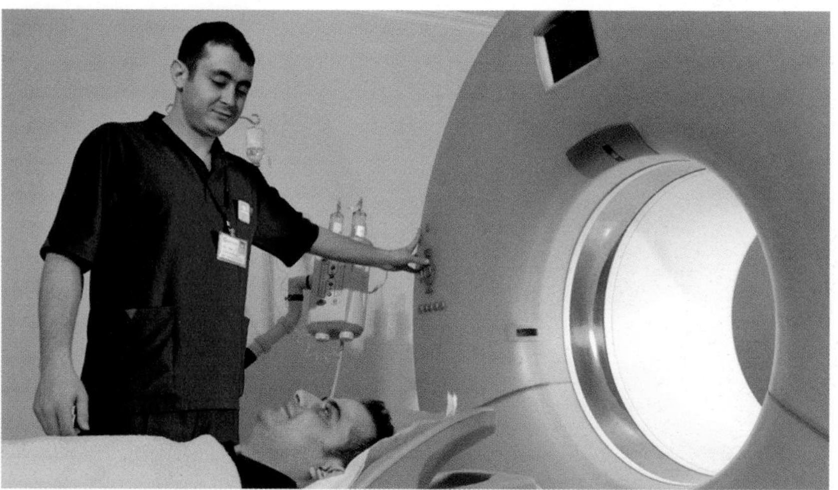

P3 Understanding developmental norms

Gessell's theory of maturational development (see page 373) formed the basis of an assessment scale that was designed to identify whether an individual's development at specific points is age-appropriate. The scale can be used to identify developmental delay and problems.

Various cognitive and social skills are assessed, as well as physical and motor abilities. The value of this tool is that it can provide care practitioners with hard data (based on scientific theory) about an individual's development relative to others. Identification of developmental problems can then quickly lead to treatment or other interventions to support the child or young person.

P2 Understanding genetic predisposition to illness and health disorders

Evidence suggests that genes have a role in behaviour, but there is little knowledge of the precise role that they play. The biological perspective has established an association between an individual's genes and conditions such as autism, schizophrenia and asthma. However, the detailed genetic factors that predispose people to these conditions, and the genetic mechanisms that lead to their development, are currently not known.

Research studies involving **concordance** rates of twins have enabled researchers to assess and identify genetic links to some of these disorders. These conditions don't appear to be genetically determined (twins would have 100 per cent concordance in cases of genetic determination). However, a genetic component is evident for autism, schizophrenia and asthma because the concordance rate for monozygotic (identical) twins is higher than for dizygotic (non-identical) twins. Health-related behaviours (such as diet, exercise and screening, for example) can help protect people who are predisposed to a disorder, enabling them to limit the impact of a **predisposition** on their own health.

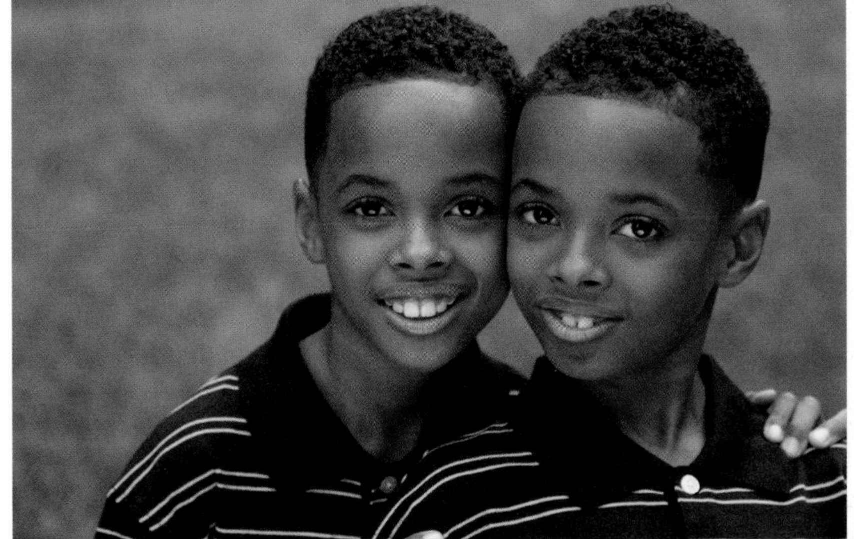

Twin studies have played an important role in biologically based psychology.

Investigate

Using internet or library sources (such as psychology textbooks) find a health-related research study that involved twins as a source of data. Summarise the purpose and findings of the study, focusing particularly on any claims made about the genetic basis of the disorder or condition being investigated.

Key terms

Concordance: *the presence of the same trait in both members of a pair of twins*

Predisposition: *a sensitivity or susceptibility towards something*

P2 Understand the effects of shift work

Biological psychology has been helpful in explaining the impact of shift work on health and wellbeing. People who work nightshifts have to reverse their 'normal' sleep pattern, resisting the urge to sleep at night and then sleeping during daylight. Some shift workers experience unpleasant physical and psychological effects because of this disruption to their **circadian rhythms**. Circadian rhythms determine the cycle of physiological processes that, in turn, affect alertness and normal body function. Higher body temperature, for example, leads to alertness; lower body temperature leads to feeling sleepy. Shift workers have to be alert and functioning, overcoming the urge to sleep, when their body temperature is naturally at its lowest. Then, they need to sleep when their body temperature is rising and causing alertness. For long-term shift workers, this can lead to psychological difficulties (such as stress) and physical health problems (especially digestive disorders).

Your assessment criteria:

P2 Explain different psychological approaches to health practice

M2 Compare two psychological approaches to health and social care service provision

D1 Evaluate two psychological approaches to health and social care service provision

Key terms

Circadian rhythm: *a roughly 24-hour cycle in the biochemical, physiological and behavioural processes of the human body*

M2 Comparing the cognitive and biological approaches

Figure 8.29 A comparison of cognitive and biological approaches to health and social care provision.

Cognitive approach	Biological approach
1. Uses a scientific approach to investigate and explain human psychological issues.	1. Uses a scientific approach to investigate and explain human psychological issues.
2. Has been widely used in health and social care to develop assessment and treatment approaches.	2. Has many medical applications in the health care field.
3. Has increased understanding of the links between thinking, emotion and behaviour in disorders such as depression, anxiety and PTSD.	3. Has increased understanding of aggression, abnormality and the role of biochemical factors in human behaviour.

Discuss

Do you think that the cognitive and biological perspectives offer complementary or contrasting approaches to psychological issues in health and social care settings?

D1 Evaluating the biological approach to health and social care provision

Figure 8.30 An evaluation of the biological approach to health and social care provision.

What does it offer?	What are its limitations?
1. A rigorous scientific approach to psychology.	1. It is sometimes seen as too simplistic, suggesting that biological factors are the key to understanding complex human psychology.
2. A range of practical applications that are used in the treatment of health and social care problems – particularly mental illnesses, autism and other brain-related disorders.	2. Reductionist and deterministic, reducing the complexities of human experience to simple, predictable biological processes.
3. Evidence that nature (biology) does play an important part in human experience and that this links to nurture (environmental) influences.	3. Ignores individual psychological differences that result from social, cultural and personal experiences.

Reflect

On balance, are you persuaded that the biological perspective has a useful part to play in health and social care settings? What, for you, are its main strength and its main limitation?

What do you know?

1. Identify two uses of the cognitive psychology perspective in health and social care practice.
2. Describe how the cognitive perspective can be used to understand and treat either depression or post-traumatic stress disorder.
3. Identify two ways in which the biological perspective in psychology has contributed to understanding or interventions in the health and social care field.
4. Describe an example of the link between genetics and a health disorder.
5. Explain how biological psychology has contributed to an understanding of the health problems experienced by shift workers.
6. Outline two ways in which the cognitive and biological perspectives in psychology are similar and two ways in which they differ.

Assessment checklist

Your learning and level of understanding of this unit will be assessed through assignments given to you and marked by your teacher or tutor. Before you submit your assignment work for assessment you should make sure that you have produced sufficient evidence to achieve the grade you are aiming for.

To pass this unit you will need to present evidence for assessment which demonstrates that you can meet all of the pass criteria for the unit.

Assessment Criteria	Description	✓
P1	Explain the principal psychological perspectives.	☐
P2	Explain different psychological approaches to health practice.	☐
P3	Explain different psychological approaches to social care practice.	☐

You can achieve a merit grade for the unit by presenting evidence that also meets all of the following merit criteria for the unit.

Assessment Criteria	Description	✓
M1	Assess different psychological approaches to study.	☐
M2	Compare two psychological approaches to health and social care service provision.	☐

You can achieve a distinction grade for the unit by presenting evidence that also meets all of the following distinction criteria for the unit.

Assessment Criteria	Description	✓
D1	Evaluate two psychological approaches to health and social care service provision.	☐

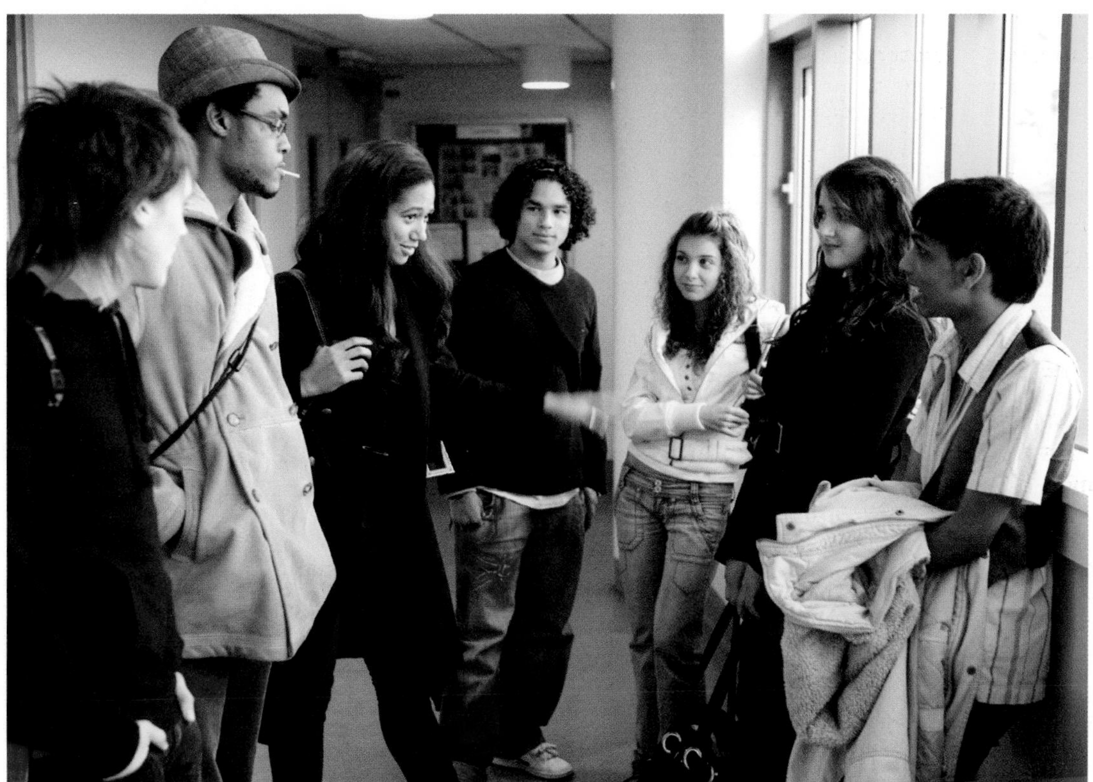

References

Asch, S. (1956) 'Studies of independence and conformity: a minority of one against a unanimous majority', Psychological Monographs, 70(9), No.416, p.70

Bandura, A. and Walters, R.H. (1963) *Social learning and personality development*, New York, Holt, Rinehart and Winston

Deutsch, M. and Gerard, H.B. (1955) 'A study of normative and informational influence upon individual judgement', Journal of Abnormal and Social Psychology, 51, pp.629–36

Erikson, E. (1968) Identity: *Youth and Crisis*, New York, Norton

Freud, S. (1920) *A General Introduction to Psychoanalysis*, New York, Basic Books

Maslow, A. (1943) *Motivation and Personality*, New York, Harper and Row

Rogers, C. (1961) *On becoming a person: A therapists view of psychotherapy*, London, Constable

Index